Winter Blues

Winter Blues

Everything You Need to Know
to Beat Seasonal Affective Disorder

REVISED EDITION

Norman E. Rosenthal, MD

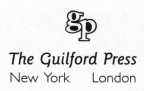

The Guilford Press
New York   London

Published by The Guilford Press
A Division of Guilford Publications, Inc.
72 Spring Street, New York, NY 10012
www.guilford.com

Printed in the United States of America

This book is printed on acid-free paper.

Last digit is print number: 9   8   7   6   5   4   3   2   1

Library of Congress Cataloging-in-Publication Data

Rosenthal, Norman E.
    Winter Blues: everything you need to know to beat seasonal affective disorder / Norman E. Rosenthal.—Revised ed.
        p.   cm.
    Includes bibliographical references and index.
    ISBN 1-59385-116-2 (pbk.) — ISBN 1-59385-214-2 (cloth)
    1. Seasonal affective disorder—Popular works.   I. Title.
RC545.R67 2006
616.85′27—dc22

                                                        2005013114

For Leora, Josh, and Liana

Contents

Part III
Celebrating the Seasons

Part IV
Resources

Acknowledgments

Space doesn't permit me to acknowledge all those who helped make this book possible. Many others contributed their stories anonymously and therefore must be thanked off the record. Special thanks, however, are due to Drs. Thomas Wehr and Dan Oren, my colleagues at the National Institute of Mental Health (NIMH), for our many creative interactions that helped shape my thinking. Other NIMH colleagues are listed in the Afterword. Other colleagues who have been exceptionally generous in sharing their thoughts and research findings are Michael and Jiuan-Su Terman, Siegfried Kasper, Kelly Rohan, George Brainard, Charmane Eastman, Barbara Parry, Jack Modell, and Elizabeth Wehr. Thanks to my editors at The Guilford Press, who have been uniformly outstanding and supportive: Seymour Weingarten, Kitty Moore, and Chris Benton. Nutrition counselor Bette Flax provided recipes and expertise. The light box companies whose products are shown in Chapter 7 and who are mentioned in Part IV were unfailingly helpful. I am grateful to all my colleagues in the field of seasonal affective disorder and light therapy, who have provided inspiration and fellowship over the past two decades. Many are mentioned in this book. Finally, I owe a huge debt to Leora and Josh for their support over the years and to my friend Michelle for her encouragement and unfailing good humor.

The following publishers have generously given permission to use extended quotations from copyrighted works:

From *Collected Poems 1909–1962*, by T. S. Eliot. Copyright 1963 by Faber and Faber. Reprinted by permission of Harcourt Brace Jovanovich, Inc., Orlando, Florida.

From "A Depression Which Recurred Annually," by George Frumkes, *Psychoanalytic Quarterly*, 65: 351–364, 1946. Reprinted with permission of *The Psychoanalytic Quarterly*.

From *The Letters of Henry Adams, Vol. II*, edited by J. C. Levenson, Ernest Samuels, Charles Vendersee, and Viola Hopkins Winner. Copyright 1982 by the Massachusetts Historical Society. Reprinted by permission of the Belknap Press of Harvard University Press, Cambridge, Massachusetts.

From "Little Gidding" in *Four Quartets*, by T. S. Eliot. Copyright 1943 by T. S. Eliot and renewed 1971 by Esme Valerie Eliot. Reprinted by permission of Harcourt, Inc.

From *The Poetry of Robert Frost*, edited by Edward Connery Lathem. Copyright 1936 by Robert Frost. 1964 by Lesley Frost Ballantine. 1969 by Henry Holt & Company. Reprinted by permission of Henry Holt and Company, Inc.

From *Selected Letters of Gustav Mahler*, edited by Knud Martner. Copyright 1979 by Faber and Faber Ltd. Reprinted by permission of Farrar, Straus and Giroux, LLC.

From "The Snow Man" in *Harmonium*, by Wallace Stevens. Copyright 1923 by Wallace Stevens and renewed 1982 by Holly Stevens. Reprinted by permission of Alfred A. Knopf, a division of Random House, Inc.

From "These" in *Collected Poems: 1909–1939, Vol. I*, by William Carlos Williams. Copyright 1938 by New Directions Publishing Corp. Reprinted by permission of New Directions Publishing Corp.

The photographs in Figures 3 through 8 were generously provided by and used by permission of the SunBox Company, Gaithersburg, Maryland; BioBrite, Inc., Bethesda, Maryland; Gary Regester for the Center for Environmental Therapeutics, *www.cet.org*; and Apollo Health, Inc., Orem, Utah.

Preface

When I decided to update *Winter Blues* for this revised edition, I imagined that this new version would involve only minor updates. I am excited to report that I was wrong. A great deal has happened in the seven years since the previous edition appeared, much of it of great relevance to those affected by the changing seasons.

I have substantially updated the entire treatment section, reflecting the maturation of the field. In the two decades since my colleagues and I first described seasonal affective disorder (SAD), there have been many new therapeutic developments. Several types of light therapy devices are now available, and consumers need to understand the distinctions between them to make informed choices. The science of light therapy has also advanced, and I am very pleased to share the research results with you. Just as exciting, however, are new developments in other forms of treatment: antidepressant medications, psychotherapy, and a variety of things you can do yourself to enjoy all seasons fully.

An enormous study of SAD, sponsored by a pharmaceutical company, finds that starting a specific antidepressant in the autumn can actually prevent the development of winter symptoms in many people. Chapter 10 describes this study and outlines the medical options available for treating SAD. A vigorous form of psychotherapy, known as cognitive-behavioral therapy (CBT), may rival in efficacy the gold standard, light therapy, or so a preliminary pilot study would suggest. I have crafted a vastly updated psychotherapy chapter that draws on the actual manual used in this study. Amazingly, machines that spew charged particles called negative ions into the air appear to have a potent effect in banishing the winter blues. Read all about it in the chapter that goes "Beyond Light Therapy." And for those wishing to avoid the dreaded winter weight gain, I have totally revamped my dietary recommendations, which are accompanied by a variety of enjoyable and healthful recipes.

Though much has changed since the last edition, I have retained much of the essential material from earlier editions. Some things don't change, such as the history of SAD and the many ways to celebrate the winter season, SAD notwithstanding, and the numerous writers and other famous people who, for better or worse, were exquisitely sensitive to the slant of the light or the cruelty of a particular month.

At the core of the book, however, are the stories of many ordinary people with extraordinary responses to the revolving year and the changing seasons. They serve as a continued source of inspiration to me, as I hope they will to you. I want to thank the many readers who have found *Winter Blues* meaningful over the years and have written to tell me so. I hope that you will find the new material in this book as enjoyable and useful as what came before. I hope also that new readers will join your ranks and find delight and comfort in these pages on a dark winter day.

Part I
Seasonal Syndromes

ONE

Introduction

Discovering SAD

Whoever wishes to pursue the science of medicine in a direct
manner must first investigate the seasons of the year and
what occurs in them.

—HIPPOCRATES

Four seasons fill the measure of the year;
There are four seasons in the mind of man.

—JOHN KEATS

When the dark days of winter approach, do you feel slowed down
and have difficulty waking up in the morning? Are you tempted to
snack more on those holiday foods, and do you find the pounds begin
to creep on even as you valiantly try to diet? Maybe you find it hard to
focus at work or in your relationships or feel down in the dumps or,
worse still, really depressed. If you answered yes to one or more of
these questions, you may be one of the millions of people who have
problems with the changing seasons. One of the astonishing facts to
emerge from recent research is that most people in the northern
United States and Europe experience seasonal changes in mood and
behavior, also known as seasonality.

In its most marked form, affecting an estimated six percent of the U.S. population, seasonality can actually cause a great deal of distress and difficulties in functioning both at work and in one's personal life. These estimated fourteen million Americans are said to be suffering from seasonal affective disorder, or SAD, a condition now generally accepted by the medical community and the public at large. Another fourteen percent of the adult U.S. population is estimated to suffer from a lesser form of SAD, known as the winter blues. Though these people are not usually affected severely enough to seek medical attention, they nevertheless feel less cheerful, energetic, creative, and productive during the dark winter days than at other times of the year.

For the last twenty-five years, I have studied the seasons and their effects on myself and others. I have loved them and hated them. I have helped others struggle with and master them, even as I have often struggled with them myself. This book is written for all of you who are intrigued by the changing seasons and their effects on our minds and bodies, whether this interest derives from medical necessity, a wish to understand or help a loved one, or plain and simple curiosity. Like the bears, squirrels, and birds, humans have evolved under the sun. We incorporated into the machinery of our bodies the rhythms of night and day, of darkness and light, of cold and warmth, of scarcity and plenty. Over hundreds of thousands of years, the architecture of our bodies has been shaped by the seasons and we have developed mechanisms to deal with the regular changes that they bring. Sometimes, however, these mechanisms break down and cause us trouble.

The effects of the seasons on humans have been well known through the centuries to artists, poets, and songwriters. Shakespeare, for example, observed that "a sad tale's best for winter," while Keats wrote of a nightingale singing of summer "in full-throated ease," and the singer of a modern ballad calls his beloved the sunshine of his life. They have also been part of our ordinary language and culture. A person might be said to have a warm and sunny disposition or a dark and icy nature. The weather reports that are part of every television news program may be as much a way of helping viewers gear their mind-set accordingly as advising them on how to dress or whether to wear a raincoat.

In recent years, science and medical practice have caught up to some extent with language, culture, and the arts, and the medical importance of the seasons is starting to be appreciated. Signs of this are everywhere in evidence. For example, on January or February evenings, after the Christmas lights have been removed, a blue-white light can be seen streaming through the blinds and shutters of some of the homes in neighborhoods throughout the North, penetrating the inky darkness of the winter night. The fanciful might mistake this strange illumination, brighter than the incandescence of an ordinary electric light and of a different hue, for an alien spaceship landed in suburbia to investigate our peculiar human ways or conquer our planet. The real explanation is more mundane. Thousands of people across the country are sitting in front of light boxes, specially made fixtures that emit far more light than is ordinarily available indoors, to treat their symptoms of SAD or its milder variant, the winter blues. Such boxes are springing up in offices as well, as many people, unashamed of their hibernating status, are treating their symptoms while at work.

But it is not only those who suffer badly as a result of the changing seasons who are becoming more cognizant of the importance of light. Having an office with a window has taken on a new importance as workers, who always wanted a view, now realize that there are medical and psychological benefits as well to having access to natural light. The "energy-efficient" buildings with tinted-glass windows, constructed in earlier decades, are now regarded with displeasure by many workers who must labor in the unnatural glow of the light transmitted through the yellow panes. In fact, in one government building near Washington, the workers mutinied and pulled the tinted "weather stripping" off the outside of the windows to let in the sunlight unimpeded.

In this book, I will describe in detail how you can use light therapeutically as well as many other ways to treat SAD or the winter blues. I must emphasize, though, that depression can be a serious illness: painful, debilitating, and, in some cases, even fatal. While identifying depression and taking steps to combat it are a critical first step, if this step does not promptly take care of the problem, a professional should be consulted sooner rather than later. There are so many things that can be done to alleviate depression, and a skillful practitioner can be an invaluable and sometimes essential ally in helping to implement these strategies. Along with specific suggestions for ways to recognize SAD or the winter blues and help yourself with these problems, I will direct you to various resources for additional help.

An enormous amount of research into the effects of the seasons and of light on human beings has appeared over the last few decades. Much of this research is based on the dramatic seasonal changes that occur in animals. I will describe some of these exciting new advances, which explain why some people experience seasonal changes so much more profoundly than others. I will also discuss the research conducted to explain how light therapy and other treatments may exert their dramatic therapeutic effects.

But it would be a shame if the seasons were considered merely a source of suffering and distress. Aside from their capacity to induce symptoms, the seasons fascinate in their own right. The predictable changes that come with the shortening and lengthening of the days, the marked shifts in weather, and the rhythmic alternation between the barren landscape of winter and the vivid colors of summer are a continuing source of wonder.

The seasons of the mind are not the same for everyone. Autumn enchants some with its grand colors, but for others it carries the menace of winter. For certain people, winter, cheerless and forbidding, is associated with stagnation, decay, and loss. But others experience a different type of winter—one that finds them snug and cozy by the fireside, with chestnuts popping. Spring brings buds and blossoms, rebirth, with sap stirring, feverish urges, and a longing to go on pilgrimages. But we are also told that "April is the cruelest month . . . mixing memory and desire." Summer yields a harvest of fruit and flowers, but according to Shakespeare, "sometimes too hot the eye of heaven shines."

In Part III, "Celebrating the Seasons," I discuss how the seasons can be a rich source of inspiration and how some of our most creative writers and artists have been intensely seasonal and have included their seasonal responses in their art.

In the final chapter, "Winter Light," I discuss life beyond SAD. By now, there are many of us who have suffered winter difficulties in the past, but have successfully treated ourselves for years and have largely overcome the problem. I regard myself as lucky to be living after the recognition of SAD and the discovery of light therapy and other effective treatment strategies. Many people with SAD enjoyed the winters of their childhood before their symptoms first appeared. Then they suffered for years until they understood the nature of their problem and found successful treatments for it. After their SAD symptoms had been treated for several years, they began to rediscover the quiet pleasures of winter and to feel reconnected with their childhood. I relay some of their stories—and my own—and celebrate the joy of winter that has eluded so many of us for so long.

SAD and Light Therapy: The Early Years

Although individual cases of SAD have appeared in the psychiatric literature for over a hundred years, and although the use of light to treat depression was suggested even in ancient times, the description of SAD as a syndrome and the systematic development of light therapy to treat it occurred relatively recently. These developments took place at the National Institute of Mental Health (NIMH) in the early 1980s and involved several individuals, each of whom made an important contribution to the story. I consider myself fortunate to have been at that place at that time and to have played a part in these events, which I describe below. And since each of us experiences our world from our own particular vantage point, it seems easiest to begin this tale of scientific discovery with my own SAD story.

My Own SAD Story

I trained as a doctor in South Africa, a country that, for all the turbulence of its politics, can truthfully boast about its climate. In Johannesburg, where I grew up, there were really only two seasons: summer and winter. During summer, one could swim outdoors and eat summer fruit: peaches, papaya, mangoes. During winter, one could not do these things. It was warm outdoors during the day, though at night you needed a sweater. Spring and autumn were transition times. After several months of winter, the blossoms would appear, and you knew it was spring. Similarly, when the long summer was over, the leaves would turn a simple brown and fall off the trees without much fuss or fanfare, and winter was there. But despite the mildness of the seasons, I was aware at some level of the effect they had on my mood. I had even considered writing a novel in which the mood of the central character changed regularly with the seasons. The novel was never written, but the seed of the idea stayed with me, germinating quietly. It required the intense seasonal changes of the higher latitudes to which I moved to activate that kernel of thought, as well as my encounters with some inspiring people, who are central to this story. I arrived in the United States in the summer of 1976 and began both my psychiatric residency at the New York State Psychiatric Institute and research into disorders of mood regulation. The summer days felt endlessly long, and my energy was boundless. I had never experienced such long summer days in Johannesburg, which is much nearer to the equator than New York City.

As the months passed, I was struck by the drama of the changing seasons. I had been unprepared for the brilliant colors of the autumn leaves in the North, the crisp days and cold nights, and most of all, the disappearance of the light. I had not anticipated how short the days would be. When the sun shone, its rays struck the earth at a strange, oblique angle, and I understood what Shelley meant when he wrote:

> Bright Reason will mock thee
> Like the sun from a wintry sky.

Then daylight savings time was over and the clocks were put back an hour. I left work that first Monday after the time change and found the world in darkness. A cold wind blowing off the Hudson River filled me with foreboding. Winter came. My energy level declined, and I wondered how I could have undertaken so many tasks the previous summer. Had I been crazy? Now there seemed to be no alternative but to hang in and try to keep everything afloat. I understood for the first time the stoic temperaments of the northern nations. Finally, spring arrived. My energy level surged again, and I wondered why I had worried so over my workload.

I registered all these impressions, but I did not put them together into a cohesive story—and I probably would never have done so had it not been for the events that followed and the remarkable people I was to meet. At the end of my residency I went to the NIMH in Bethesda, Maryland, to undertake a research fellowship with Dr. Frederick Goodwin, whom I had heard speak on the topic of manic–depressive illness from both biological and psychological points of view. Dr. Goodwin made the subject come alive, describing how our shifting moods and fluctuating perceptions of the world correspond to certain changes in our brain chemistry. Since mind and brain seemed equally fascinating frames of reference, I wanted to use both models to try to understand mood disorders.

Shortly before my first visit to the NIMH, I met Dr. Alfred Lewy, one of several psychiatrists working with Fred Goodwin at the time. Dr. Lewy had just developed a technique to measure the hormone melatonin, in collaboration with Dr. Sanford Markey. Melatonin is produced by the pineal gland, a pea-sized structure tucked underneath the brain. Each night, like clockwork, the pineal gland releases melatonin into the bloodstream in minute quantities and continues to do so until dawn. The secretion of melatonin signals the duration of darkness and thus serves as an important seasonal time cue in animals. Although it is unclear whether melatonin is instrumental in causing seasonal changes in humans, the research in this area proved to be a critical step in the description of SAD and the development of light therapy.

Dr. Lewy and I spoke about our common interests and the various directions in which our research might take us. On occasion, we chatted over a mass spectrometer, the instrument he had used to develop his technique for measuring melatonin. It looked like a very large washing machine. He injected samples of clear fluid into a small hole in the top, and reams of paper rolled off it, while inked pens traced out a graph upon the paper. He pointed to one blip on the graph and said, "That's melatonin." I was suitably impressed.

After I joined Dr. Goodwin's group, I was assigned to work most closely with Dr. Thomas Wehr, an outstanding clinical researcher, who had for some years been studying biological rhythms in an attempt to learn whether abnormalities in these rhythms might be at the basis of the mood disturbances in depression and mania. Shortly before my arrival at the NIMH, Lewy and Wehr had shown that bright light was capable of suppressing the secretion of human melatonin at night—a finding that was to have great influence over the events that followed. There was a buzz in Goodwin's group at that time—a sense of excitement—and I felt certain I had come to the right place.

A Light-Sensitive Scientist

Although many people were responsible for the discovery of SAD, our steps toward this end can all be traced back to the actions of one man: Herb Kern. In some ways, Herb might have appeared to be an unlikely person to initiate a new area of medical investigation, for he was not himself a medical professional, but a research engineer with a major corporation. I met Herb a year after arriving at the NIMH. At sixty-three, he was a youthful-looking man with a wiry build, a crew cut, and a twinkle in his eyes. He was intensely curious, and he had noted in himself a regular pattern of mood and behavior changes going back at least fifteen years. A scientist by nature and training, he had kept careful notes of these changes in numerous small notebooks. He observed that each year, from July onward, his energy level would decline and he would withdraw from the world. At these times, he lacked energy, had difficulty making decisions, lost interest in sex, and felt slowed down and "ready for hibernation." He found it difficult to get to work in the morning, and once there, he would sit at his desk, fearful that the telephone would ring, obliging him to have a conversation with someone. It is typical for a depressed person to withdraw—to have neither the desire nor the energy to interact with others. In fact, in many cases, he or she may feel it is an impossible task. People who are depressed simply want to be left alone.

More bothersome to Herb than his social isolation was the decrease in his creative powers during his depressed periods. He would procrastinate at work because "everything seemed like a mountain" to him, and his productivity decreased markedly. It was only by grim perseverance that he was able to write up his studies from the previous spring and summer. His sleep was disrupted, and his characteristic enthusiasm for life evaporated.

The months would drag on like this for Herb until mid-January, when, over a two-week period, his energy would return. As he put it, "The wheels of my mind began to spin again." He had ample, even excessive, energy at these times and needed little sleep. Ideas came freely, and he was eager to communicate them to others. For five or six months he was very confident of his abilities and felt that he could "tackle anything." He was very efficient and creative, needed only four hours of sleep per night, was more interested in food and sex, and admitted to a "tendency to go overboard" in buying luxuries.

Herb had observed that his mood improved as the days lengthened and declined as they shortened, and he had actually developed a theory that this might be due to changes in environmental light. He attempted to interest several people in his hunch that his mood and energy levels were related to the time of year. One of these, Dr. Peter Mueller, a New Jersey psychiatrist in private practice, who had a research background, listened to Herb and subsequently looked for other patients with a similar history. Herb was treated with several different antidepressant medications, all of which resulted in unacceptable side effects without correcting his symptoms. Herb read about the work of Drs. Goodwin, Wehr, and Lewy and found his way to the NIMH, where he asked us to work with him on his seasonal difficulties.

Dr. Lewy suggested that we treat Herb by lengthening his winter day with six hours of bright light—three before dawn and three after dusk—in an attempt to simulate a summer day. He reasoned that since bright light is necessary for melatonin suppression in humans, it might similarly be necessary for altering mood and behavior. This reasoning was based on two pieces of information: first, the secretion of melatonin is an important chemical signal for regulating many different seasonal rhythms in animals; second, the nerve pathways involved in the suppression of melatonin secretion by light pass through parts of the brain that we believe are important in regulating many of the physical functions that are disturbed in depression, such as eating, sleeping, weight control, and sex drive. If the suppression of melatonin required much brighter light than ordinary indoor fixtures provided, then perhaps bright light might also be necessary for the brain to perform other mood-related functions.

We asked Herb to sit in front of a metal light box, about two feet by four feet. The box emitted as much light as one would receive while standing at a window on a spring day in the northeastern United States. We chose full-spectrum fluorescent lights—a type that mimics the color range of natural sunlight coming from a summer sky—to replicate the conditions that appeared to bring Herb out of his winter depressions. We covered the lamps in the light box with a plastic diffusing screen to create a smooth surface. Modern light boxes differ to some degree from the one we originally used in treating Herb. We now realize that it is unnecessary to use full-spectrum light and that, in fact, the ultraviolet rays present in some full-spectrum lights may actually be harmful to the eyes and the skin. In addition, newer light box models are smaller and more portable. Some models are angled toward the patient's eyes, an arrangement that has been found to have advantages over the original upright version. Specific details about light boxes are provided in Chapter 7, "Light Therapy," and Part IV, "Resources."

Within three days, Herb began to feel better. The change was dramatic and unmistakable. He was moving into his spring mode several weeks ahead of schedule. Did we dare to hope that we might have found a new type of treatment for depression? Intriguing as this possibility was, our excitement was immediately tempered by our scientific instincts. After all, Herb had been heavily invested in the light therapy. Might his response not have been due to something other than the light—the wish to feel better, for example, or the emotional impact of entering an experiment in which three research psychiatrists were studying the outcome of a treatment based on his ideas? The so-called placebo effect had to be considered seriously. The placebo effect has dogged behavioral researchers for years, and we could not rule it out in evaluating the antidepressant effects of light therapy on Herb.

A Human Bear

During the same winter that Herb was receiving light treatment at the NIMH, Dr. Peter Mueller, a private practitioner, in consultation with Al Lewy, tried artificial light treatment with another patient, whom we will call "Bridget." She also appeared to benefit from light and had an unusually good winter that year. The following summer, as luck would have it, Bridget moved to the Washington metropolitan area, and Dr. Mueller suggested that she contact us. Bridget's history and ingenuity in fitting the details of her seasonal problems into a coherent story were as remarkable as Herb's.

She was a professional in her mid-thirties, who had been aware of disliking winter since childhood. But it was not until her early twenties that a regular pattern of seasonal changes emerged. Bridget's problem would begin each year in August or September, as she anticipated the forthcoming winter with increasing anxiety. She was mystified about what subtle cues might have caused her premonitory dread, since this feeling began during the summer, when the days were still warm. She wondered whether it might be the fall catalogs, with their pictures of winter clothes, that triggered the memories of unpleasant winters of earlier years. Regardless, when the leaves began to turn, she would have a strong urge to take out her winter clothes and stock her cupboards with food, "like a squirrel getting ready for winter."

As winter approached, Bridget experienced many symptoms similar to those described by Herb, such as feelings of extreme fatigue—a leaden sensation that made her want to lie down and sleep all day long. She would overeat at these times and observed a marked craving for sweets and starches. As in Herb's case, Bridget continued to struggle in to work each day, though her productivity declined markedly. In addition to her seasonal mood problem, Bridget felt depressed and irritable for a few days before each menstrual period, regardless of the season. When spring arrived, her depression lifted and was replaced by elation. In her earlier years, she would forget her winter difficulties once they were over. "I was like the grasshopper," she remarked, "singing and playing all summer long," indifferent to the next winter that was to come.

Bridget had also observed that other changes in the environment besides the seasons seemed to affect her mood. She had visited the Virgin Islands during the two winters before her first light treatment. Both times, she had been impressed by the marked improvement in her mood just days after her arrival on the islands and the relapse a few days after her return to the North. She had lived for some years in locations at different latitudes: Georgia, New York, and Quebec. The farther north she lived, the earlier her depression began, the more depressed she felt, and the later was her remission in the spring. She began to suspect that something in the environment was influencing her mood and that perhaps it was the light. Why else did she seem to crave it so? Why else did she hate her poorly lit office? She made up any excuse to seek out the brightly lit photocopying room. Light treatment made good sense to Bridget. She was eager to try it and was delighted to find that it worked for her.

In Search of SAD

Unusual individual cases have historically played an important role in medical research in general and psychiatry in particular. We wondered whether Herb's and Bridget's symptoms might be examples of a special seasonal kind of depression and whether they might help us understand how others respond to the changing seasons and environmental light.

Although single cases may be of great importance in generating new hypotheses, we generally need groups of patients to test them experimentally. Dr. Mueller said he had encountered several other patients with seasonal depression. We wondered how common the problem was. Were there any other such patients in the Washington, DC, area who might be interested in participating in a research program? I called a few local psychiatrists who specialized in treating depression, but they said they had not encountered the problem. I concluded that it must be quite rare and that the only chance we had of finding such a group was by publicizing our interest in *The Washington Post.*

Sandy Rovner, a journalist who specialized in health issues, sat across the room from me, tape recorder in hand, and listened to my story. She decided it would be of interest to her readers and wrote an article for the *Post,* which launched an entire field of research. Rovner's article began with Bridget's own words: "I should have been a bear. Bears are allowed to hibernate; humans are not."

The response to the article took us all by surprise. Instead of our hearing from a handful of afflicted people, the phones rang for days and we received thousands of responses from all over the country. We sent out screening questionnaires, which were returned by the hundreds. I read them with a growing sense of excitement. In psychiatric research, heterogeneity *is* a major problem. In other words, the same condition may differ greatly in character from one patient to another, which has proven to be an enormous obstacle to psychiatric researchers, especially in the area of schizophrenia. As I read the questionnaires, it seemed as though Bridget had been cloned, as one person after another reported the symptoms of the condition that we went on to call SAD. I wondered whether this similarity in symptoms might correspond to a similar underlying disturbance in brain chemistry, which might imply a favorable response to light, as we had observed with Herb Kern and Bridget.

We interviewed many people and admitted into our program all those with clear-cut histories of winter depression. During that summer, as expected, all the participants felt well and showed an unusually high level of energy. This generated considerable skepticism among some of my colleagues, who speculated that we might be dealing with a group of suggestible people who had read the article and persuaded themselves that they had the syndrome. That seemed unlikely to me, but I had no way of disproving it and could not help feeling slightly uneasy when one of my colleagues pointed out that if none of the participants became depressed when winter arrived, we would all look a little foolish.

The First Controlled Study of Light Therapy for SAD

The days grew shorter, and in October and November, right on schedule, the participants began to slow down and experience their winter syndromes, just as they had described. Although clearly not affected to the same degree as my seasonal patients, I noticed that I, too, had to push myself harder to get anything done. It was more difficult to get up in the morning, and even the project did not seem so exciting as it had the previous summer.

We planned to treat the patients with light as soon as they became moderately depressed—just enough so that we would be able to measure an effect of the treatment, but not to a degree where they felt incapacitated. We decided to use full-spectrum light, as we had with Herb Kern, for three hours before dawn and three hours after dusk. In any experiment designed to show the effectiveness of a treatment, it is important to have a control condition—one that incorporates all the ingredients of the "active treatment" condition except the one believed to be crucial for achieving the desired effect. In this study we believed that the brightness of the light would be crucial, so we used dim light as a control. To make the control treatment more plausible, we chose a golden-yellow light—a color associated with the sun.

We treated each patient with two weeks of bright light and two weeks of dim light, then compared the effects. This type of treatment design—called a "crossover" because the individual is "crossed over" from one treatment condition to the other—has since been used widely for light therapy studies. We presented the two conditions to the patients in random order. In other words, some began with the bright white and others with the dim yellow light, so as not to bias the outcome. It is also important for psychiatrists evaluating the effects of a treatment not to be aware of which treatment a patient has received, so that their prejudices cannot be reflected in their ratings. For this reason, treatment conditions were known only to me, not to my collaborators in this study, Drs. Thomas Wehr, David Sack, and J. Christian Gillin.

I will never forget the first patient who underwent the bright light treatment—a middle-aged woman, markedly disabled by SAD. During the winter she was barely able to do her household chores, get to work, or attend her evening classes. After one week of treatment, she came into our clinic beaming. She was feeling wonderful, keeping up with all her obligations, and mentioned that her classmates were regarding her with a new competitive respect as she answered questions in her evening classes, as if to say "Where have you been hiding all this time?"

The second patient who was exposed to the bright light was treated around Christmas. I called the ward from New York City, where I was spending the holiday with friends, and asked Dave Sack how things were going with the study. He replied, "I don't know what treatment 'Joan' is receiving, but she's blooming like a rose."

And so it went. Nine patients responded to bright light, and the dim light proved ineffective. I began to use the lights myself and was sure that they made me feel better. Some of my colleagues requested them, too. After a few weeks I had to put a big sign in front of the dwindling stack of light boxes, asking anyone who wanted to borrow a fixture to discuss it with me first so that we would have enough for the study. A local psychiatrist, whom I had initially polled about the existence of people with SAD, and who had told me that he did not know of any, called to say that he had realized that he himself had the syndrome and asked about how he might use the lights himself.

Many questions were raised by the results of our first study. Was it really possible that light was affecting mood? Could there be some explanation for the improvement other than the light itself? Was it all a placebo effect? And if it was the light, how was it working? These were all important questions, and in due course, we and other researchers would address them, one by one. But as we reviewed the study in the spring of 1982, we delighted in its two main findings. The patients had become depressed during fall and winter as they had predicted they would, and the light treatment had worked more dramatically than we had ever hoped it might. The azaleas and the dogwoods were in bloom. Spring had arrived, and at that moment, nothing else seemed to matter very much to either our patients or us.

Twenty Years of SAD

In the two decades since the appearance of our initial description of SAD and light therapy, we and other researchers have made tremendous strides in understanding and treating this fascinating condition. A recent survey of the literature showed almost a thousand publications on these topics. Throughout the United States, Europe, and Asia, scientists have found large groups of people suffering from the very same symptoms as our initial study subjects. We now know that SAD is common, affecting up to nine percent of U.S. adults in the northern part of the country and in other northern regions such as Scotland. As one might imagine, it is far less common in the South, affecting an estimated one and a half percent of Floridians and those in other southern regions. To date, dozens of population studies have been undertaken to establish the frequency of SAD in different parts of the world.

In many instances the charge to educate people about SAD has been led by patients themselves. The highly successful patient support group SADA (Seasonal Affective Disorder Association) has been operating in the United Kingdom since the early days of SAD research. To date, unfortunately, efforts to organize similar SAD support groups have been less successful elsewhere. Despite the wealth of literature, market research indicates that clinicians still often fail to recognize SAD, thereby losing opportunities to alleviate the suffering that goes along with the condition. A recently conducted large-scale study indicated that patients with SAD on average had suffered fourteen winter depressions before entering the program. Of these, fewer than half had received any previous treatment for their symptoms. Why the lingering ignorance about the subject? Nobody knows for sure, but it may have something to do with light therapy itself, which continues to be viewed by many clinicians as outside the mainstream. This problem was highlighted by a recent lead article in the prestigious *American Journal of Psychiatry*. One encouraging development is that pharmaceutical companies have begun to take SAD seriously.

Three recent very large studies, encompassing collectively almost a thousand patients with SAD, indicate that the antidepressant Wellbutrin XL, if given before the onset of winter symptoms, can prevent an attack of SAD. These are exciting findings not only because they offer a novel approach to preventing symptoms, but also because they signify the entry of a large pharmaceutical company into this area. Historically, such corporate involvement has been important for the optimal recognition and treatment of other emotional conditions.

In 1987, the American Psychiatric Association recognized a version of SAD in its diagnostic manual, the DSM-III-R, and it can be found in the most recent version, the DSM-IV-TR. Now what we need is greater awareness among clinicians as well as the general public. My hope is that this book will continue to disseminate the valuable information that researchers have painstakingly garnered, fact by fact. The chapters that follow outline what we have learned so far about how the seasons affect us, what we can do to modify these influences, and some of the questions that have yet to be answered.

TWO

All About SAD

What exactly is SAD? What are its symptoms? Who tends to get it and when? How long does it last? How does it affect the way people function at home, at work, and in their relationships? How does SAD relate to the "winter blues" or "February blahs" that so many people complain about? In this chapter I will introduce some key elements of these conditions as well as a few people who have suffered from them in their mild and severe forms and triumphed over them.

We now know that the great majority of the population experiences some seasonal changes in feelings of well-being and behaviors, such as energy, sleep, eating patterns, and mood, to a greater or lesser degree. At one end of the spectrum are those who have few, if any, seasonal changes. Then there are those who experience mild changes that can easily be accommodated in the course of their everyday lives. Yet another group finds these changes a nuisance—not worth taking to the physician, but troublesome nonetheless. This group may be suffering from what is commonly known as the winter blues or February blahs. At the far end of the spectrum are patients with SAD, whose changes in mood and behavior are so powerful that they produce significant problems in their lives.

Such changes were well expressed by Jenny, who suffers from a typical case of SAD. She has observed that she feels like "two different people—a summer person and a winter person." Between spring and fall she is energetic, cheerful, and productive. She initiates conversations and social arrangements and is regarded as a valuable friend, coworker, and employee. She is able to manage everything that is expected of her with time and energy to spare. During the winter, however, her energy level and ability to concentrate are reduced, and she finds it difficult to cope with her everyday tasks. She generally just wants to rest and be left alone, "like a hibernating bear." This state persists until spring, when her energy, vitality, and zest for life return. It is easy to understand why she thinks of herself as two different people and why her friends wonder who the "real Jenny" is.

This theme is echoed by a variety of other seasonal people I have encountered. For example, a man from Missouri writes:

> I feel as though I "live" only during the sunny months. The rest of the time I seem to shut down to an idle, waiting for spring, enduring life in general. This is no joking matter to those of us who are like this. We, in effect, live only half our lives, accomplishing only half of what we should. It is really rather sad, when you think of it.

One woman wrote about her elderly mother, who has suffered from SAD for her entire adult life:

> In late spring or early summer, she is full of energy, requiring only five or six hours of sleep. She talks incessantly and tries to do too many things. Then in late fall (occasionally she makes it to Christmas), her personality takes a complete turn. She sleeps twelve hours at night, cries all morning, and then takes a nap. She won't drive the car, seldom leaves the house, and won't answer the telephone.

Who are the victims of SAD? All sorts of people. The hundreds of patients with SAD I have known have come from all different walks of life: different races, ethnic groups, and occupations. One fact that has intrigued researchers for years is that the disorder is about four times more common among women than among men. Although people in their twenties through forties appear to be most susceptible, SAD occurs in all age groups. I have encountered children and adolescents with the problem (see Chapter 5), as well as the elderly. In addition,

SAD may affect different ethnic groups to a different degree (see Chapter 4).

Just as the degree of seasonal difficulties may vary from one person to the next, so may the timing of the problem. For example, one person may begin to feel SAD symptoms in September, whereas another will feel well until after Christmas. The more severely affected person might emerge from the winter slump only in April, whereas a mildly affected one may feel better by mid-March. Many people can predict almost to the week when they will begin to experience their winter difficulties and when they will begin to feel better in spring, almost as one can predict when different flowers will begin to bloom.

The timing of the appearance of symptoms also depends on where a person lives. My colleague Dr. Carla Hellekson, when she worked in Alaska, noticed that the patients in her SAD clinic became depressed about a month earlier, on average, than my patients in Maryland and began to feel better, on average, about a month later. Terry, a thirty-eight-year-old realtor, is typical of many who have lived at different latitudes when she reports that during her years in Canada and New York, her problems began earlier than when she moved south to Washington, DC.

Merrill, a vocational guidance counselor, sits in front of me, checking off on her fingers the symptoms she has during successive months. She has come to know her internal calendar well over the last eighteen years during which she has suffered from SAD. Since she is thirty-two years old now, these problems have been going on for more than half of her life.

I feel good for only two or three months: May, June, and July. By August my energy level has already begun to slip. I begin to sleep later in the morning, but I can still get to work on time. In September, things are a little worse. My appetite increases, and I begin to crave candy and junk food. By October I begin to withdraw from friends, and I tend to cancel engagements. November marks the onset of real difficulties for me.

I become sad and worry about small things that wouldn't bother me at all in the summer. My thinking is not as good as usual, and I begin to make stupid mistakes. Other people notice that I am not looking well. Preparing for Christmas is always an enormous chore. I am bad about getting my cards off and my gifts wrapped. I tend to avoid the usual round of parties: I don't want people to think I am being rude, but I find it very difficult to pretend to be cheerful and make conversation when all I feel like doing is going home and sleeping.

January and February are my worst months. On many days it's all I can do to get in to work, and often I don't. I call in sick. Once I'm there it's very hard to get my work done. I procrastinate as much as possible and hope that I'll be able to handle things later.

In March and April, my energy begins to come back, and that's a relief, but my thinking is still not back to normal, and I continue to feel depressed at times. They are tricky months, because you never know what the weather will be like. You can feel good for a few days and then, wham, you're down again. And then it's late spring and summer, and once again I feel myself: friendly and happy. I can do my work and can be available to the people I care for. But it's so hard to have to cram everything you want to do into three months.

In Washington, DC, the three months during which most patients with SAD feel like going into hibernation are December, January, and February. These months could well be called the SAD months. Then comes the thaw of March, April, and May. People emerge from their low winter state in different ways. Some glide gracefully through April and May into feeling cheerful and well in June and July. Some have a bumpy course over the spring, especially in places where it is dark, stormy, and unpredictable. Others emerge into an exuberant state where they may be excessively energetic, needing little sleep and feeling "wired" or "high." At times this state of excessive energy, known clinically as hypomania, can constitute a problem in its own right. A final group of people with SAD never quite emerge completely from their winter depressions and remain somewhat down all year round, though less so in the summer.

Elsewhere the pattern of SAD symptoms may differ. For example, in some more northern areas, symptoms may begin earlier, but may also end earlier if the ground is covered with bright snow, reflecting vast amounts of light on sunny winter days.

In Chapter 11, "A Step-by-Step Guide Through the Revolving Year," I will describe how many people with SAD feel during the different months and offer advice as to how best to cope with the effects of the changing seasons.

Profiles of SAD

Following are profiles of four patients with SAD and one with subsyndromal SAD, or the winter blues. Their symptoms include the full range of seasonal changes. Neal and Angela suffered from milder and more common forms of SAD, which is why I profile them first, whereas Peggy and Alan, whom I profile second, suffered more severely. Finally, I profile Jeff, one of the first people with the winter blues to be studied and treated at the NIMH.

As you read these stories, bear in mind a couple of changes that have occurred since they were written for the original edition of this book over a dozen years ago. First, although they focus exclusively on light therapy, many other forms of treatment, fully detailed later in this book, have emerged in the intervening years. Second, the commonly held idea that the winter depressions of SAD are necessarily mild has been challenged. A recent Scandinavian study compared the symptoms of depression in patients with SAD to those in people with nonseasonal depression who had recently been hospitalized following a suicide attempt. The surprising finding was that patients with SAD actually reported more depressive symptoms than their nonseasonal counterparts.

Neal and Angela:
Light for a Living and Light to Write By

Neal Owens is currently the president of the SunBox Company, which sells lights for the treatment of SAD. He is in his late forties and has had difficulties during the winter for the last several years. His problems occurred in both his personal and professional life and affected the way he felt about himself.

Twice divorced, he feels now that his first marriage crumbled in part as a result of his seasonal changes. During the winter he was little fun to be around. He moped and withdrew into himself, was unable to enjoy the holidays, and was not available to his wife when she needed him. Then, single once again, he felt very bad about himself, and this was not helped by the fifteen to twenty pounds he would gain each fall and winter. He would find it impossible to exercise at this time, losing yet one more source of enjoyment and means of reducing his weight and feeling good about himself.

In his work as a sales representative, he found his productivity declining markedly in the winter months. He would sleep late, cancel appointments, and spend much of the day at home, depressed. When he was able to get to work, he came home exhausted and would collapse on the couch for the rest of the evening. It is not surprising that for a salesman, who needs to be upbeat, energetic, and eager to interact with others and promote his product, the symptoms of SAD would be rather disabling.

He consulted a psychiatrist at the urging of his girlfriend and was given a series of antidepressants, none of which proved helpful. After seeing a television documentary about SAD, he mentioned light therapy to his doctor, who was not supportive of the idea. He then obtained information about it from the NIMH, constructed his own light box, and began therapy on his own. He switched therapists and improved noticeably, using a combination of light and psychotherapy. Neal's positive experience with light therapy inspired him to change careers and start a business to help others by selling light boxes and providing information on SAD. Neal now feels well all year round and is very hopeful about the future since his winter depressions are under control.

Angela is a sixty-year-old writer with a long history of winter difficulties too mild either to meet criteria for a diagnosis of SAD or to lead her to seek medical help. Since her childhood, she has disliked winter and dark climates and places, which she has avoided whenever possible. She thought of herself as entering a "little hibernation" in the winter, when she would feel less creative than usual and "slightly melancholy," if not actually depressed. She had never consciously associated her low energy states with the quality of winter light, but when she first heard about SAD, she immediately identified herself as having a minor version of the condition.

Angela first found out about light therapy when she was writing a magazine article on the subject, for which she interviewed me. But she did nothing about her own winter problems until four years later, when she had strenuous writing deadlines to meet. She installed a set of lights on her desk, and they have been there ever since. She uses the lights in both summer and winter, whenever she happens to be working—at least when she is living in Washington, DC. She observes:

Since I started using the lights in winter, my brain seems to
be clearer, I seem to be happier, and the writing goes better.
Not only am I much more productive, but I also seem to be
much more creative. The words come more easily and I seem
to get more images. I also don't mind being at my desk and
writing as much as I did before. When I used to think of having to write in the winter, it was a great effort. I felt almost as
though I would have to pull the resistant words out of my
head by force and sheer will. Now I have a much lighter feeling about it. It's more fun.

In the last few years Angela has been so successful in her writing that
she has purchased a second home in a popular Florida resort, where she
spends much of her time—and she's happier and more creative than ever.

Peggy: Forty-One Grim Winters

Peggy is an attractive, youthful-looking woman in her late fifties, with
blue eyes, fair skin, and silver-gray hair. Retired now, she worked as a
medical statistician for many years. She was married twice and now
lives alone. She grew up in the Midwest and has had difficulty with the
winter since she was eleven years old. She was always an excellent student. She would start out particularly well in the fall semester, but
when winter came, there were always problems. Her teachers, who regarded her as one of their best students, would register surprise and
dismay at the sudden change in her work. Her parents would also become "disgusted" with her performance, which would decline for no
apparent reason.

   This seasonal problem in school performance increased over time.
In her senior year of high school she was an honors student and was
given the responsibility for keeping a log of student aid contributions.
The task involved simply putting a check mark next to the name of every student who had donated a nickel. Although she applied herself to
the job enthusiastically in the fall, by the time November came, she
found it overwhelming. Having such difficulties with so simple a task
was confusing for Peggy but typical of her state of mind every winter.
She scored above the ninety-ninth percentile on intelligence tests, but
when she had difficulties with simple things, she believed she was a
fraud and that the test results must have been wrong, that teachers
must have given her good grades just because she was a nice person.

Peggy is sure that her mother had SAD as well. During the winter, her mother would nap most of the day, whereas in summer she was energetic and vivacious. Both Peggy and her sister were conceived in August. Winter seemed like a low time for the whole family, and Peggy's own difficulties went unnoticed by the other family members. These troubles reached a crisis during her junior year of high school:

It was mid-January. There had been a string of gray days, but nothing bad had happened. I hadn't failed any exam or lost a boyfriend, but I felt so weighed down and in such a state of despair that I saw no future for myself. Everything I looked at was wrong. I went down into the basement, found a water pipe, got a piece of clothesline, and tried to make a noose out of it, but I was unable to do so. I just didn't have the energy to figure out how to do it properly or the strength to do it.

I went back upstairs to the bedroom I shared with my sister and lay down on my bed crying, disgusted that I couldn't even commit suicide properly. I kept the whole thing to myself. The next day was sunny and I said to myself, "Had you committed suicide yesterday, you wouldn't be alive to see this beautiful day," and I felt better. I always thought that it was a miracle that the sun was shining the next day. I wonder what would have happened had it been cloudy. That experience taught me not to try to predict the future—that one day can be bad and the next day good.

Although Peggy had thoughts of killing herself on several subsequent occasions, that was the only time she ever came close to trying.

During adulthood, Peggy's seasonal cycles continued. She would begin to prepare for winter in September, buying a six-month supply of toilet paper and all other nonperishable goods, "like a squirrel about to hibernate." In November, she notes:

The physical difficulties start first: eating more, sleeping more, and the slowing down of brain functioning. Initially, I'm not sad. I can still sit down and laugh with friends and enjoy my favorite TV shows. As it becomes obvious that I'm less able to function at work or with friends, mental depression starts taking over. I have trouble writing Christmas cards, which adds to my depression, since I am unable to

communicate with people I really care about. Even though I
really don't want to lose touch with them, I simply want to
be left alone from December until April.

Needless to say, this wish to withdraw caused Peggy difficulties
both at work and in her personal relationships:

I worked in an office where there was a lot of gift giving. I
would feel very upset with people who got their gifts out before December 20. I would wonder, "Why can't I get my
gifts out on time?" By then I was closing the door to my office. I didn't want anyone to come in, and I would select only
those phone calls I wanted to take. It was okay if people just
wanted to chat, but I would hate it when they wanted me to
dig up data or, worse still, to do a computer run. In the summer, doing that stuff was like a game. It was fun to sit in front
of the computer. But in the winter any task was daunting.

The winter changes also caused problems in Peggy's relationships
with men, in part due to her irritability and fault finding—common
early signs of her winter depressions. She would drive to work in the
winter "cussing out the other drivers." It was hard for her to believe
that this was the same morning commute that she found enjoyable
during the spring. The same relationships to which she was open in
the summer seemed unappealing in the winter:

I had several relationships with men I met in the fall, during
the beautiful, sunny October days, and managed, because of
the early passion of the relationship, to make it through the
first winter. Summer was great. Then the next winter came
along, and the relationship would collapse. During the winter, when someone canceled an evening social engagement, I
generally felt relieved and spared the guilt of having canceled
the engagement myself.

The memory and thought-processing problems that troubled
Peggy during her school and college days continued to cause difficulties later on. She would forget to set her burglar alarm, or where she
had put the keys, or have problems with other things that she would

take for granted in the summer. Every chore seemed to take much longer in the winter, and complex tasks, which were easy for her in the spring and summer, were quite impossible during the winter months. She would become anxious about her failures, irritated by her ineptitude, and accuse herself once again of being a fraud.

She would eat more in the winter, particularly carbohydrates. When she lived in the Northeast, she would have to drive home from work for an hour each evening through the gray New England landscape, and when she finally reached home, as she confessed to the minister at her church one Lent, she could not resist gorging on cookies. Was she not guilty of gluttony?

Her energy level stayed low all winter long. Over the years she developed strategies for coping. For example, she would buy lots of winter clothes and let the laundry pile up for months until the spring, when she could finally face doing it all.

Peggy's sex drive was low during the winter. She recalls with amusement how there were two workmen in the house one winter. In the late afternoon she was unable to stay awake, so she retired to bed and asked them to tell her husband that he could find her there when he got home from work. When he returned, he was incensed, "as though I were this terrible seductress who had gone to bed, tempting the workmen in the house. He felt as though I had destroyed his honor. I laugh when I think of it now. All I wanted to do was sleep, and the last thing I was interested in was seducing those men."

Peggy was in classical psychoanalysis for three years, "five days a week, every month of the year except for August," but the seasonal pattern of her problems never emerged as an issue for discussion in the analysis. She had no other formal treatment for her seasonal difficulties.

During the summer, she would often feel even more energetic and enthusiastic than the average person. Her high energy level would keep her working in the garden till nine at night, and she would stay awake until two in the morning. She required only six hours of sleep. She recalls with amusement the summer day when she went rowing on a lake with a very large man. She felt so energetic that she did all the rowing, and the sight of a small woman rowing a 200-pound man across a lake caused a group of passing fishermen to whistle catcalls at him.

It was her winter depressions, not her summer highs, that

brought Peggy to the NIMH Seasonal Studies Program. She was beginning to enter her November decline when she received a tax audit notice. The thought of having to collect and submit all the necessary records threw her into an intense depression and induced her to seek psychiatric help. She was fifty-two at the time and had suffered regular winter depressions for forty-one years, though she had never recognized them as such. On being asked how that could have happened, she replied, "I thought it was normal to feel like that in the winter."

Peggy was treated successfully with light therapy. Shortly after treatment was started in January, she managed to refinance her house within a week—something she would never have been able to do before during the winter. After finding out about her seasonal problem, Peggy learned to take winter vacations in the sun. She moved into a house with large windows and decorated it in light colors. She entered weekly psychotherapy to deal with a variety of psychological issues. Having retired from her former job, she undertook a new career, working with elderly people. As a result of her treatment, Peggy now feels fulfilled and much happier with her life than ever before.

When she thinks of what her understanding of SAD and her light treatment have given her, Peggy concludes:

> Now I don't have to blame myself for what happened in past winters. It's liberating to know that SAD is a physical disorder—not my fault. I can give myself some leeway for what happens now. I don't have to be so critical of myself. I have a tool to make myself feel better.

Alan: Too Low or Too High

Alan is a divorced electronics technician in his late thirties. Well built, dark, and handsome, he has a wry smile, a twinkle in his eyes, and a cynical attitude toward life. This view of the world may have been shaped partially by his SAD and its consequences. Since about age seven, he has had winter difficulties—times when he didn't want to be around people, accompanied by changes in sleep and appetite. He was considered a "moody" child, and his greatest early difficulties were related to school, where his dyslexia was aggravated during the winter. He remembers reversing numbers and letters, writing on the wrong side of the page, and having great difficulty spelling. Yet somehow he managed better in the summer and fall. In winter, his increasing difficulties made him panicky about going to school, which he perceived as "an institution where I would have to go to be humiliated."

By age twelve, he was refusing to go to school on a regular basis. He was taken to a psychiatrist and given electroshock therapy, apparently to cure him of his "fears, phobias, and dread of going to school." Not only was it unhelpful, but Alan has grim memories of the experience. By thirteen, the problem was so severe that reform school was considered, and, later, when his parents agreed to go regularly to see a psychiatrist with him, the county provided him with a tutor a few days a week. With this help, Alan was able to pass seventh and eighth grades. Eventually the tutor was dropped, and Alan played hooky regularly until he was fifteen. By then, he was aware that his problems were related not only to school but in some way also to the changing seasons, since he continued to feel bad in the winter.

At fifteen, Alan began to work and, after a series of jobs, became an electronics technician. He dated girls extensively in his late teens and at age nineteen entered into a stormy marriage that was to last eight years. The turbulence in his work and domestic life was dictated to a large extent by his dramatic responses to the seasons:

> By October, I would definitely start to feel a little gray. My performance at work would start falling off, as would my strength, and my sleep would begin to increase. At work, my output would suffer and I'd begin to start charging less for the same job. I lost confidence in the quality of my work. I'd start worrying about everything and ask myself, "Why the hell am I doing this? What's the use?" It was somewhere between apathy and panic, because I knew something was going wrong but had no idea at the time what the heck it was.

His difficulties at work caused Alan to lose jobs on a regular basis, usually around Christmas. Four to five months of unemployment would follow, when he would live on the money he had earned and saved.

> During that time I would feel very depressed. My wife would do all the grocery shopping. In the early years she was worried and panicky and would try to come home and be a cheerleader. I was usually so disagreeable to be around that she didn't say anything about my behavior. If anybody said,

"What's the matter? Why aren't you up getting a job?" I would get very upset, scream, and yell. Usually, after one of those encounters, people would stay clear of me.

If money ran out, Alan would "get some kind of job, moving pianos, driving semis, fixing cars, collecting loans, or bouncing at nightclubs"—anything except working at electronics repairs. He was unable to figure out the logic of the circuitry, diagnose a problem, and find a solution to it—all things that came easily to him during the summer.

In winter, Alan found little pleasure in anything. Occasionally he would forget himself and his misery for a few minutes but would soon be engulfed again by helplessness and despair. He considered suicide many times. Standing by the roadside, he would think of walking in front of a truck; or he would stand on a balcony or bridge and consider "flopping over onto the asphalt below." While taking a bath or shaving himself, he would contemplate his razor and think of cutting his wrists. On one occasion, in the winter, Alan actually tried to kill himself. His winter problems had been getting worse during his late twenties and early thirties, and during that particular winter, he felt the worst ever—"incapacitated, hospital material." One day, he sat for a long time with the barrel of a gun in his mouth, the hammer cocked and his finger on the trigger. He still doesn't know exactly what stopped him from pulling the trigger.

By mid-March, Alan would be aware of a difference in the way he was feeling, and by mid-April, he would begin to emerge from his depression. Between spring and summer, he would move "along a pretty even curve" from depression to exuberance or even mania.

Usually by the time something was green, I was beginning to feel better. It's frightening at first. You begin to wonder, "Is it a teaser? Am I going to feel better for a few days and then bad again?" By May I was feeling pretty damn good. By June and July I was feeling like it was very urgent to do things. With a lot of enthusiasm and exhilaration, I'd think, "I beat the beast again." I felt fantastic compared with how hellacious I had felt in the winter.

By July 4, I would really begin to accelerate, to feel extremely strong and healthy, definitely virile, much more likely to be at all the parties. I'd work as much overtime as I could get. I was on top of the world. By August, things were going even faster, and I was needing less sleep. A lot of people thought I was doing speed during the summer, especially at that time, when a lot of people *were* doing speed. People were amused, shocked, or irritated. For example, at the beach or a party, if I wanted to go into the water nude, I would just do it. But I wasn't using drugs; my mood was simply high—it was summer, after all.

My sex drive would increase and become just about my reason for being. Trying to find one individual who had the same drive was kind of tough. I usually ended up seeing a lot of people during the summer months.

By August, my temper was much worse. If nothing drastic happened, I would generally get through the summer with just a couple of fights. If I really got speeded up, which happened one particular year, I got into trouble with the police. By September, I'd mellow out a little. I'd usually be licking my wounds from what happened in July and August.

Although Alan had made a connection between his changing behavior and the seasons, he had never specifically connected his behavioral changes to the light. But he had always been fascinated by light: "colored light, sunlight, white light, reflections, and, in the sixties, strobe lights." He even built some colored strobe lights for himself. However, he was skeptical when his psychiatrist recommended the NIMH Seasonal Studies Program to him. It sounded "absolutely bizarre—right up there with shock treatments and sleeping under the full moon. It was kind of a lunatic idea." But antidepressants, lithium, and psychotherapy had been of no help to him, so he thought he had little to lose.

His first light treatment was given as part of a study on an inpatient unit. He recalls that "about the third day I said to one of the nurses, 'I feel kind of funny, light-headed. Something's happening.' I got the dose of light that night, and I knew what the feeling was—exhilaration. It was like compressing two or three months into four days. By the fourth day, I asked a nurse to marry me or something, and by five days, I was higher than a kite."

Although individual cases cannot prove the effectiveness of a treatment, it was hard for me to believe that Alan's response was anything other than real and specific. A highly skeptical individual, who had been treated unsuccessfully with a wide range of potent interventions, Alan seemed like the last person to respond to a placebo. In addition, when he was asked to stop using the lights on a number of occasions as part of the research program, he became depressed each time. When Alan restarted light treatments, he observed that the effects were not immediate; rather, it took a day or two before he began to feel good again. If he used them for too long, he would get a tingling feeling in his hands and feet and become "wired" and overactive.

Alan has used lights for the last several years. He has special sets at work, where he has no windows, and at home. After starting light treatment, he functioned well at his job and worked consistently. Financially, it made a big difference for him to be working twelve months a year instead of nine. He was able to establish friendships and hold on to them "without having to start over again in the spring because I've insulted people or disappointed them or just felt too bad to have anything to do with them." He was able to spend time on hobbies he enjoys, such as carpentry. Curiously, he was no longer troubled by manic symptoms in the summer, probably because his light environment was more constant across the seasons. Because Alan's mood was more even all year round, he found life easier and less unpredictable. He became more optimistic and was able to enter into more stable, long-term relationships.

Jeff: A Case of the Winter Blues or February Blahs

Soon after we first encountered patients with SAD, it became clear that there were many people with a milder form of the condition. These people generally would not seek out medical help for their winter difficulties but, when asked specifically about them, would recall having some problem each winter—for example, lack of enthusiasm or decreased productivity. To study these people, Dr. Siegfried Kasper and I undertook a study of what we called subsyndromal SAD, or the winter blues, at the NIMH. We established criteria for this condition, which are outlined in Chapter 3, and set out to find people who met the description.

Jeff, a typical victim of the winter blues, read a newspaper article that provided a checklist of symptoms that people with the winter blues typically experience: low energy, difficulty concentrating and getting one's work done, and tiredness; in short, a syndrome that was milder than the winter depressions we had previously shown to respond to light therapy. Jeff is in his mid-forties and is a well-informed mental health professional, but he had never quite recognized the basis of his seasonal problem.

Looking back on his difficulties, it was clear to him that his ability to concentrate would decline each winter. A self-declared workaholic, he was always less productive during the winter months than during the rest of the year. In winter, he felt tired and attributed it to a lack of sleep, even though he was actually sleeping more than he did during the summer. He had never been treated formally for this winter problem. Instead, he treated his low energy level with cups of coffee and found that if he put several very bright lamps on his desk, it helped him concentrate. He also found that if he had to meet a deadline, he could sometimes do so by sleeping from 7:00 P.M. to midnight and working straight through the night and the following day. Sleep restriction is a known treatment for depression, which I discuss later in this book.

Curiosity led Jeff to take part in the NIMH research program—curiosity and a hope that maybe there was an explanation and a simple treatment for his recurrent winter difficulties. He entered the program with great skepticism. His expectations of the effects of the light treatment were very low. But the treatment worked dramatically for him, and he has used bright light at his desk ever since.

Kasper has shown that bright light is effective for most people with the winter blues, which seem to affect at least twice as many people as SAD. While the effects are not as dramatic, this milder winter syndrome does interfere with the quality of life in those who suffer from it and decreases their productivity. Since it is easily reversible in most cases, it is important to identify these milder symptoms and consider treating them.

Scientists believe that SAD and the winter blues are two broad categories of problematic seasonal change (also known as seasonality) to which many people are susceptible. Although some clearly fall into one category or another on the basis of the severity of their winter problems, many fall into a gray zone between the two. The important point is that bright light or other forms of treatment can help those in either category. The distinction between the two is that those who are depressed should seek professional help, whereas those who are more mildly affected might reasonably consider trying to treat the problem themselves. Guidelines are provided in Chapter 3 to help readers decide when self-help alone might be reasonable and when to consult a physician.

Diagnosing SAD

When clinicians or researchers diagnose a psychiatric condition, they use a set of standardized criteria. When we first described SAD, we needed to develop such a set of criteria. More recently, the American Psychiatric Association has established a different set of criteria, which are laid out in the DSM-IV-TR (see Table 1). While these criteria are useful guidelines for clinicians and researchers, I would encourage you not to take them too seriously. If you experience some of the seasonal changes described in this chapter and find them problematic, you may well have SAD or subsyndromal SAD and may benefit from the treatments described in Part II of this book.

TABLE I
Criteria for Seasonal Affective Disorder

SAD criteria of Rosenthal et al. (1984)	DSM-IV-TR criteria for major depression with "seasonal pattern"
There is a pattern of winter depressions, at least two of which developed during consecutive winters.	There has been a regular temporal relationship between the onset of major depressive episodes and a particular time of the year.
At least one of these depressions was severe enough to meet the criteria for major depression.	In the last two years, two major depressive episodes have occurred that demonstrate the temporal seasonal relationship, and no nonseasonal major depressive episodes have occurred during the same period.
There are nondepressed periods in spring and summer.	Full remissions (or a change from depression to mania or hypomania) also occur at a characteristic time of the year (e.g., depression disappears in the spring).
No other major psychiatric disorder is present.	
There are no clear-cut recurring social or psychological reasons to account for the recurrent winter depression.	There is no obvious effect of seasonal-related psychosocial stressors (e.g., regularly being unemployed every winter).

DSM-IV-TR criteria reprinted with permission from the *Diagnostic and Statistical Manual of Mental Disorders* (4th ed., text revision). Copyright 2000 by the American Psychiatric Association.

Core Symptoms of SAD

Although the individuals profiled earlier had very different experiences with seasonal difficulties, each had some manifestation of the core symptoms of SAD, described below in a little more depth.

SAD as an Energy Crisis

Jenny, a middle-aged housewife, makes the point succinctly:

> I don't really feel depressed. I just feel like all my systems have been turned off for the winter. I feel leaden and heavy and just want to lie about all the time. It's only when I am expected to do something out of the ordinary, and I realize I cannot do it, that I feel my mood being pulled down.

Jenny's description provides us with an important clue to the understanding of SAD and of depression in general. Many of the symptoms of depression involve physical functions: sleeping, eating, activity levels, sex drive. Disturbances in these functions produce physical symptoms, and their presence is an important clue that someone is suffering from a clinical depression and not just ordinary sadness. Often, in fact, the sadness and gloom that we associate with depression are not the most prominent part of the general picture. So important are the physical symptoms that modern diagnostic systems do not permit the diagnosis of depression if there has not been a history of at least some physical symptoms.

Almost all people with SAD have problems with their energy level, and they often express it in similar ways. Here are a few of their voices:

> The fatigue is agony. I feel I have to drag myself from one place to the next.

> Everything seems like more of a chore in the wintertime.

> I have to use all my willpower just to get up in the morning, go to work, be pleasant to people, pay my bills, and put my dishes in the dishwasher.

Changes in Eating, Sleeping, and Sex Drive

Most people with SAD eat more in the winter and report a change in their food preference from the salads, fruits, and other light fare of summer to high-carbohydrate meals: breads, pasta, potatoes, sugary foods. Many have told me that eating carbohydrates actually makes them feel better, more energetic. Laura, a musician in her forties, describes her seasonal change in eating patterns:

> By September and October, I feel like I am constantly feeding and gnawing. My winter diet consists mainly of pastas, macaroni and cheese, rice casseroles, and chicken and mushroom soup—heavy, heavy food. Things that take a long time to cook so you smell them. Stews and pot roast with potatoes and gravy . . . lots of gravy on everything. And dessert— heavy dessert.

Two research groups have actually tried to record the eating habits of people with SAD at different times of year. Dr. Judith Wurtman at MIT and Dr. Anna Wirz-Justice in Basel, Switzerland, have confirmed that the increase in carbohydrate consumption reported by so many patients does, in fact, occur. This pattern seems to be an exaggeration of the eating patterns in the population as a whole. One study performed in the cafeteria of the NIMH found that people eat more carbohydrates in winter and more salads in summer. The same patterns were also found in a study conducted in Montgomery County, Maryland.

People with SAD report that eating carbohydrates seems to give them *more* energy, which is surprising because research with people who do not have SAD shows just the opposite. Dr. Bonnie Spring, now professor of psychology at University of Illinois at Chicago, showed that carbohydrates actually make nondepressed people feel more drowsy. In an NIMH study, my colleagues and I gave high-carbohydrate meals (six big cookies) and high-protein meals (a plate of turkey salad) to people with SAD and nonseasonal people. We found that our patients' reports had been accurate, for the high-carbohydrate meal did indeed make the SAD group feel more energetic, whereas the nonseasonal group felt more fatigued. This suggests that there is a basic difference in the brain chemistry of seasonal and nonseasonal individuals, resulting in a difference in response to carbohydrates.

We don't know for sure what this biochemical difference is, but studies of serotonin, a nerve chemical messenger that is of widespread importance in brain functioning, may provide some answers. Drs. John Fernstrom and Richard Wurtman of MIT showed that in animals dietary carbohydrates increase the production of serotonin in the brain. Further studies show that this mechanism may also occur in humans. One reason patients with SAD crave carbohydrates and consume them in excessive quantities may be that they are responding to an instinct to correct a deficiency in brain serotonin transmission.

Another reason people crave carbohydrates may be that they secrete too much insulin, a hormone released from the pancreas. Insulin drives down blood sugar levels, which, in turn, may result in cravings for sweets and starches.

There is now evidence from researchers in Basel, Switzerland, that patients with SAD do indeed secrete too much insulin in response to dietary carbohydrates. When their depressions improve, during summer or after light therapy, this tendency to oversecrete insulin appears to subside. It is known that a tendency to oversecrete insulin can be quite unhealthy over time. It may signal a greater risk of diabetes, obesity, and heart disease in later life. It is therefore possible that treating SAD properly can be beneficial not only psychologically but also physically. In fact, there is an accumulating literature suggesting a connection between depression and cardiac disease.

Considering the change in diet and the low level of activity that occur in the winter in SAD, it is not surprising that patients tend to gain weight, often quite dramatically. One physician with SAD tells me that his winter trousers are two sizes larger than his summer ones, and that is not unusual. I have seen people gain up to forty pounds in the winter and lose it all the following summer. Unfortunately, some people do not lose it all and become steadily heavier from year to year. This yo-yo pattern of weight loss and weight gain has in itself been associated with serious medical conditions, such as diabetes and heart disease. Besides the strategies for treating SAD, which I outline later in the book, I provide specific dietary advice to avoid the carbohydrate binges and weight gain to which SAD sufferers are so often vulnerable.

People with SAD complain as much about changes in their sleep patterns as they do about their eating. Common problems are difficulty getting up in the morning, being tardy at work, and not getting the children off to school on time. People with SAD generally sleep more but don't feel refreshed on waking. Sleep is often interrupted and "low quality." Laura, the musician mentioned earlier, recalls seasonal changes in sleep patterns from her school days:

> I can remember being unable to get up in the morning during the winter as I was growing up, during high school, junior high. My mother would scream at me to get up and get ready for school. I would drag myself up. In contrast, during the spring, I would go out in the yard every morning before school started and look for a flower to wear in my hair or in my buttonhole. Obviously, I had to get up early enough to go and get the flower and have the desire to do that. In winter, I'd have a terrible time staying awake. . . . I used to work in the cafeteria, and I would get these baking powder biscuits at dinner. You could take home whatever was left over after dinner. So I would take a pile of these biscuits and a Coke. If you put a bite of biscuit and a sip of Coke in your mouth, it reacts and fizzes—that was how I stayed awake to study in the evening after I would get back. I gained a lot of weight, but in the summer, the weight would come off—without dieting.

Flora, an editor in her forties, describes somewhat different sleep patterns:

> I'm tired all the time during my depressions, but I do have a little trouble going to sleep, so I'll read in bed for a long time. I never knew how often I woke up in the middle of the night until I started keeping track of it, but untreated, that's what I do. Then I would find it impossible to get up in the morning and would sleep through the alarm clock. Once, in college, I slept through a fire drill, which made my dorm mates very angry. The bell was right outside my room, and they all went out in the cold and stood there. But since I didn't go out, they had to repeat the fire drill. . . . This was in the winter.

Studies performed at the NIMH actually showed differences between the way people with SAD and nonseasonals sleep at different times of the year. In the winter, people with SAD sleep longer, as measured by electrical recordings of their brain-wave activity. They also have a decrease in a type of deep sleep called slow-wave sleep. The decrease in this component of sleep, as well as the tendency toward more sleep disruptions in SAD patients during the wintertime, may account for their daytime fatigue, despite their increased duration of nighttime sleep.

In most people with SAD, sex drive decreases markedly during the winter. Many people report not wanting to be touched or to exert themselves in any way, but rather wanting to curl up and be left alone. I have heard many reports of women who wear long flannel nighties to bed during the winter. While these garments are worn mainly for warmth and comfort, they send out a strong signal to the partner that the person with SAD has little interest in sex. Male patients with SAD may be similarly affected by a lack of sexual interest. Of course, marked changes in sex drive affect not only the person who experiences them but also his or her partner. The partner can easily feel rejected by the lack of sexual interest shown by the person with SAD. When spring and summer arrive and the SAD patient's sexual interest picks up again, the couple will have to adjust to the new equilibrium, which is often difficult. The patient with SAD, forgetting that he or she has been uninterested in sex for several months, may be surprised at the aloofness of his or her partner. The partner, having felt rejected or, at the very least, frustrated during the winter months, may eye the renewed sexual interest with suspicion or anger. An understanding that marked shifts in sexual interest are a common feature of SAD—together with communication between the partners about this problem—can greatly ease the tensions that tend to result.

Sylvia and Jack are a middle-aged couple who have learned to deal with Sylvia's seasonal changes over twenty years of marriage. Their sex life suffers in the winter, when Sylvia just wants to be left alone. She retires to bed before Jack does, and by the time he gets there, she's asleep. He has learned to let her sleep at those times because, as she puts it, "I wouldn't be much fun if he woke me up." For the rest of the year, the couple enjoys an active and satisfying sex life.

The effect of SAD on relationships is not confined to the sexual arena. People with SAD often just want to be left alone. A woman who may be a social butterfly in the summer often wants no company in the winter. Conversations are avoided and invitations turned down. Anything that requires expending the energy involved in social contact is experienced as an overwhelming demand, to be avoided if at all possible. Many people with SAD compare themselves to hibernating bears. Although this is not a scientifically sound comparison, it accurately conveys the feeling of wanting to be left alone.

As one might expect, there are considerable social costs to such behavior. Friends become annoyed. Marriages come under strain as the spouse experiences withdrawal and distancing on the part of the seasonal person. Lovers are lost, although, at the time, this may be experienced by the SAD sufferer as a relief, since it results in a welcome decrease in personal and sexual demands. I know many seasonal people who have consistently started relationships in spring and summer but failed to keep them through the winter.

Cognitive Problems

As the seasonal people you have already met in this book will testify, problems in thinking are among the most troublesome symptoms of SAD. Generally, we concentrate and process information automatically. It is only when we are unable to do these things that we really notice them. I am sure you can remember a time when you were not thinking properly—for example, when you have been very tired. That is how people with SAD often feel during the winter months. They tend to have problems thinking clearly and quickly. It's very difficult, if not impossible, for them to summon up the information and knowledge needed for their work—or even casual conversations. They are not able to keep up with what is going on around them or what needs to be done.

A scene from Chaplin's *Modern Times* comes to mind. A factory worker is toiling away quite well on an assembly line when suddenly the conveyor belt begins to move faster. The worker rallies in an attempt to keep up with the increased challenge, but eventually, the rate at which he is called upon to perform is accelerated so rapidly that it is impossible for him to continue. This provides a wonderful vehicle for Chaplin's madcap antics. In reality, however, the feeling of having information coming at you faster than you can handle it can be an overwhelming, and even frightening, experience.

In SAD, the ability to concentrate and process information varies greatly over the course of the year. In summer it's a snap; everything goes "click, click, click" and gets done. In winter, it's a drag, with minor tasks taking on major proportions. I have heard many patients say, "I begin to make stupid mistakes in the fall."

These mistakes can become apparent even in the performance of relatively simple tasks. Routine chores such as doing the shopping or cooking a meal involve several steps that need to be performed in a certain sequence. People with SAD often feel unable to focus on the task, to remember all its different parts and to carry them out in the correct sequence. Patients often say, "I just can't get my act together. Simple things seem so difficult." In all the patients profiled in this chapter, a combination of low energy, low motivation, and, especially, difficulty in thinking impaired their ability to function at work, which was a major complaint. In children, this combination of symptoms results in school difficulties, which may be the first problem to come to a parent's attention. The effects of SAD in children and adolescents are discussed in Chapter 5.

Many business executives and professionals with SAD complain that during the winter they are unable to take the necessary steps to handle the tasks that await them. Instead, they hide behind their office doors, shuffling papers around on their desks, creating the appearance of getting work done. Secretaries and assistants, who aren't fortunate enough to have personal offices in which to hide, often call in sick and say they have the flu, a more acceptable excuse than depression.

Tasks involving logic are often especially difficult, but some people complain of difficulties even in estimating distances. One woman reported that while driving during the winter, she had a hard time estimating the distance between her car and the one in front of her. A young tree surgeon with SAD found it hard to estimate the length of a branch he was sawing off and injured himself as a result.

Dr. John Docherty, who has had extensive experience with SAD in Boston and New Hampshire, has estimated the frequency of the different work-related problems encountered by his patients with SAD. They are, in order of frequency, decreased concentration, productivity, interest, and creativity; inability to complete tasks; increased interpersonal difficulties in the workplace; increased absences from work; and simply stopping work. Quite a staggering list of problems.

To measure the cognitive difficulties in SAD objectively, Dr. Connie Duncan and colleagues at the NIMH recorded the brain-wave pattern responses to visual stimuli in SAD patients and others. They showed that a part of the brain-wave response that corresponds to a person's ability to attend to a stimulus increases in strength in patients with SAD after they have been treated with light therapy. This change occurs at the same time as people begin to feel better and their ability to think improves. It should be reassuring for people with SAD to realize that their ability to think can be measured objectively and shown to change after light therapy. It helps them realize that they are suffering from a temporary problem in brain function during their depressed phase and that the problems that arise from their thinking difficulties are not their fault.

Mood Problems

As I mentioned earlier, many people with winter problems may experience physical changes long before any feelings of sadness occur. In fact,
some people may experience only physical changes with the changing
seasons and never feel depressed. These people are comparatively
lucky, because the emotional aspects of depression are among the most
painful experiences known to humans.

John is an engineer who has just turned fifty. A well-groomed
man, with gray hair and blue eyes, he sits in my office, trying to control himself, as he has always been told he should. But the depression
breaks through his mask and the tears begin to roll down his cheeks.
He feels sad, he says, but doesn't know why. Life has no meaning for
him anymore. His wife, children, and job have all ceased to give him
any pleasure. He feels he is just a burden to his family and that they
would be better off without him. He feels guilty—he has let them
down, been a bad father and husband. He thinks back on his childhood and feels that even then he failed to come through for his parents when they needed him. He goes to work each day racked with
anxiety—small problems become overwhelming. How will he get it all
done? Perhaps the best thing would be to end it all, but that is against
his religion. He contemplates a spot on the freeway where the road
veers sharply to the right and there is a steep decline to the left. Sometimes he thinks about driving his car over the edge if the pain gets too
bad. That way, he reckons, his suicide might look like an accident and
not be a source of shame to his family.

John expresses feelings that are typical of depressed people and,
indeed, he is severely depressed. His thoughts—that he is a failure as a
father, husband, and worker—are not shared by his children, his wife,
and his supervisor, all of whom feel he is caring, devoted, and hard-
working. They can legitimately be regarded as distortions of reality,
though they certainly feel real to him. A serious symptom of severe depression is losing touch with reality in this way.

A college student in her late twenties described the loss of perspective that occurs in depression:

> A patient with diabetes knows that his pancreas is disordered,
> and that's not so hard to understand. But when you're de-
> pressed, your mind and heart and soul are disordered—every-
> thing that makes you a human being—and that's not so sim-
> ple to understand, especially when you are in the middle of it.

The anxiety that John reports often occurs in depression, and treatment often helps it, as well as the sadness. Sometimes the unpleasant feelings that depressed people experience are directed outward to others. People with SAD often recognize that they are being snappy, irritable, and unpleasant toward others but are unable to restrain themselves. It is important for the friends and family of a person with SAD to recognize that if these behaviors are confined to the autumn and winter, they are almost certainly symptoms of the condition. This recognition helps the affected person's friends and family not to take angry or snappy comments too personally.

Depressed people—including those with SAD—often distort reality by blaming themselves unfairly. Another type of cognitive distortion that may occur involves blaming others—or one's life circumstances—for problems that are really the result of SAD. A woman might say, for example, "My marriage is going wrong because my husband is inconsiderate and too demanding," while the major reason may be that she is depressed and unable to meet his needs. Another might say, "This job is not right for me. It's causing me distress and feelings of failure." While a difficult job can aggravate the symptoms of SAD, the main cause of the problem at work may be the SAD itself. I often counsel patients not to make important decisions while they are depressed if they can possibly avoid doing so. Decisions made hastily by a depressed person are often the result of mistakenly attributing one's problems to one's life circumstances, and they are often regretted later. The best way for a depressed person to handle problematic life circumstances, either at work or at home, is to have the depression treated first and then to decide on the best course of action.

Physical Illnesses and SAD

People with SAD may suffer all sorts of physical problems during the winter months, from backaches, muscle aches, and headache to different types of infection. Many people with SAD feel as though they have suffered from the flu all winter long. We don't really know whether having SAD or being depressed actually makes you more likely to get the flu, or whether it just feels worse to be sick when you are already suffering from SAD. Fibromyalgia, a condition of muscular aches and pains occurring especially in the neck and shoulder areas, typically gets more severe in the winter, is associated with sleep difficulties, and responds to treatment with antidepressants. Researchers have speculated that it may be some-

how related to SAD, and it would be interesting to find out whether it responds to light therapy. The idea that the mind or brain exerts an influence on the body in general and the immune system in particular is
gaining increasing acceptance in scientific circles and is an exciting new
area of developing research. The possible relationship between SAD and
physical afflictions has yet to be explored fully.

Premenstrual Difficulties

At least half of all menstruating women with SAD report that they
have suffered from emotional and physical problems related to their
periods, usually in the week before the period begins. This condition,
premenstrual syndrome (PMS), also known as premenstrual dysphoric
disorder (PMDD), may occur all year round, but most severely in winter. Others have PMS only in the winter. Many women say that during
their premenstrual period, they feel a bit like they do when they have
SAD.

Sharon is a housewife in her early thirties and the mother of two
teenagers. She is aware of eating too much, craving sweets and starchy
foods, gaining weight, and sleeping more during the four or five days
before her menstrual period. At these times, she tends to retain fluid,
and her rings feel tight on her fingers. She also has abdominal cramps.
But most distressing to her and her family is her irritability during
these days. She will tend to pick fights with her husband, with whom
she normally gets along rather well. This was especially bad before
they recognized the cyclicity of their arguments and their biological
origin. Now they have learned to beware during the week before her
period and have resolved to postpone all contentious discussions until after it has passed. Even her children have learned to tread carefully during those premenstrual days. Irritability is more typical of
PMS than SAD, where people more commonly feel lethargic and sluggish. One woman pointed out to me in colorful terms that "My
premenstrual problem is like a black cloud hanging over me; the winter problem is more like being in a blue funk—it's a condition inside of
me that I walk around with."

Not every episode of PMS is necessarily the same. During some
cycles, a period may arrive unexpectedly without any symptoms of
PMS. Yet at other times, unpredictably, these difficulties may be rather
severe. In a similar fashion, the severity of episodes of SAD may also
vary from cycle to cycle, from one year to the next.

Hunger for Light

Even before any formal studies of light therapy had been performed, some patients had made a connection between light and mood. For example, one woman would routinely sit in front of her plant lights because she found she felt better there. Another would wander through brightly lit supermarkets at night, while still another would seek out the photocopying room because it was well lit. It is common for people with SAD to want to turn on all the lights in the house during the dark winter days. One middle-aged woman was nicknamed "Lights" by her husband because of this habit. For some, the wish to turn on all the lights in the house has led to arguments about the high cost of electricity from spouses who have not understood the biological nature of their partners' needs.

In their search for light, some people have instinctively chosen winter vacations in the south, year after year. Others have relocated permanently. In many instances, the people involved may not have realized how medically important it was for them to move—they may just have done so instinctively. Not all patients with SAD have made the association between their symptoms and the amount of available environmental light. Some have reacted by lying down in darkened rooms, thereby inadvertently aggravating their symptoms. It is important to recognize that SAD is a condition where the patient's behavior can have a profound effect on how he or she feels. Light-seeking behavior can do much to alleviate symptoms. Conversely, avoiding the light can make matters much worse.

Self-Treatment with Drugs:
Alcohol, Caffeine, Nicotine, and Others

> Stay me with flagons, comfort me with apples
> For I am sick of love.
> —*Song of Songs*

Since biblical times, people have realized the mood-altering effects of food and wine. In an attempt to feel better, depressed people often resort to commonly available drugs, some of which may compound the problem. I have already discussed the use of sugar and starches as mood regulators by people with SAD, but, obviously, the effects of food go beyond its carbohydrate content. Many people specifically crave chocolate, perhaps seeking the combination of sugar and caffeine that it contains. Others crave stews, pastas, "heavy," and "crunchy" foods. One woman with SAD actually craved broccoli in the wintertime. We cannot explain these idiosyncratic choices, but it is possible that these cravings may represent the physiological need for a particular nutrient. Gratifying that need may result in an improved sense of well-being, if only for a short while.

Caffeine is a mood-altering drug that often appeals to people who feel sluggish, lethargic, and unable to get things accomplished. Flora, mentioned earlier, recalls caffeine addiction during her depressed times:

> I used to drink eight, ten, or twelve mugs—tremendous amounts of coffee steadily all day: espresso, made by drip method. At times, the amount of coffee it took to keep me going was enough to upset my stomach.

Caffeine is such a widely available and accepted stimulant that patients with SAD naturally gravitate toward the coffeepot or the teakettle. When these are not available, caffeinated sodas are a common substitute. People often drink many more cups of tea or coffee in the winter than in the summer. Although the immediate stimulant effect of caffeine can be quite useful in certain circumstances, it also has distinct problems and limitations. These are becoming more widely appreciated, as evidenced by the growing number of calls for decaffeinated coffee. Besides indigestion and abdominal cramps, caffeine can cause jitteriness, palpitations, and insomnia. In addition, people frequently become tolerant of its effects, so they may have to drink increasing amounts to get the same energy boost. Nevertheless, the problems associated with caffeine should not be overstated: Many people drink it with impunity, and for them, a few cups of tea or coffee a day may be helpful. I should remind those who want to stop drinking tea or coffee that doing so abruptly can cause withdrawal symptoms, such as sluggishness and headaches.

Alcohol is another substance to which depressed people at times resort—"drowning their sorrows in drink," as the saying goes. One patient who comes to mind is John, an engineer in his early fifties. During the fall and winter, he feels increasingly depressed as he becomes less able to function effectively at work. His regular routine of exercising usually falters at this time, and he tends to drink to obliterate his painful feelings of failure. Not surprisingly, the heavy drinking becomes a problem in its own right and causes him further difficulties at work and at home. Drinking too much alcohol can, of course, cause many problems, a detailed description of which goes beyond the scope of this book. It is well known that excessive alcohol use can be physically harmful, disrupt relationships, kill others (as in driving while intoxicated), and ruin the life of the addicted individual. What is less well known, however, is that in depressed people, even small amounts of alcohol, which are easily tolerated by many people, tend to aggravate the symptoms of depression, sometimes days after the drinking has occurred. At times, it has taken me a while to convince patients of this relationship between alcohol and the worsening of their depressive symptoms. The patient and I have had to observe the sequence of drinking and mood exacerbation several times over before he or she is finally persuaded that there is a cause-and-effect relationship.

I have also seen people turn to marijuana in the winter. One young man—a tennis instructor greatly concerned with his physical health—takes up marijuana each winter, despite his awareness of its potential physical dangers. He is an enthusiastic and upbeat person in the summer, sought out by friends and employees for his support, understanding, and counsel, but he feels desolate and bleak in the wintertime. Life loses all of its charms, and nothing seems to give him any pleasure. At these times, he smokes marijuana to escape into a haze in which his daily cares seem far removed. He does not feel happy with this solution to his problems and is eager for alternative approaches.

Even smoking tobacco may seem more appealing in the winter. One physician in his mid-forties, who hardly needs any lectures on the harmfulness of tobacco, takes up smoking during the winter, even though he has given it up the previous spring.

So it is that many people seek refuge from the pain of SAD in commonly available substances. Some, like pasta and cookies, may be innocuous unless eaten to great excess. Others, like alcohol, can be more destructive, creating problems that far exceed those for which it is consumed. Why some people resort to alcohol, while others resort to cookies or chocolates, is not understood at all. It may be a feature of our peculiar individual biochemical makeup, or a result of what we were conditioned to associate with comfort from childhood. For example, one friend of mine recalls being comforted with sips of brandy when she woke up at night as a child feeling sick. In other families, ice cream or candy may be the standard remedy. In general, these "drug" solutions are regarded as unsatisfactory by those who adopt them. For better solutions, I refer you to Part II on treatments for SAD.

Other Conditions That May Resemble SAD

In medicine, it is always important to question a diagnosis. Could you be suffering from a condition other than (or in addition to) the one you suspect? In a suspected case of SAD, we need to consider other conditions that produce similar symptoms, such as lethargy, overeating, carbohydrate craving, weight gain, and depression. Many physical illnesses can cause lethargy and depression, which is why it is important for people who think they are suffering from SAD to be checked out by a physician. However, it is unusual for other conditions to appear in the winter and leave in the summer, year after year. Even so, it is better to be on the safe side and have a physical examination and the necessary blood tests, since you could have another illness as well as SAD.

Specific illnesses that need to be considered are the following:

1. *Underactive thyroid function (hypothyroidism)*. In this condition, people feel sluggish and cannot tolerate the cold weather. The thyroid gland, situated centrally in the front of the neck, is responsible for producing hormones that regulate the rate of metabolism. Underactivity of the thyroid can usually be treated simply by taking thyroid hormone in the form of pills.

2. *Low blood sugar (hypoglycemia)*. People with this condition feel weak and light-headed at times, usually one to two hours after a meal. They may feel very hungry and crave sweets. This condition can usually be treated by dietary regulation. People with hypoglycemia should avoid foods containing high concentrations of sugar in forms that are rapidly absorbed into the system. Examples of these "simple" carbohydrates are candies and other very sweet things. Instead, people with this condition should eat combinations of proteins and complex carbohydrates, such as fruit and legumes.

3. *Chronic viral illnesses*. SAD symptoms can resemble those of the Epstein–Barr (E-B) virus (which is responsible for infectious mononucleosis) or even the flu, which may be most prevalent during the winter. It is not uncommon for people to feel lethargic and debili-

tated for some time after a bad attack of flu. Similarly, the E-B virus may cause long-term lethargy and fatigue.

Unfortunately, chronic viral illnesses are very difficult to diagnose precisely, and there are no specific treatments for them. Blood tests showing antibodies against the E-B virus simply indicate that a person has been infected in the past—not that the virus is necessarily responsible for the present symptoms. Luckily, however, most cases of chronic E-B virus infection get better with time.

Although viral conditions may masquerade as SAD, the occurrence winter after winter of typical SAD symptoms, which improve in spring and summer, points strongly to SAD. In any event, since the presence of viral infections is difficult to document and there are no specific treatments for them, and since there are specific treatments for SAD, it usually makes sense to treat the problem as SAD.

4. *Chronic fatigue syndrome (CFS)*. This disabling condition is thought to occur following viral infections, at least in some cases, but its causes are poorly understood. Whatever its cause, the patient is often left in a state of disabling fatigue. My colleagues and I at the NIMH surveyed a group of CFS patients for a history of seasonal variations in mood and behavior and found that they reported changes that were even less prominent than those occurring in the general population. This suggests that CFS patients suffer from a condition quite separate from SAD that troubles them all year round. It is unknown at this time whether light therapy is of any benefit whatsoever in these individuals.

Importantly, however, some cases of CFS have a specific basis—such as Lyme Disease—and can be treated. It is therefore important to fully explore this condition with your doctor and, together, search diligently for a cure.

SAD Plus: The Problem of Comorbidity

Although researchers have sought out "pure" cases of SAD in which problems are confined to the criteria described earlier, the real world is not usually so tidy. Having more than one psychiatric condition, which is called comorbidity, is commonplace. Often the symptoms of SAD are superimposed on top of other conditions, such as chronic depression, also known in its milder form as dysthymia; PMS (as already described); and eating disorders such as anorexia nervosa and bulimia.

While it is beyond the scope of this book to go into each of these conditions in detail, it is important to look for any seasonal component to them as this may suggest that treating the SAD elements could be of some benefit. I deal with this in greater detail in Part II.

As we have seen, there is a great deal of variability in the degree to which people respond to the changing seasons, even among those for whom these changes are a problem. One of the most important reasons for recognizing how seasonal you are is that it helps you understand so much about your behavior that might previously have seemed inexplicable. Another reason is that it helps you determine whether to take steps that will alleviate the effects that the changing seasons have on you.

All of the people described in this chapter benefited from therapy with bright light. Peggy, Alan, and Jeff received this in a formal treatment setting, whereas Neal and Angela undertook treatment on their own. Both Neal and Angela believe that they made mistakes as a result of not having had their treatment properly supervised. Neal used the lights for too many hours each day. As a result, he felt "wired"—excessively activated and uncharacteristically irritable. Through trial and error, he finally found out how much light he needed. Angela did not realize that she should sit within three feet of the fixture and thus did not experience the full benefit of the light for some time.

The five people described in this chapter are very different individuals, united by one particular trait—their marked physical and emotional responses to the changing seasons. Although their symptoms will sound familiar to all SAD sufferers, individual experiences are colored to a large degree by a person's particular personality and life situation. The following chapter will show you how to evaluate your own degree of seasonality and whether you might benefit from light therapy.

THREE

How Seasonal Are You?

> "It is certainly very cold," said Peggotty.
> "Everybody must feel it so."
> "I feel it more than other people," said Mrs. Gummidge.
> —CHARLES DICKENS, *David Copperfield*

Most people are seasonal, though some are more so than others. In fact, my colleagues and I at the NIMH were astonished to find that over ninety percent of all those who responded to a survey we conducted in Maryland, about thirty-nine degrees north, reported that they felt some difference in mood, energy, or behavior with the change of seasons. In this chapter, I will show you how to determine how seasonal you are by means of the Seasonal Pattern Assessment Questionnaire (SPAQ), which we developed for research purposes but which turns out to be very easy to administer and interpret once you have the key. Using the SPAQ, researchers have established that seasonality is actually a genetically transmitted trait and have estimated the prevalence of SAD and the winter blues in many parts of the world. (See Chapter 4.)

To understand the pattern and extent of your seasonality, complete the SPAQ, shown in Figure 1. To obtain a stable and accurate assessment, you will have to think back over a period of time—say, three years—when you have lived continuously in one climatic region. Since

The purpose of this form is to find out how your mood and behavior change over time. Please fill in all the relevant circles. Note: We are interested in your experience; not others you may have observed.

1. In the following questions, fill in circles for all applicable months. This may be a single month ●, a cluster of months, E.G., ●●●, or any other grouping.
   At what time of year do you . . .

	J a n	F e b	M a r	A p r	M a y	J u n	J u l	A u g	S e p	O c t	N o v	D e c
A. Feel best	○	○	○	○	○	○	○	○	○	○	○	○
B. Tend to gain most weight	○	○	○	○	○	○	○	○	○	○	○	○
C. Socialize most	○	○	○	○	○	○	○	○	○	○	○	○
D. Sleep least	○	○	○	○	○	○	○	○	○	○	○	○
E. Eat most	○	○	○	○	○	○	○	○	○	○	○	○
F. Lose most weight	○	○	○	○	○	○	○	○	○	○	○	○
G. Socialize least	○	○	○	○	○	○	○	○	○	○	○	○
H. Feel worst	○	○	○	○	○	○	○	○	○	○	○	○
I. Eat least	○	○	○	○	○	○	○	○	○	○	○	○
J. Sleep most	○	○	○	○	○	○	○	○	○	○	○	○

   OR ○○○○○○○○○○ No particular month(s) stand out as extreme on a regular basis

2. To what degree do the following change with the seasons?
   (ONE CIRCLE ONLY FOR EACH QUESTION)

	0 NO CHANGE	1 SLIGHT CHANGE	2 MODERATE CHANGE	3 MARKED CHANGE	4 EXTREMELY MARKED CHANGE
A. Sleep length	○	○	○	○	○
B. Social activity	○	○	○	○	○
C. Mood (overall feeling of well being)	○	○	○	○	○
D. Weight	○	○	○	○	○
E. Appetite	○	○	○	○	○
F. Energy level	○	○	○	○	○

3. If you experience changes with the seasons, do you feel that these are a problem for you? . . . . ○ No ○ Yes

   If yes, is this problem . . . .
MILD	MODERATE	MARKED	SEVERE	DISABLING
○	○	○	○	○

4. By how much does your weight fluctuate during the course of the year?
   ○ 0–3 lbs.
   ○ 4–7 lbs.
   ○ 8–11 lbs.
   ○ 12–15 lbs.
   ○ 16–20 lbs.
   ○ Over 20 lbs.

5. Approximately how many hours of each 24-hour day do you sleep during each season? (Include naps)

   Hours slept per day   OVER 18 HOURS
   ○ WINTER (Dec 21–Mar 20) ⓪①②③④⑤⑥⑦⑧⑨⑩⑪⑫⑬⑭⑮⑯⑰⑱   ○
   ○ SPRING (Mar 21–June 20) ⓪①②③④⑤⑥⑦⑧⑨⑩⑪⑫⑬⑭⑮⑯⑰⑱   ○
   ○ SUMMER (June 21–Sept 20) ⓪①②③④⑤⑥⑦⑧⑨⑩⑪⑫⑬⑭⑮⑯⑰⑱   ○
   ○ FALL (Sept 21–Dec 20) ⓪①②③④⑤⑥⑦⑧⑨⑩⑪⑫⑬⑭⑮⑯⑰⑱   ○

6. Do you notice a change in food preference during the different seasons? . . . . ○ No ○ Yes

   Please specify:
   _____
   _____
   _____

FIGURE 1. Questionnaire for evaluating your degree of seasonality.
   Modified from the Seasonal Pattern Assessment Questionnaire (SPAQ) of N. E. Rosenthal, G. Bradt, and T. Wehr (public domain).
   Note to scholars and researchers: Over the years, many have written to me to ask for permission to use this questionnaire. The SPAQ was developed under the aegis of the NIMH, a government institution, and is therefore in the public domain and can be used freely by scholars and researchers. Notifying its authors of your planned usage of this instrument in a research project is merely a courtesy. The "Further Reading" section in this book lists those articles that may be of assistance in the scoring and interpretation of this instrument.

52

seasonality can change over time, and the most recent years are generally clearest in one's memory, think of the most recent three years during which you have lived consistently in one area when considering the questions posed by the SPAQ.

How to Interpret Your Scores on the SPAQ

I. What is your seasonal pattern?

The first step in determining how seasonal you are is to rate your seasonal pattern (see question 1 on the SPAQ). Based on the analysis of many SPAQ responses, we came up with definitions for different patterns of seasonality. How you filled out the questionnaire will give you an idea of which one applies to you:

• *If you feel worst in December, January, or February, you have a winter seasonal pattern.* Almost half of all people in the northern United States report that they feel worst during the winter and can be said to have a winter pattern of seasonality. This pattern is more marked among people who live at higher latitudes. For example, a higher percentage of people dislike winter in New Hampshire (forty-two degrees north) than in Sarasota, Florida (twenty-seven degrees north). On the other hand, the closer people are to the equator, the more they dislike summer. In south Florida, for example, more people report disliking summer than winter, presumably because of the heat and humidity.

Most winter types report eating most, sleeping most, and gaining the most weight in the winter months and, conversely, eating and sleeping least and losing weight during the summer months. They also find it easiest to socialize during the summer. Although they often join in the round of parties that takes place at Christmas, they find it hard to muster up the spontaneous pleasure of summer get-togethers, where they feel a true desire to mix with people. Rather, winter celebrations often take on the quality of a chore, a command performance, asked of people who would much rather be left alone with a dish of sweets. Indeed, people with SAD often report a strong preference for sweets and starches during the winter months—an exaggeration of an eating trend observed in the general population. People also commonly report preferring "heavy" foods—stews and casseroles—during the winter months, whereas salads, fresh fruit and vegetables, and protein-rich foods are preferred in the summer months.

• *If you feel worst in July or August, you have a summer seasonal pattern.* Interestingly, in the United States and Europe winter types are far more common, while in Japan and China, more people dislike the summer. At this time, it is unclear whether these differences are genetic or related to the more widespread availability of air conditioning in warm regions in the West. People who dislike summer may tend to socialize least at that time. Unlike winter types, they often do not overeat, oversleep, and gain weight during the time of year when they feel the worst. Instead, they tend to eat less, lose weight, and sleep less.

• *If you feel worst during December, January, or February and July or August, you have a summer–winter pattern.* Summer–winter types may enjoy only the spring and fall.

• *If there is no time of year when you generally feel best or worst, you have a nonseasonal pattern.* Some people report very few seasonal changes at all. These people will generally mark most of the items in question 2 as not changing with the seasons.

There are other, less common seasonal patterns. For example, some people feel worst in the spring; others in spring and fall. Note that the patterns discussed here refer to those who have been living in the northern hemisphere; the opposite months would apply to those in the southern hemisphere.

The pattern of sleeping and eating more and gaining weight in the winter is often seen even in those who do not have SAD. What distinguishes people with SAD and the winter blues from the general population is the overall seasonality score, which is greater in the first two groups than in the population at large.

2. How seasonal are you?

The severity of your seasonality is determined by examining the degree to which you experience seasonal changes in sleep length, social activity, mood (overall feeling of well-being), weight, appetite, and energy level (see question 2 of the SPAQ).

To derive your overall seasonality score, add up your scores for all six items, for a possible range of 0 to 24. This overall seasonality score would be expected to vary depending on where you live. For example, the same person who has a very high seasonality score during years spent in Alaska is likely to find the score greatly reduced after living for several years in Hawaii. Likewise, successful treatment is also likely to reduce one's overall seasonality score. In general, the six functions measured vary seasonally most markedly in people with SAD, but also in those less severely affected and in the general population. The extent to which they vary is reflected in the overall seasonality score.

Your overall seasonality score can provide you with a rough guideline as to whether you may be suffering from seasonal problems. For example, most people who do not experience seasonal problems have overall seasonality scores of 7 points or less. Most people with full-blown SAD have seasonality scores of 11 or more, while people with the winter blues may have scores of 8, 9, or 10. Remember, these are just rough guidelines, not hard-and-fast rules. Use these guidelines together with the other factors outlined in Table 2 to help you determine whether you may be suffering from SAD or the winter blues.

TABLE 2
Diagnosing SAD and the Winter Blues on the Basis of the SPAQ

	SAD	Winter blues
Question 1		
Seasonal pattern: During which months do you feel worst?	Winter type (feel worst in months between December and February)	Winter type (feel worst in months between December and February)
Question 2		
Overall seasonality score: To what degree do the following change with the seasons: sleep length, social activity, mood, weight, appetite, and energy level? (Obtain score as indicated above.)	11 or more	8–10
Question 3		
If you experience changes with the seasons, do you feel that these are a problem for you? If yes, is the problem mild, moderate, marked, severe, or disabling?	Yes; moderate or greater	If score on question 2 is 8 or 9: Yes; mild or greater If score on question 2 is 10: No or Yes; mild or greater

According to a population study conducted by Dr. Siegfried Kasper and colleagues at the NIMH, women in their late thirties tend to have the highest seasonality scores, which tend to decrease as they get older. There is less evidence that seasonality scores change with age in men.

3. Are seasonal changes a problem for you, and, if so, to what degree?

If seasonal changes are a problem for you, you may regard them as mild, moderate, marked, severe, or disabling (see question 3 of the SPAQ). Your answer to this question should be related to your overall seasonality score. The higher your score, the more likely it is that the changing seasons are a problem for you. Almost all people accepted into the NIMH programs as either SAD or subsyndromal SAD patients rated their seasonal changes as being at least a mild problem. Approximately twenty-five percent of the general population surveyed in the northern United States report the changing seasons are a problem for them. Most of these complain of winter rather than summer difficulties and could benefit by increasing their environmental light exposure during the winter months.

Questions 4, 5, and 6

These questions about the weight you gain and lose during the year, the number of hours you sleep during different seasons, and any changes in food preference you experience through the year are not taken into account for scoring purposes but are of interest to clinicians and researchers who treat SAD and may be of interest to you as well. We have found that patients with SAD report sleeping an average of two and a half hours more in winter than in summer. Corresponding figures for people with the winter blues and the general population in the northeastern United States are 1.7 hours and 0.7 hours, respectively.

In interpreting how you filled out the SPAQ, it is important to remember that the questionnaire was developed as an instrument for population surveys as well as to screen patients in a clinical setting, but not as a diagnostic test. For that reason, you should not depend on the test results alone as a guide to diagnosis. If, after completing this questionnaire, you think you may have a significant problem with the

changing seasons, I encourage you to follow up by scheduling a detailed clinical evaluation. Guidelines on the following pages will help
you decide when it may be appropriate to consult a doctor. First, however, use Tables 2 and 3 to evaluate whether you may have SAD or the
winter blues.

Estimating Whether You Are Suffering from SAD or the Winter Blues on the Basis of the SPAQ

Remember that a person may have the winter blues when living in one
type of climate (say, southern California), but this may develop into
full-blown SAD after the person moves north (say, to Michigan). The
same person may be free of all symptoms after relocating permanently

TABLE 3
Clinical Guide to Distinguishing SAD from the Winter Blues

	SAD	Winter blues
Winter changes last at least four weeks	Yes	Yes
Regular winter problems (at least two consecutive years)	Yes	Yes
Interferes with functioning (work or interpersonal)	To a significant degree (productivity decreases markedly; marked loss of interest or pleasure; withdrawal from friends and family; conspicuous changes in energy, sleeping, or weight)	To a mild degree (less creative; slightly less productive; less enthusiastic about life; less enthusiastic about socializing; slight decrease in energy or bothersome weight gain)
Have seen doctor or therapist about winter problem (or others have suggested it)	Yes	No
Have felt really down or depressed in winter for at least two weeks	Yes	No

to an equatorial climate, such as Venezuela. In providing diagnostic guidelines based on a questionnaire, we decided on cutoff scores that include most people who have the condition in question and exclude most people who do not have the condition. The guidelines outlined in Table 2 tend to be a little on the strict side, especially for diagnosing the winter blues. In other words, studies have shown that some people may not meet SPAQ criteria for these conditions but may be found to have SAD or the winter blues on the basis of clinical evaluation. Those people with SAD will generally, at the very least, meet SPAQ criteria for the winter blues; however, they may not qualify for any diagnosis according to the SPAQ criteria. People tend to rate themselves differently—more or less strictly—which may account for some of the discrepancies between self-rating and clinical evaluation. If your diagnosis, based on your SPAQ responses, differs from your perception of yourself as someone with SAD or the winter blues, remember that the SPAQ is only a guide. Table 3 shows how clinicians go about making the diagnoses of SAD and the winter blues and may provide you with further insight into whether you may be suffering from one of these conditions.

When to Seek Medical Advice

It is likely that in the future, more and more people will become aware of comparatively minor, subtle seasonal difficulties and will attempt to modify their environmental lighting to cope with them. A self-help approach is reasonable as long as symptoms are mild. Those who score 12 or more on the SPAQ or consider their seasonal problem to be at least of moderate severity, however, may well benefit from a professional's care.

You should definitely seek medical help if:

1. *Your functioning is impaired to a significant degree.* For example, if you develop problems at work that are marked enough for others to notice, such as:

- Difficulty getting to work on time on a regular basis
- Marked reduction in your ability to think and concentrate so that you make frequent errors or take much longer than normal to finish a task
- Difficulty completing tasks that you could previously manage

Be sure to catch the problem before your supervisors or clients do and turn it around by getting appropriate help.

The problem can also occur in your personal life. For example, you may feel that you want to be left alone and withdraw significantly, which can cause difficulties with friends or family. Your spouse or partner may feel that you are distant and unavailable. It may be worth asking significant people in your life to what degree they feel your winter difficulties interfere with feeling close to you. If the degree is significant, it would pay to get help for the problem rather than to risk damage to important relationships.

You should also suspect that your ability to function is slipping if you begin to fall behind with bills and other necessary chores. Marked seasonal changes in thinking and getting things done can result in chaos in the administrative areas of one's life, which further amplifies feelings of depression and hopelessness and often consumes the spring months with digging out from under the winter mess.

2. *You experience significant feelings of depression.* This includes the following:

- Regularly feeling sad or having crying spells
- Feeling that life is not worthwhile, or wishing you would not wake up in the morning
- Thinking negative thoughts about yourself—that you are a bad person, incompetent, unreliable, an impostor—which you would regard as inaccurate descriptions of yourself at other times of the year
- Feeling guilty much of the time
- Feeling pessimistic about the future

3. *Your physical functions are markedly disturbed during the winter.* For example:

- You require several more hours of sleep per day or have great difficulty waking up in the morning.
- You would like to lie around for much of the day.
- You feel you have no control over your eating and weight.

All of these symptoms are indications that you should have the situation checked out and treated, if necessary, by an appropriate professional. If your symptoms of depression are severe, and especially if you have suicidal thoughts, you should seek out a qualified professional as a matter of urgency. On the other hand, if your symptoms are mild, you may choose to enhance your environmental light levels on your own either with the help of special fixtures or by generally increasing the lighting in your home or workplace. I discuss light therapy and other useful strategies for turning around the winter problem in Part II.

Besides seasonal changes, some people react strongly to a variety of climatic conditions. Most people enjoy sunny days and dislike gray, cloudy days; most prefer dry to humid weather. The difference between seasonal types is primarily in the degree to which they dislike certain types of weather or climate. Winter types strongly prefer long, sunny days and abhor short, dark ones. Summer types, on the other hand, strongly dislike the heat and greatly prefer cool weather.

Obviously, some external factors that can produce changes in mood or physical symptoms on a seasonal basis do not imply SAD. For example, people with allergies have trouble during certain seasons. Pollen appears in high concentrations at different times of the year, and your specific allergy may determine when you are most miserable. I mention this mainly to point out that a seasonal problem simply provides a clue that some seasonally changing variable may be causing distress or difficulty. This might include a psychological or work-related factor. For example, an accountant may be most stressed at tax season and a landscaper during the summer. In all of these cases, the changing seasons are like some giant shape sorter, sorting out different types of people according to their specific biological or occupational vulnerabilities.

FOUR

What Causes SAD?

While the other chapters in this section are of practical use, this chapter is intended for the curious, those who are not satisfied with knowing how to diagnose and treat SAD but who want to know more. Why do some people get SAD while others don't? Why are the symptoms of SAD worse at certain times than at others? And how might the various treatments outlined in this book work their seemingly magical effects? If you're seeking answers to these questions, read on.

There are three keys to the development of depression in SAD:

- Inherent vulnerability
- Environment, specifically light deprivation
- Stress

Inherent Vulnerability

Although SAD affects all types of people, women are most vulnerable, and the twenties through the forties seem to be prime time for this problem. SAD runs in families, and most patients have at least one close relative with a history of depression (often SAD). An example of familial transmission is described by a woman in Tennessee who has had a long history of SAD: "We have identified [my SAD] as coming to me through my paternal grandmother, being carried by her seven sons, and showing up as active illness in the females of my generation."

In a study of thousands of twin pairs in Australia, Pamela Madden and colleagues found that seasonality is heritable. Although her sample did not include enough patients with SAD to comment on the genetic basis for SAD, we have since found certain genetic variations that are associated with this condition. My colleagues and I have found at least two separate genetic variants associated with SAD, both in genes involved in the transmission of nerve signals by means of the neurotransmitter (nerve chemical messenger) serotonin. I discuss these new discoveries later in this chapter.

We really don't know why women are more vulnerable to SAD than men, but we suspect that it is related to the cyclical secretion of the female sex hormones, estrogen and progesterone. Support for this theory comes from population surveys in both adults and children. Dr. Siegfried Kasper and I, in our survey of adults in Maryland, found that women showed a greater tendency to seasonal changes between their twenties and their forties—in other words, during their reproductive years. After menopause—when there is a profound decrease in the cyclical secretion of female sex hormones—the tendency to experience seasonal changes was no greater in women than in men.

Support for the relationship between seasonal changes in women and the secretion of female sex hormones was also provided in a survey of Maryland schoolchildren by Dr. Susan Swedo and colleagues. Young girls report a marked increase in seasonal changes after puberty. In boys, on the other hand, there is not such a clear-cut relationship between seasonal changes and the onset of puberty. Female sex hormones may predispose affected individuals to seasonal changes by acting directly on certain brain centers. There is good evidence that receptors for sex hormones are present in the brain, and hormones may act on these centers to differentiate the responses of men and women to the type of light deprivation that occurs during the winter.

Environmental Considerations

The most important environmental factor to consider when someone with SAD becomes depressed is light deprivation, in all its forms. Many people experience feelings of low energy and sadness similar to

those that SAD patients report in the winter months as a result of light
deprivation, regardless of the time of year. A change in latitude is a
common cause of light deprivation, triggering winter depressions that
may not previously have been a problem. For example, a young physician who moved from Texas to New York City and became depressed
the following winter might have been suffering from light deprivation
and SAD, rather than from problems of adjustment to big-city life.
The following letter provides a good description of how one middle-
aged woman looks back on her experiences at different latitudes:

> The last two winters have been miseries of depression for me.
> About February I begin to regain hope as spring approaches
> (in Florida), and I am truly euphoric by May. Yet even now,
> as I revel in July's bright days and in my own comfortable sta-
> bility, I am inwardly dreading next winter.
>
> I grew up in Canada, and of course it is worse there—it
> depresses me even to visit there now. But even in Florida,
> there is a different quality to the daylight in winter: It seems
> as though it takes something really wonderful to make me
> happy during the winter, whereas in summer it takes some-
> thing pretty bad to make me sad.

Population surveys conducted at different latitudes have shown
that those who live farther from the equator are more likely to develop
SAD, as shown in Table 4. As you can see, this tendency is most apparent in the United States, where Dr. Leora Rosen, currently at the National Institute of Justice in Washington, DC, found approximately
nine percent of those living in New Hampshire (forty-two degrees
north) report symptoms of SAD while only five percent of those living
in southern Florida (twenty-seven degrees north) report similar symptoms. In other parts of the world, the relationship between latitude
and frequency of SAD is looser. Although some studies in northern
climes, such as Scotland, show the predictable high proportion of
SAD sufferers, and other correspondingly southern locations such as
Australia and Thailand show low frequencies, other studies do not
obey this general rule. Of particular interest are the inhabitants of Iceland and Canadians of Icelandic extraction, who show a low frequency
of SAD despite their northern locations, according to studies performed by Dr. Andres Magnusson, currently at the University of Oslo.
This may reflect some genetic protection in these people, who evolved

TABLE 4
Prevalence of SAD and the Winter Blues by Latitude

City/state/country	Latitude	Prevalence (% of sample)		
		SAD	WB	Total
Sarasota, Florida	27°	1.4	2.6	4.0
Maryland	39°	6.3	10.4	16.7
New York City	40°	4.7	12.5	17.2
Nashua, New Hampshire	42°	9.7	11.0	20.7
Fairbanks, Alaska	65°	9.2	19.1	28.3
Stockholm, Sweden	59°	3.9	13.9	17.8
Helsinki, Finland	59°	7.1	11.8	18.9
Oslo, Norway	59°	14.0	12.6	24.6
Reykjavik, Iceland	64°	3.8	7.6	11.3
Tromsö, Norway	69°	13.7	10.7	24.4
Nagoya, Japan	35°	0.9	0.8	1.7

in the North and represent a relatively insulated gene pool. It is easy to imagine how having SAD in the North could be a significant disadvantage to the extent that those afflicted with winter symptoms might have failed to thrive and reproduce over the centuries. It is also possible that there may be other ethnic differences in vulnerability to SAD. For example, low frequencies of SAD were found in Japan by Dr. Norio Ozaki, currently at the University of Nagoya, and in China, by Dr. Ling Han, formerly a fellow at the NIMH.

Another cause of light deprivation, which often goes unrecognized, is a move from a brighter to a darker home. For example, a thirty-year-old secretary who moved from her twentieth-floor apartment, where the sun streamed in every morning, to a basement apartment suffered the effects of diminished environmental light and became depressed. Recognizing this relationship between mood and the environment, a student from Minnesota writes:

I have often wondered over the last several years why it is that when I go home I lose all energy and have a strong desire to sleep. This occurs all year round for me, although it is more pronounced during the winter months. My house is exposed to very little direct sunlight and is quite gloomy. I have also noticed that when I go and stay at a certain friend's house that is exposed to a lot of sunlight my mood lightens drastically.

People with SAD are particularly susceptible to moving into dark places in the summer, when the prospective home may seem quite adequately illuminated and the memories of SAD may be far away. Bob Wilhelm, a professional storyteller, who suffered from SAD for many years until he discovered the nature of his condition and how to treat it, describes how he moved to the Pacific Northwest during the summer and purchased a house in the middle of a forest of evergreens. During the summer days, when he signed a contract to buy the house, the sun's rays streamed down between the trees, making the cottage seem like an ideal place for Bob and his wife. Unfortunately, he did not realize that when winter arrived, the sun would be low on the horizon and the small amount of available sunlight would be blocked by a dense screen of conifers. The winter that followed was marked by one of the most severe depressions that Bob can recall, and he identified literally and figuratively with the poet Dante, who, centuries before, had written about finding himself in midlife in a dark wood from which he didn't know how to escape.

Moves from a well-lit to a darker workplace can also bring on depression. One schoolteacher from Minneapolis writes:

> In many of our area schools, windows are being closed over to conserve energy, bringing the effect of winter darkness all year round. No wonder I found my classroom depressing after the windows were sheeted up; it was darker.

Even in sunnier places, however, working people are often exposed to very little bright light. For example, Dr. Dan Kripke and colleagues in sunny San Diego measured light exposure in working adults and found that on average they were exposed to only half an hour of bright light per day. In recent years, there has been a tremendous increase in the number of windowless buildings, apparently designed in response to concerns about energy conservation. Even in offices with windows, the glass is often coated with a light-absorbing substance— again, in an attempt to conserve energy. Unfortunately, electrical energy is conserved at the expense of human energy, at least in those who suffer from SAD or even in those with less severe degrees of low energy in the winter.

Apart from changes in season, latitude, and indoor lighting environment, certain weather patterns, regardless of when they occur, may deprive us of light. It is fascinating too for one who deals with many patients with SAD to see how their mood and energy level behave like a living weather vane. If there has been a sunny streak, all will be fine. If there has been a long spell of cloudy days, all will be amiss. Small inconveniences will feel like major disruptions, and there will be an abundance of symptoms, both physical and psychological. These symptoms may occur even in the summer if there has been a string of rainy days. Conversely, a clear snap in the winter may result in unseasonable remissions.

A woman who writes to me from the Northeast clearly associates light deprivation, rather than season, with her symptoms:

> On gray or stormy days (no matter the season!), I become very depressed. The longer the duration of this weather, the lower I feel. As soon as the sun appears, my mood drastically improves. I do not like a dark environment and will seek out bright areas. Dark rooms are oppressive to me.

I have received several letters from San Francisco, where fog abounds and obliterates the sunlight in many areas of the city. One street may be foggy, while over the next hill it may be sunny. Apparently the price of real estate depends in part on these patterns of sunlight and fog, and given the powerful effect that light can have on mood, this is not surprising. For individuals who live and work in fog-ridden pockets, it might as well be winter all year round. One self-diagnosed "sun worshiper" wrote to me:

> I live in the coastal region of San Francisco, where it is often foggy, overcast, and windy. I often feel depressed about the lack of sun in our area. While this depression is not strong enough to be incapacitating, it does make me irritable and somewhat of a "complainer." My husband simply cannot understand my feelings. When we spend a day or two in an area such as Sacramento, where the temperatures remain in the hundreds during most of the summer, I feel alive. But my husband can hardly wait to get back to San Francisco, to what he and many others refer to as the "naturally air-conditioned city." It is encouraging to find support for my

theory that fog, wind, and cold can get some people down while others can thrive on it.

Light deprivation is a problem in many parts of the world. As one might expect, SAD has been described in Scandinavian countries, where recognition of the problem was accepted as part of the culture even before the disorder was described in modern times. In Iceland, for example, the condition of *skamdegistunglindi,* or short-days depression, was described in medieval epics. In Tromsö, a Norwegian city 125 miles north of the Arctic Circle, all manner of ills are blamed on the *morketiden,* or murky days—those forty-nine days of total darkness around the winter solstice (see Chapter 14). Light deprivation is not confined to these countries of legendary darkness, however. Though it may be less common elsewhere, SAD has been described in sunnier countries, such as Italy and Japan, and in the southern hemisphere: Brazil, Australia, and South Africa. Even in tropical countries where winters are sunny, there is frequently a cloudy, wet monsoon season, during which the country's inhabitants are often light-deprived and may experience the symptoms of SAD. Even in Hawaii, which many of us think of as eternally sunny, colleagues have reported cases of SAD, especially in residents of those parts of the islands less well known to tourists, which are often covered with clouds.

An unusual cause for the emergence of SAD symptoms came to my attention recently when I was consulted by an engineer in his early sixties, who had developed SAD some three years earlier. It is rather extraordinary for a man of that age to develop such symptoms out of the blue, and I quizzed him about all the usual triggering factors. Had he moved north recently, changed homes or his working environment? "No," he answered. It was only toward the end of the consultation that it emerged that he had injured one eye about four years previously and a cataract had grown across the lens. This greatly decreased the amount of light entering the eye and had apparently pushed him over his threshold of vulnerability for SAD. I have since seen other people for whom visual problems were followed by the development of SAD symptoms.

No studies have yet been performed on the rate of SAD among the visually impaired. Such research would certainly be worthwhile, for the more we understand about the many different effects of light deprivation on brain function, the more likely it seems that in understanding and treating the blind we will need to take into account not only their loss of vision but also the loss of these other light-related functions.

Researchers have shown that some SAD patients display subtle abnormalities in light processing that may contribute to their symptoms.

Stress in SAD

Light deprivation is not the only environmental factor that can trigger feelings of depression in the winter. Stressful events may also contribute to them. For example, a young sales manager had a sales conference scheduled in January, just at a time when the extra hours of work and preparation required for this major event were most difficult for him. During previous winters, he had felt quite well, experiencing only mild drops in his energy and productivity. But this time, the high level of stress and the demands of his work, coming in the middle of the winter, combined to precipitate him into the depths of a depression.

A young mother with SAD was required to start a stressful new job during December. Although she was normally a quick study, she was unable to learn the new skills that the job required, in addition to running her household and coordinating her day care arrangements. She became progressively more depressed, and when she was able to analyze the difficulties, she concluded that she would have been able to handle all those stresses during the summer, or the household and family ones during the winter, but the combination of stresses, occurring in winter, rendered her unable to function adequately either at work or at home.

What We Now Know About the Biology of SAD

Although nobody knows for sure why some people get SAD, we have many clues, as knowledge has accumulated rapidly. Between that and the decoding of the human genome, it is a fair bet that within twenty-five years we will understand SAD as clearly and completely as we currently do, say, heart attacks. If you already know as much as you care to about brain chemistry, turn to Part II, where I discuss treatments. But gaining an understanding of the biological underpinnings of SAD—

the pieces of a jigsaw puzzle as yet unfinished—will help you understand why available treatments are effective.

Are There Animal Models of SAD?

One aspect of SAD that has captured the imagination is how the symptoms of SAD seem to resonate with the seasonal changes seen elsewhere in the animal world.

To the urban dweller, signs of seasonal change in the birds, animals, and insects around us may be subtle, muted by the myriad stimuli that emanate from a bustling city. At the onset of winter, we may see geese winging their way overhead in V formation and squirrels scurrying about to store away the last of nature's bounty for the year. The winter landscape, relatively lifeless for the most part, may yield the occasional reward—the scarlet of a cardinal on a holly bush, a bushy-tailed fox darting across a field. But for the most part, only the crows seem to thrive, their blackness blending in perfectly with the darkness of the season. And then in spring, the ebb of winter is accompanied by a return of rabbits, birds, and bugs. This urban or suburban seasonal tableau is but a dim reflection of the amazing array of changes taking place outside the bounds of the city, especially in the temperate and boreal regions of the world, where a host of species undergo their annual cycles. I describe a few of these species since they offer special insights into different aspects of the study of SAD.

Lessons from Algae

Gonyaulax polyhedra is a single-celled alga that has attracted the attention of scientists in part because it is a nuisance and in part because of its physiology. It is one of the species responsible for the so-called red tides that have been observed off the west coast of the United States, where they have been responsible for food poisoning. To scientists, however, the alga has been a source of fascination because of its clear-cut daily and seasonal rhythms. Its daily rhythms appear to be governed by at least two internal clocks, one responsible for its movement through the water and another for its ability to bioluminesce—to glow in the dark. It also has a seasonal rhythm according to which it alternates between two forms, a motile creature that flits through the water during the warm summer days and the round, immobile cystic form into which it metamorphoses at the approach of winter. This capacity to turn into cysts is thought to protect *Gonyaulax* against the cold winter waters.

One reason the seasonal rhythms of *Gonyaulax* are of interest to SAD researchers is that its seasonal cycle appears to be mediated by the hormone melatonin, a substance of widespread importance in coordinating seasonal rhythms in a multitude of species. Melatonin is secreted by the pineal gland, a small structure tucked underneath the brain, when it is dark, and its secretion is suppressed by light. During the long nights of winter, melatonin is produced for a long time, which is the stimulus that induces *Gonyaulax* to turn into its cystic form. During the shorter nights of summer, on the other hand, the duration of melatonin secretion is shortened, which induces the alga to return to its motile form.

This biological system, by which the duration of day and night is translated into the duration of nocturnal melatonin secretion, which is the signal that elicits seasonal changes in behavior, has been conserved throughout millennia of evolution. As we shall see, there has been much speculation about the potential importance of this mechanism in inducing the symptoms of SAD.

Understanding the "Night Within"

The transition between day and night, which we experience every day with the alternation of light and dark, is perceived not only in relation to such external events as dawn and dusk but internally as well. People (or other animals) kept in conditions that isolate them from all outside clues about time of day will still show an alternation of sleepiness and wakefulness and all the other biological changes associated with night and day. These day-and-night states of mind, which the late famous biologist Colin Pittendrigh called "the day within" and "the night within," are part of our biological programming, determined by the body's clock. As the night expands in winter, so does "the night within" and all the biological changes associated with it—for example, sleepiness and the secretion of the hormone melatonin. If we are to appreciate the psychological impact of winter, we must try to understand the effects of the expanding night on our minds and bodies.

Melatonin has been called the hormone of darkness because it is secreted almost exclusively during the night. The onset of melatonin secretion begins in the late evening and is influenced by the timing of dusk; its offset occurs in the morning and is influenced by the timing of dawn. The duration of melatonin secretion can therefore be used as a biological marker of our internal day and night. The capacity to track dawn and dusk and thus measure the duration of night and day, though long recognized to occur in animals, has only recently been shown to occur in humans as well, by Dr. Thomas Wehr at the NIMH. Inspired by a movie about primitive humans, who lived before the onset of artificial lighting, Wehr wondered about their lives. How did they sleep, and how did they feel during their waking hours?

Wehr and colleagues set out to study this question by having volunteers spend extended periods of time on an inpatient unit at the NIMH. In an attempt to re-create the winter conditions of light and dark to which primitive humans were exposed, the researchers asked these volunteers to expose themselves to ordinary lighting conditions and go about their normal lives for ten hours each day, but to lie in a restful state in complete darkness for the other fourteen hours. They measured their sleep patterns and blood levels of melatonin and other hormones. For comparison purposes, these researchers then asked the volunteers to adhere to a summer light–dark cycle: sixteen hours per day of exposure to ordinary outdoor lighting during the summer day and eight hours per day of restful time in complete darkness. Once again, they examined sleep and hormonal measures.

When he compared the profiles of melatonin secretion in the artificial winter and summer conditions, Wehr found a pattern of seasonal change that strikingly resembled the seasonal changes seen in so many of the other species that have been studied, from the lowly single-celled *Gonyaulax* to sheep and cattle. During the long winter nights, the duration of melatonin secretion expands, whereas during the short nights of summer it contracts. One important implication of this finding is that the biological underpinnings for seasonal response—the capacity of melatonin secretion to be influenced in a predictable way by the length of the night—is intact in humans. At this time we do not know what effects, if any, these changes in duration of melatonin secretion may have on human physiology, mood, or behavior.

Wehr and I and our colleagues reached certain intriguing conclusions from a series of studies in which we extended the duration of night:

• During the winter, patients with SAD undergoing their normal light–dark routine show the same type of expansion of plasma melatonin duration seen in nonseasonal volunteers kept in artificial darkness for fourteen hours per day. In other words, despite the presence of artificial lighting, patients with SAD appear to vary seasonally with respect to this important biological variable.

These results have profound implications as they imply that people with SAD do not "see" light in the same way as nonseasonal people. Although there is no evidence of any visual problems in SAD sufferers, there may be more subtle problems with processing light either at the level of the eyes or within the brain itself.

Other intriguing findings to emerge from Wehr's experiments include:

• During extended nights, sleep breaks up into two components, an early and a late one. Such first and second sleep periods were recorded in historical documents written before bright indoor lighting was widely available.

• People slept far longer on average than is the norm in our society and reported a "crystal-clear consciousness" when awake. This finding suggests that many modern people may walk around in a less wide-awake state as a result of chronic sleep deprivation.

• During the extended darkness, there was an increased level of the hormone prolactin in the bloodstream. This hormone has been reported to increase during meditative states. It may explain why the subjects in Wehr's study were not anxious when awake in the dark—in contrast to the way insomniacs often feel—but experienced instead a peaceful stillness. Prolactin secretion may also explain the serene demeanor of certain polar animals as they rest peacefully in the frozen Arctic wilderness, patiently awaiting the return of the light. These creatures are described in more detail later.

Winter as an Energy Crisis: Lessons from Svalbard

The Northern Arctic archipelago of Svalbard or Spitzbergen must surely have one of the most inhospitable climates for sustaining life, especially among complex creatures. Located halfway between Norway and the North Pole, the islands are immersed in darkness for over two months of each year. All vegetation on the islands grows in the two months of summer, during which it is light for twenty-four hours a day. Foraging during the winter season is made more difficult in Svalbard because temperatures are less extreme than in other parts of the region, causing melting and refreezing, resulting in a relatively thin crust of ice, which is dangerous for animals to cross. Despite these extremely severe conditions, two species, the Svalbard reindeer and the Svalbard ptarmigan, a plump white bird, have succeeded brilliantly in colonizing the islands.

Although these species eat more during the autumn, storing extra body fat against the winter, researchers have calculated that this extra fat is quite inadequate to sustain their energy need throughout the winter of frigid temperatures and food deprivation. Instead, they rely on slowing down their activity to an extreme degree. People often comment on the apparent tameness of the reindeer or ptarmigan when approached by humans. Instead of running away, they stand still or lie in the snow and ice, staring into space. The appearance of having given up, which has been called arctic resignation, is in fact a life-saving strategy. By slowing down all movements, for example, the reindeer reduces its energy consumption to one-fourth of what it would expend if it were trotting. Such apparent tameness may have evolved because in the arctic regions, winter, with its subzero temperatures, is a far more dangerous enemy than any natural predator, and saving energy by lowered metabolism and levels of arousal is more valuable to the animal than vigilance, swift reflexes, and being ready to run off at a moment's notice. It is more adaptive to "resign" and conserve energy than to flee and squander it. It is this sort of decision—to be active or passive—the calculation of which varies with the terrain and the season, that is a key to survival in the harsh winters of the Far North.

Is SAD a Form of Human Hibernation or Arctic Resignation?

I often encounter variations of this question, usually from people who feel a strong identification with hibernating bears. The desire to be recumbent, to be a couch potato, to loll the day away, to be left alone in some dark space, inevitably brings to mind a bear in his cave. Biologists scoff at such analogies. They point out that small hibernating mammals show marked drops in temperature that are not seen in patients with SAD. Nor are SAD patients really like bears that while away their winter months in a sleeplike state. But these dismissals don't address what people who ask this question often really want to know: Is SAD an adaptive state that might actually be a useful energy-conserving mechanism for some people during the winter months in the same way hibernation is for bears? In other words, is it our society rather than our biology that is at fault for expecting us to function fully all year round in a manner that is contrary to the ways of nature?

It is possible that differing historical roles of women and men in society might account for the greater levels of seasonality and SAD occurring in women. In tribal life, women stayed at home, bearing and nursing children, while men hunted for food and protected the tribe against marauders. During the winter, when food is scarce, it might have been adaptive in such tribes for women to increase their food intake and decrease their level of activity and for men not to show these seasonal changes and to be alert and active all year long.

We have no good answers to these speculations at this time. It may be that certain SAD symptoms are exaggerations of adaptive responses to the changing seasons that might have conferred an advantage to an individual or to a society under certain circumstances. On the other hand, it can be argued that SAD is a maladaptive response—perhaps a breakdown in normal physiological systems—that might have been a liability even in societies beyond our own. In support of this second line of reasoning is the low prevalence of SAD in Iceland, which suggests that those with a genetic vulnerability to SAD did not reproduce as effectively as those without such genes. In addition, it has been pointed out that states of hibernation and winter energy conservation in animals are often preceded by increased eating and fat deposition in anticipation of the season of scarcity. In SAD patients, this overeating and weight gain generally continues throughout the winter—a pattern that would be maladaptive in times of scarcity.

When to Have Sex: Seasonal Rhythms of Reproduction

In the movie *Alien Nation,* one alien insults another by declaring, "Your mother mates out of season." This sensitivity toward mating in the right season is shared by many species on our own planet, and for good reason. It is clearly advantageous for offspring to be born during the spring, when the weather is more hospitable and food is more freely available. Thus, depending on the gestation period of a species, conception should be timed accordingly if this is to happen. In hamsters, for example, which have a short gestation period, conception occurs optimally as the days are getting longer. For sheep, on the other hand, the optimal time for conception is during the winter, given their four-month gestation period.

To accommodate these seasonal rhythms of fertility, nature has contrived ingenious methods of contraception in certain seasons and maximum fertility in others. These seasonal adaptations differ in males and females. For example, rams show a certain level of sexual interest in ewes all year round, whereas the ewes are entirely unresponsive to their approaches until autumn. At that time, influenced by the decreasing duration of the days, they go into estrus and become fertile. This is a period of sexual excitement for ewes. The ewe becomes generally nervous, and there is swelling of the vulva, the opening to the vagina. The end of a ram's penis is slender and twisted so as to be able to enter the cervix of the ewe's uterus for more effective fertilization of the ovum. The cervix of the ewe, however, is closed for most of the year except for the breeding season, and only then can it be penetrated by the ram's penis. Seasonal changes in the ram's sexual functioning are also apparent. For example, testicular weight is at its lowest level during the spring and reaches its maximum in late summer.

These changes in reproductive functioning have also been found to be mediated to a large degree by the secretion of the hormone melatonin. Once again, the length of the night has been found to influence the duration of melatonin secretion, which signals to the animal whether it is summer or winter and initiates a cascade of biological events that results in the appropriate seasonal reproductive behavior.

There is evidence that humans also vary seasonally in relation to their sex drive and fertility. There is a general increase in sexual interest and activity in the spring. There is also a clear-cut seasonal rhythm in births, with peaks occurring in spring, though there is evidence that this rhythm has become less marked over the last century as our lives have become more insulated from the effects of the seasons. These tendencies may be exaggerated in patients with SAD. For example, I have treated certain women with SAD who stopped menstruating during the winter months but began to menstruate once more after receiving light therapy. Dr. Erick Turner and I reported this connection between light and reproductive functioning in a patient we treated at the NIMH. The patient was a woman at the verge of menopause who developed hot flashes only during the winter. These hot flashes, which are believed to result from the deficient estrogen that accompanies ovarian failure, disappeared following light therapy. This suggests that light therapy can provide a stimulus to the reproductive system, possibly via its effects on melatonin, which might have certain therapeutic applications.

Growing a Winter Brain: The Chickadee

Chickadees, dressed in their black bibs and black bonnets, bustle about in easy view on the leafless branches of the yellow birches in winter. All the bird-watcher needs to do to get a closer look at them is to make a "pish, pish" sound and they dip down to the lower twigs to investigate. To obtain enough food in the barren winter landscape, they need to forage over a territory four times greater than they do in summer. They have managed to survive the deprivations of the winter season by using an ingenious biological strategy that allows them to keep track of this greater foraging territory and to remember where they have stored their food caches—they grow more brain cells. Research by Dr. Fernando Nottebaum of Rockefeller University has shown that in black-capped chickadees, the hippocampus, a part of the brain believed to be involved in memory and spacial learning, grows each October.

It is exciting to contemplate the adult brain not as rigid and unchanging but as capable of continued growth under certain circumstances. To what extent these observations may apply to humans as well is unclear at this time, but there is evidence that certain neurons in the suprachiasmatic nuclei, the body's clock, which produce a substance known as vasopressin, are present in greater numbers in the winter than in the summer. Dr. Paul Schwartz at the NIMH has shown that the size of the pituitary gland, which is located behind the eyes and is responsible for secreting a large number of hormones, varies across seasons in humans. In addition, the nature of this variation is different in men and in women. These findings from human studies suggest that there may be a certain seasonal plasticity in the adult human brain that is reminiscent of that found in chickadees.

Behold a SAD Horse: Clues to Individual Vulnerability

There is no reason to assume that diversity among individuals in their responses to winter exists only among humans. Very probably other animals show these varied responses too, and they might be easy to detect if one had a mind to look for them. I was called, for example, by Dr. Deborah Marshall, a veterinarian in Miami, Florida, who consulted me about the seasonal changes in one of her favorite horses. The young gelding, Tango, was capable of managing the most complex of jumps during the summer, but in February, according to Dr. Marshall, "he just packs up. He cannot solve complex problems. His mind is in a fog. Whatever is a normal stress for him in summer becomes over-whelming in winter. He can't handle jumps that he would easily have managed the previous summer."

On one occasion, while Dr. Marshall was riding Tango during the winter months, the horse threw her and she was seriously injured. Sadly, she contemplated putting him down until she remembered that she had experienced similar seasonal difficulties with his mother, a dearly beloved twenty-eight-year-old mare, who would become very erratic and aggressive in the late winter.

The similarity between the seasonal difficulties experienced by both the mother and her foal led Dr. Marshall to consider the possibil-ity that Tango might have inherited from his mother an equine form of SAD. Horses are known to breed during the long days. Their repro-ductive capacity shuts down in November and reawakens again in the spring. Dr. Marshall consulted me about Tango, and we decided to put a bright light in his stall in the morning and the evening from Septem-ber through April. To Dr. Marshall's delight, this intervention im-proved Tango's winter difficulties "about eighty-five percent." He was able to solve complex problems for the first time during the winter months and to execute several difficult jumps in sequence. "It is like riding the horse I've always dreamed of riding," Dr. Marshall says, "a horse with wings." Dr. Marshall's coworkers now question whether there is anything wrong with the horse at all, but Dr. Marshall knows better. Tango is now, happily, a successfully treated SAD horse.

And as to the old mare, she has been put out to pasture after her long life of service. Since little will be asked of her in the form of jump-ing or other behavioral demands, she will be permitted to experience her seasonal changes without interruption.

There might be much to learn from examining animals such as Tango, especially since it is now possible to detect the genetic variation responsible for such behavioral differences. Such an approach has been helpful in determining the genetic basis of circadian rhythms and might similarly be valuable in helping us understand the genetic basis of seasonality.

The Chemistry of SAD

The human brain, a three-pound structure no larger than a cantaloupe, contains a hundred billion cells or neurons that communicate with each other by means of chemical messengers called neurotransmitters.

Researchers have explored these neurotransmitter systems for possible clues to the disturbances that occur in depression in general and SAD in particular. The three neurotransmitters that have received the most attention are serotonin, dopamine, and norepinephrine. These neurotransmitters communicate with adjacent neurons by means of special receptors, specific to the neurotransmitter in question.

An early Scandinavian study of the brains of people who died at different times of year found that in the hypothalamus, that portion of the brain responsible for so many essential functions like eating, sleeping, and biological rhythms, levels of serotonin plummeted during the winter. That was perhaps the first clue suggesting a role for serotonin functioning in the symptoms of SAD. Since then, many other clues have been discovered. Here are some of them.

- The amount of serotonin in the blood coming from the brain varies directly with the amount of sunlight on that particular day.
- People with SAD show exaggerated responses to a drug that stimulates serotonin receptors.
- During the summer or after successful light therapy, this response becomes normal, suggesting that light therapy may work by influencing serotonin transmission.
- Feeding people with SAD a mixture that lowers brain serotonin reverses the beneficial effects of light therapy.
- Medications that work by influencing serotonin transmission, such as Prozac, Zoloft, Celexa, and Lexapro, may help people with SAD.
- Carbohydrate-rich meals can boost levels of brain serotonin. That may be why people with SAD are so inexorably driven to gorge on sweets and starches in the winter. In the summer, when they are feeling better and when serotonin levels in the hypothalamus are higher, these cravings subside. The huge appetite for high-calorie foods in the winter leads to the predictable but unwelcome weight gain that is so common in SAD. I discuss how best to deal with that in Chapter 8.

A second important neurotransmitter that may go awry in SAD is dopamine, which is responsible for pleasurable experiences and human interactions, among many other functions. In a recent series of large studies conducted at many centers across North America, my colleagues and I found a very useful role for the antidepressant Wellbutrin

XL in the prevention of SAD. This antidepressant works largely on dopamine systems, although it also influences the neurotransmitter norepinephrine. By giving patients with SAD Wellbutrin XL, 150 to 300 milligrams per day, before they developed their typical winter symptoms, we were able to prevent the onset of SAD in many cases and delay its onset in others. Other clues that dopamine systems may be involved in SAD relate to temperature regulation and ocular functioning, which depends in part on dopamine.

Of the three key neurotransmitters, there is the least evidence for norepinephrine as instrumental in SAD. It is important to remember, though, that these neurotransmitters often work in concert with one another and it is difficult to disentangle their individual roles. For example, the secretion of melatonin, another chemical that almost certainly plays a part in the dance of chemicals responsible for SAD, is under the direct influence of norepinephrine.

How Does Light Therapy Work?

Knowing how light therapy works may provide a window into our understanding of SAD. So far there have been more theories than facts in this regard. To find out about some of the leading theories, read on.

As we have seen, the duration of nocturnal melatonin secretion is of widespread importance as an informational cue about day length, season, and the appropriate seasonal response. It was therefore logical that our first hypothesis about SAD was that it was related to melatonin secretion and that light therapy worked by decreasing the duration of melatonin secretion, as it suppressed the secretion of the hormone at dawn and at dusk. We and others have tested this theory in a number of ways and obtained mixed results. Here are some of the most important findings:

• The studies by Wehr and colleagues have shown that the duration of melatonin secretion expands at night in people with SAD but not in nonseasonal controls living in modern conditions where there is artificial light. This opens the possibility that it is the melatonin itself that triggers symptoms in SAD patients. An alternative explanation might be that the seasonal changes in melatonin simply reflect an abnormality of information processing either in the eyes or in the brain and may not in itself be causally important.

• Blocking melatonin secretion by means of the common blood

pressure medication propranolol, administered in the early morning hours, may help patients with SAD, according to researcher Dr. David Schlager at the State University of New York at Stony Brook. Earlier work by my colleagues and me at the NIMH found that administering a similar drug at night was less effective. These findings are in keeping with observations that light treatment used early in the morning is more effective than similar treatment used later in the day.

• Some exciting new research by Dr. Alfred Lewy and colleagues suggests that administering very small amounts of melatonin in the afternoon may be helpful for people with SAD. Melatonin used in this way can shift daily (circadian) rhythms earlier. Lewy had earlier hypothesized that such a rhythm shift might be therapeutic for people with SAD. He theorized that morning light therapy might work best because it shifts rhythms earlier, and some research backs that up. On the other hand, light therapy used in the evening, which would be expected to shift circadian rhythms later, also seems to be effective, though less so. This last observation argues against Lewy's hypothesis.

Light therapy may also work by its influence on the three key neurotransmitters mentioned above—serotonin, dopamine, and norepinephrine. Those interested in an extensive scholarly discussion of the research into the effects of light therapy and the biological abnormalities in SAD will find a wealth of relevant information on my website, *www.normanrosenthal.com*, and in Part IV of this book.

Often, the existence of many theories about how something works means we cannot be certain of any of them. That is the situation when it comes to SAD and light therapy. The good news, however, for those who suffer from this potentially serious condition is that we don't have to have these answers to treat SAD effectively. In the section that follows I discuss the many things that you can do to reverse the symptoms of SAD and even, believe it or not, make winter a season of joy and wonder.

FIVE

SAD in Children and Adolescents

Some time ago, a middle-aged woman walked into the NIMH Clinical Center and asked me if I knew of any articles on SAD in children. I said I did indeed have an article and wondered why she was interested in the subject. "My son asked me to stop by and find out more about the condition," she said. "He thinks he has it." It emerged that her twelve-year-old son had seen a television program on the subject and had identified with the patients.

I was reminded of Jason, another smart twelve-year-old, who had seen both of his parents suffering from SAD and being treated with light therapy. That winter he approached his father, saying that he thought he was also suffering from SAD, since he had noticed that he was eating more candies. His father dismissed this observation with a psychological explanation—the boy was clearly identifying with his parents, and what child doesn't eat too much candy? But Jason, normally a fine student, began to have increasing difficulties with his schoolwork. One day his father, finding him dozing over his homework, asked him again what the problem was. "Dad, I think it's the winter," Jason replied. And he was right. Light therapy has since reversed the problem to a large degree.

While some children are able to recognize that they have a seasonal problem, many children with SAD do not understand what is wrong. Often they are not even aware that the change is internal, but blame it instead on the world around them, which they experience as having turned cruel and uncaring. In their view, teachers have become excessively strict and parents unfairly demanding. Many adults similarly misperceive the source of their SAD symptoms and seek external explanations to account for the dramatic difference in the way they feel when depressed.

I first started looking for children and adolescents with SAD because about one-third of our adult patients reported winter symptoms going back to these early years. In addition, many of the adult patients reported similar symptoms in their children, which is not surprising, considering the high familial incidence of the disorder. SAD in children has many similarities to the adult form—for example, there is often difficulty waking up on time in the morning and accomplishing tasks, particularly schoolwork. One difference is that children appear to show more irritability during their winter depressions than do adults.

How Common Is Childhood and Adolescent SAD?

Dr. Susan Swedo and colleagues at the NIMH surveyed children in middle and high schools in Montgomery County, Maryland, and found that seasonal problems are by no means uncommon in these age groups. Although SAD appears to affect only about one percent of children in the lower grades, there is a dramatic increase in frequency in the last three years of high school. This marked increase corresponds to the onset of puberty and is more pronounced in girls than in boys, suggesting that cyclical secretion of female sex hormones may be one factor in the development of the symptoms of SAD.

By the senior year of high school, approximately five percent of schoolchildren in this mid-Atlantic suburb report seasonal problems severe enough to qualify them as suffering from SAD, which makes the problem almost as common as it is for adults surveyed in the same geographical area. When all the schoolchildren from ages nine to seventeen in the United States are considered together, about three percent—about a million children and adolescents—are estimated to suffer from SAD. This makes the problem about as common as attention-deficit disorder (ADD). Yet unlike attention-deficit/hyperactivity disorder (ADHD), which is often associated with hyperactivity and learning difficulties, which are easier to spot, the symptoms of SAD are often less conspicuous and easily missed.

In another study of seasonality in children, Drs. Mary Carskadon and Christine Acebo at Brown University surveyed the parents of children in grades four through six for a history of seasonal changes. They found that almost half of all parents reported some behavioral change with the seasons and, depending on how they calculated it, the proportion of children with seasonal problems ranged from four to thirteen percent. They also found that, as with adults, seasonal problems are more marked the farther north you go. "Given the potential therapeutic benefit of light therapy in children with such seasonal patterns," they noted, "a careful assessment of seasonality is merited when evaluating children who present with mood and behavior problems in the winter."

How Can You Tell If a Child or Adolescent Has SAD?

If you would like to find out whether a child you know meets the criteria for SAD, as developed by the researchers at the NIMH, you can do so by consulting the Seasonal Pattern Assessment Questionnaire for Children and Adolescents (SPAQ-CA), shown in Figure 2. It is important to recognize that these criteria have been used for research purposes and do not coincide fully with clinical criteria. A proper diagnosis of SAD can be made only by a qualified clinician. Nevertheless, the answers on this questionnaire do provide useful information and guidance as to whether it is worth having a child or adolescent evaluated more fully for SAD. In addition, the questionnaire tends to be conservative, underestimating rather than overestimating the likelihood of seasonal problems in children and adolescents.

How to Interpret Scores on the SPAQ-CA

1. Establishing the pattern of seasonality

If the subject is suffering from winter SAD, he or she should report feeling worst during January or February on at least one of the items noted in question 1, namely "I have the least energy," "I am the most irritable," or "I feel my worst."

1. Please circle the × under the month(s) when the following happen:

	Jan	Feb	Mar	Apr	May	Jun	Jul	Aug	Sep	Oct	Nov	Dec	All the same
I have the least energy	×	×	×	×	×	×	×	×	×	×	×	×	×
I am the most irritable	×	×	×	×	×	×	×	×	×	×	×	×	×
I feel my worst	×	×	×	×	×	×	×	×	×	×	×	×	×

2. For you, do any of the following vary with the seasons? (circle the ×)

Length of sleep	×	×	×	×	×
Getting in trouble	×	×	×	×	×
Social activity	×	×	×	×	×
Substance abuse (drinking, smoking, drugs)	×	×	×	×	×
Mood	×	×	×	×	×
School performance					
a. Difficulty	×	×	×	×	
b. Grades	×	×	×	×	×
Weight	×	×	×	×	×
Irritability	×	×	×	×	×
Energy level	×	×	×	×	×
Appetite	×	×	×	×	×

3. If you experience change with the seasons, do you feel this is a problem for you?

             Yes: _____   No: _____

       If yes, is this problem (circle one):

         Not bad   Pretty bad   Very bad   So bad I have trouble functioning

FIGURE 2. Seasonal Pattern Assessment Questionnaire for Children and Adolescents (SPAQ-CA). Adapted by S. Swedo and J. Pleeter from the SPAQ of N. E. Rosenthal, G. Bradt, and T. Wehr; public domain.

2. Establishing the degree of seasonality

The global seasonality score can be obtained from question 2 simply by adding up all the individual item scores. Since there are eleven items and each item score ranges from 0 to 4, the global seasonality score will range from 0 to 44 for each individual. In their school survey, Dr. Swedo and her colleagues used 21 as their cutoff score for diagnosing SAD. It is important to remember this score is somewhat arbitrary, and people with lower scores may also suffer seasonal problems. One of the problems with self-administered questionnaires such as this one is that it requires accurate memory and the recognition of a seasonal pattern, which may be quite difficult to reconstruct, especially for younger children. In fact, many of the children and adolescents diagnosed as suffering from SAD at the NIMH had cutoff scores lower than 21.

3. Determining whether SAD is a problem

To make a diagnosis of SAD, researchers have required that a child rate the problem with the seasonal changes to be at least "pretty bad." Here, again, researchers are tending to be strict so as not to over-diagnose the condition. From the point of view of a concerned parent, however, it might be worth taking note if a child reports that seasonal changes are a problem at all. The child may be underestimating the degree to which these changes are a problem, and even if they are minor, they may respond favorably to a simple intervention, such as making sure that the child goes outdoors for at least half an hour each day.

In summary, suspect that a child or adolescent may be suffering from SAD if you find all of the following responses on the SPAQ-CA:

- In January or February the child feels least energetic, worst, or most irritable.
- The global seasonality score is 21 or more.
- Seasonal changes are experienced as a "pretty bad" problem.

Most patients with childhood SAD first come in for treatment when they are about fifteen or sixteen, having experienced an average of six winters of symptoms. There are several reasons why it takes so long for children to get diagnosed. First, some of the symptoms of SAD fit the stereotype of what people might expect to find in adolescence, such as lethargy, irritability, and lack of motivation. Research indicates that this stereotype is a myth and that adolescence is frequently a happy and stable time. Second, many physicians are still unaware of SAD, especially in its childhood and adolescent forms. Third, it takes several years for a seasonal pattern to emerge, so that the reason for the first few difficult winters is quite likely to be missed. Fourth, children may be less adept than adults at recognizing the seasonal pattern. Fifth, it is easy to attribute school difficulties to other causes, such as psychological problems. Finally, as noted earlier, in contrast to children with ADHD, those suffering from SAD are often not regarded as troublesome by teachers. These children generally sit quietly at their desks, lost in their daydreams, and often don't get the special attention that teachers reserve for "difficult children." This is a real shame, because a timely diagnosis of SAD in a child or adolescent may save the young person many years of suffering, since the condition is so eminently treatable.

Telltale Signs of SAD in Children: A Guide for Parents

The single biggest clue that your child may be suffering from SAD is that he or she develops problems during the fall and winter each year. This particular point may be more important than the actual symptoms themselves, which may be atypical in children and may manifest, for example, as anxiety or school avoidance. Children with SAD often do well in school in the first few months after returning from their summer vacations and generally do not experience seasonal problems until December or January. When the problem does hit, however, its effects can be marked, and parents are frequently surprised to discover how much of a struggle schoolwork can become for a child who might have been a fine student in the early part of the semester. Adolescence is often a time when sleeping and eating habits are erratic, so reports of changes in these behaviors are less helpful in making the diagnosis of SAD than problems with concentration, schoolwork, energy, and mood.

Common symptoms of SAD in children and adolescents are:

- Feeling tired and washed out.
- Feeling cranky and irritable.
- Having temper tantrums.
- Having difficulty concentrating and doing schoolwork. This may manifest either as slipping grades or as the need to work harder to maintain grades at preexisting levels.
- Being reluctant to undertake chores and other responsibilities not previously regarded as a problem.
- Making vague physical complaints, such as about headaches or abdominal pains.
- Demonstrating a marked increase in cravings for "junk food."

Several children with SAD come to mind: Michael, a twelve-year-old swimming champion, had swim times that invariably deteriorated during the winter and improved during the summer. Susan, an eight-year-old with long, flowing blond hair and a wistful gaze, had suffered from pronounced seasonal rhythms since infancy. Her parents noticed marked differences between her sleep length during the short summer nights, when she would wake up with the first rays of the sun, and during the long winter nights, when she would sleep for hours and hours. Her problems began in nursery school, when teachers noticed that she would withdraw from friends and be uninterested in the usual routine of daily activities during January and February. Jeannie, a thirteen-year-old, not only had the usual difficulties with schoolwork and social activities in the winter but also became overactive in the summer. At that time, her activity level would increase, she would need little sleep, and she would tend to be impulsive and show poor judgment. On one occasion, her father found her cavorting about on the roof, enjoying the night air, apparently unaware of the danger of falling.

What Happens When Children with SAD Grow Up?

To answer this question, Dr. Jay Giedd, a fellow psychiatric researcher at the NIMH, and I followed up six of the first children who had been diagnosed as suffering from SAD in our research program an average of approximately seven years earlier. Interestingly, all reported a pattern of continued winter difficulties. They also continued to experience beneficial effects when they enhanced their environmental lighting during the winter, either with light therapy or by spending extra time outdoors. When they forgot to seek out additional environmental light in winter, however, their symptoms returned. A few of these young people had been treated with Prozac in addition to light therapy, which suggests that, just as with adults, light therapy alone is sometimes insufficient.

Treating SAD in Children and Adolescents

Dr. Susan Swedo and I at the NIMH, together with Drs. Martin Teicher and Carol Glod at McLean Hospital in Massachusetts, set out to study systematically whether a combination of two treatments that have been found to be helpful in adults with SAD would also be beneficial for younger people with this disorder. The two treatments, light therapy and dawn simulation, are described in greater detail in Part II.

In our study, we found that a combination of a two-hour artificial dawn stimulus together with one hour of bright light therapy in the afternoon was better than a control treatment in reversing the symptoms of SAD. Because of the sensitivity of the eyes of young children to light, we used less intense light sources (2,500 lux) for children eight years or younger but treated those children who were nine years or older with light of the same intensity (10,000 lux) as is generally used for treating adults.

College Freshmen: A Population at Risk

Jackie's story is a familiar one; I can think of several others like hers. She was an upbeat young woman, a good student in high school with many friends and varied hobbies and activities. Although she suffered from asthma, that condition was well controlled by medications, which she took regularly. In retrospect, winters were somewhat difficult for her, but not to the degree that they would interfere with her participation in sports, her social life, or her grades. That all changed when she went to college in New England. The beginning of the first semester went well. She enrolled in several difficult classes, participated fully in college life, and continued to thrive until December. After returning home from the Thanksgiving break, she began to have trouble waking up in time for her morning classes and fell behind in her studies. She felt exhausted in the early evening and was unable to turn in her papers on time or to prepare for examinations.

For Jackie, failure was a new experience, and it caused her to question all the assumptions she had previously made about herself, namely, that she was a competent, successful, and popular person. Could it have been that she had fooled herself and everybody else all through high school? she wondered. Now that she was in the real world, life was showing her up for what she was, a second-rate mediocrity and an impostor. She lay around in bed a good part of the day and neglected many aspects of her life, including regular visits to the health center to have her asthma monitored. When her medications ran out, she didn't refill them, became physically ill, and had to drop out of school.

A careful history revealed that her SAD had been the leading edge of the problem. After receiving appropriate treatment for it (light therapy, psychotherapy, and antidepressant medications), she returned to school in the spring, when she did very well. During the summer, she caught up on the work she had missed the previous winter and entered the fall semester armed with extensive knowledge about SAD, a referral to a knowledgeable psychiatrist close to her college, and a game plan for managing the fall and winter quarters. This game plan included the following elements: (1) a light schedule of relatively easy courses, none of which required early morning classes; (2) a light box, which she planned to use regularly; (3) a dawn simulator to help her wake up in the morning; (4) plans to exercise outdoors regularly during the daylight hours; and (5) regular scheduled sessions with her psychiatrist.

Jackie did well until mid-January, when her SAD became problematic despite all these preventive measures. At that time, her psychiatrist put her on an antidepressant (see Chapter 10), which she continued to take until the end of March. Although it would be an exaggeration to say that she actually enjoyed the winter, Jackie felt well throughout the semester, continued to take her asthma medications, had no relapse, and closed out the year with a feeling of accomplishment and a fine grade point average.

Jackie's story illustrates several points that are important to bear in mind in planning for college freshmen who have a history of problematic seasonal changes. First, the move to college often involves a change of latitude or climate, which may enhance the tendency toward SAD. Second, when at home, a young person is often awakened and bundled off to school by parents. This makes it less likely that classes will be missed and ensures exposure to natural early morning light. This support does not carry through to college, where the student, left to his or her own devices, may lie for hours in a dark dorm room and miss both classes and sunlight. Finally, the newly experienced demands of college often pose a much more stressful challenge to the freshman than the familiar routine of high school. While these stresses may be relatively easy to handle in fall and spring, they may prove too burdensome in winter, when the vulnerable student becomes less resourceful and resilient, and they may bring on or aggravate the symptoms of

SAD. Once these symptoms emerge, they compound the problem further, which frequently leads to failure and, as in Jackie's case, to dropping out of school. Although her tendency to develop asthma was specific to Jackie, many individuals have special needs that require extra attention, and these are often sacrificed when energy and concentration decline in the winter months.

It is particularly important to target vulnerable individuals in high school, since good planning can prevent predictable misfortune. I can imagine a time not too far from now when school counselors routinely screen high school seniors for a history of problematic seasonal changes and counsel those at risk. Those seniors who know they are at risk may even consider geography as one of several factors to take into account in their choice of colleges.

ADD and SAD

ADD may look like SAD in some instances, but it should not appear regularly in fall and winter unless the child has a seasonal problem as well. Indeed, I have encountered patients with both problems. One young girl I treated suffered from ADD all year round, for which she was treated with the stimulant Ritalin. During the winter she experienced typical symptoms of SAD, apparently inherited from her mother, who suffered from similar problems. Thirty minutes of treatment with bright light in the morning reversed all her symptoms and helped her wake up and get to school on time, which had previously been a serious problem for her.

In my experience, ADD and SAD seem to occur together more frequently than you would expect by chance alone, and they may be accompanied by a third problem, called delayed sleep phase syndrome, or DSPS. People who suffer from DSPS have a hard time falling asleep and waking up at conventional hours. Both DSPS and SAD respond to light therapy, administered during the morning. New research by Dr. Robert Levitan in Toronto suggests that light therapy may be helpful in the treatment of ADD. However, stimulants and other medications are usually used as first-line treatments for this condition.

Nonseasonal depression may also occur in children and may become worse during winter. Children with this form of "double depression" may benefit from light therapy.

Treatment of Children with SAD

A crucial element in the treatment of SAD in children and adolescents is the attitude of the significant adults in the life of the child. If it is difficult for adults to accept that they have psychiatric problems, it is even harder for children and adolescents, who are very eager not to seem different from their peers. If young people are to accept their seasonal problems, it is critical to present them in a nonstigmatizing way as simply a variant of the seasonal changes that affect many people and, indeed, all of the natural world.

Treating SAD optimally requires organization, which is difficult to muster when one is tired and unfocused. The child or adolescent with SAD will therefore need the help of adults in getting organized. This can easily result in a power struggle between parent and child if the matter is not handled empathically and tactfully. It is often easier to do so if one of the parents is also seasonal, since there are many opportunities to empathize with each other and share strategies for coping. But whether the parent is seasonal or not, it is valuable to point to the diversity in nature and the many ways that different people and animals adapt to our changing world.

Depending on the nature of the child, it may be sufficient to make this point in passing. If your child has an inquiring mind, however, it may be fun and useful to engage him or her in activities involving the changing seasons and the responses they elicit in nature. You could construct a sundial in the garden, for example, and chart the annual course of the sun across the sky. Projects involving plants, insects, or animals are ideal for studying the natural effects of the seasons. For example, forcing bulbs generally involves exposing them to dark and cold conditions followed by warm and sunny ones. These conditions, presented in the midst of winter, trick a tulip or daffodil bulb into behaving as though it were spring so that it blooms early. It is easy to help a child make the connection between this simple experiment and tricking the human brain with light so that it too responds as though it were spring, even though the signs of winter are everywhere in evidence. It is even possible to study the effects of seasons on human mood and behavior. In fact, the results of the NIMH survey of schoolchildren mentioned earlier resulted from a school science project, developed by a talented high school senior.

Once the presence of SAD is accepted, destigmatized, and regarded as a manageable fact of life, and once the child is recruited as a collaborator in the treatment process rather than the object of it, all specific suggestions become much easier to implement. Such specific suggestions are not in principle different from those outlined in Part II. They include the following:

- Helping the child wake up in the morning
- Ensuring that he or she is exposed to sufficient light, either natural or artificial
- Helping the child manage stress
- Reminding the child that many of the difficulties encountered are a result of the seasonal problem rather than signs of failure—that it is not the child's fault
- Encouraging the child through the difficult months
- Antidepressants when the other interventions are insufficient

A knowledgeable and sympathetic psychiatrist or other therapist can be invaluable in helping you and your child negotiate the difficult winter months and should be involved in an ongoing way if the problem does not respond to simple self-help measures. In addition, a psychiatrist should certainly be consulted before any medications are initiated.

Waking up in the morning is generally the first battle of the day for a child or adolescent with SAD (as it is for many adults). This will be much easier if the child wakes up in the light. A bright bedside lamp, set up with a timer, can be helpful. Although the more expensive and sophisticated dawn simulator or SunRise clock (see pp. 145–146), which provides a more graduated artificial dawn, may be superior and is almost certainly more pleasant than having a light go on at full intensity in the early morning, a scientific comparison between these two morning light exposures has not yet been undertaken. A radio alarm clock may also be very useful. By helping to wake the child up, this will result in earlier exposure to the light of morning, either real or artificial. It is best if the child assumes responsibility for waking up, because struggles between parent and child around this issue start the day off on a bad note.

A child with SAD either may have his or her own light box or may share a light box with other members of the family. I recall a mother and daughter, both of whom suffered from SAD, who would enjoy sitting and talking together by their light box each morning. As with adults, light treatment can be administered to good effect either in the morning or in the evening and in conjunction with homework or other sedentary tasks. Often, though, it is a better strategy not to let light therapy become associated in the child's mind with unpleasant chores. Instead, compliance is often better if the child is allowed to play video games or engage in some other favorite activity while sitting in front of the lights.

Since childhood and adolescent SAD is a more recently recognized and studied entity than adult SAD, there is less research on the use of light in children. My experience suggests that children may need shorter treatment sessions than adults—perhaps as little as ten to fifteen minutes per day. It is particularly important that the light source emit as little ultraviolet light as possible, since the lens of a child's eye does less to filter out these potentially harmful wavelengths than the lens of an adult. As far as we know, conventional light fixtures, used under the supervision of a professional, are quite safe. More information about the best type of lights to use and the potential long-term effects of bright light is provided in Chapter 7. Besides formal light therapy, children should be encouraged to spend at least a half hour a day outdoors so that they can derive the benefit of natural light as well. It may also be useful to enhance the lighting in a child's room in an informal way (see p. 151).

Activities that the child with SAD handles easily in summer and fall often become burdensome in the dark months. Gentle assistance with organizing schedules and anticipating and managing stress is often necessary at those times. A child with SAD might consider leaving demanding and time-consuming extracurricular activities, such as participating in a school play or working on the school newspaper, to the spring and fall months. Sporting activities, on the other hand, can relieve the symptoms of SAD since they combine aerobic exercise, which may be useful in itself, with exposure to outdoor light. Tasks associated with deadlines should be anticipated well ahead and tackled as early as possible to prevent last-minute crises. Just sitting down with your child and reviewing his or her schedule can be supportive and serve as an early warning system for potential trouble down the road.

A review of Part II will provide further insights and tips for helping your child. Remember, you may be working against resistance.

Your child does not want to think that he or she is suffering from an illness, so tact and creativity will help in broaching the topic. On the other hand, your child may already know that there is problem. Recognizing it, giving it a name, and outlining practical solutions will generally be appreciated. By setting an example in this way, you are instilling in your child the capacity to take charge of the problem and overcome it—a skill that will be invaluable in the years to come.

SIX

"Summer SAD" and Other Seasonal Afflictions

> Of natures, some are well- or ill-adapted for summer, and
> some for winter.
>
> —HIPPOCRATES

The Summertime Blues

Although the commonest form of recurrent seasonal depressions in northern countries is the winter pattern of SAD, it is by no means the only one. In response to the first newspaper articles on SAD, approximately one in twenty people with seasonal depressions mentioned a pattern of mood change just the opposite of those that had been described in the articles. They regularly became depressed each summer and felt better when fall arrived. Studies indicate that most people in the northern United States dislike winter more than summer. When you look as far south as Florida, however, the pattern is reversed and more people dislike the summer. In our NIMH survey of seasonal changes in Maryland, we found about five cases of winter SAD for every case of summer SAD. Whereas winter difficulties are more prominent than summer difficulties in the United States and Europe, in Japan and China more people report having problems with summer.

Dr. Thomas Wehr and I have studied several patients with summer SAD. One of Dr. Wehr's original patients with summer SAD, Marge, was a retired government administrator in her mid-sixties when she came to the NIMH for help. She had suffered from regular bouts of depression for the previous forty-five years but had not recognized that her moodiness, lethargy, and irritability were out of the ordinary until the last fifteen years. For her, summers were always the worst times, except once when she went on vacation with her family for a few weeks to the Finger Lakes in upper New York State. She recalls swimming two or three times a day, "in that deep, dark, cold water. After a few days of that, my mood lifted, and that summer, at least, the depression never came back."

Although she knew her depressions were related to summer, she was never really sure why. Perhaps, she thought, it was related to being on vacation. During the summer she was "too down and lethargic" to think about it, "and when fall came, I felt so much better I didn't bother because I had so many other things to do. When it goes away, you don't expect it to come back. But it always comes back in the spring." When she first saw Dr. Wehr in the summer, she said that her depression had apparently remitted spontaneously a day or two before the consultation. This coincided with an unusual front of cold air that had moved into the Washington, DC, area, changing its usual sweltering and humid summer days into cool and pleasant ones.

Dr. Wehr postulated that it might be the heat of the summer that was triggering this patient's depressions and that the cool air and her swims in the cold, spring-fed lakes of the North might have exerted a therapeutic influence on her mood. He observed that temperature changes had been suggested as a cause of depression since the time of Aristotle. On the basis of this hypothesis, Dr. Wehr suggested that Marge stay in her air-conditioned apartment for a week and avoid the summer heat completely. She followed his suggestion and showed a markedly positive response to this treatment.

As often happens in clinical work, it took a very interesting, prototypical patient to make researchers wonder exactly what caused these recurrent summer depressions. Marge played this role for summer SAD. Following her successful treatment, journalist Sandy Rovner ran an article in *The Washington Post* in which she described the summer version of SAD and mentioned that a new research program at the NIMH was looking into the condition. Numerous responses followed, and we evaluated the histories of these patients.

In general, there are many similarities between people with summer and winter depressions. Most of the patients are women, and feelings of low energy are once again a prominent part of the picture. Many are not aware of experiencing any actual mood changes but regard themselves as "being in a holding pattern." They just want to be left alone. As one of the patients put it, "I'm just not running on all cylinders." Just as for winter depressives, a notable proportion of family members of summer depressives have also suffered from mood disorders.

In contrast to patients with winter SAD, who tend to eat more and crave sweets and starches during depressions, summer sufferers tend to eat less and lose weight. These differences have also been observed by two Australian researchers, Drs. Philip Boyce and Gordon Parker, who sent out questionnaires to those responding to an article in a women's magazine and similarly received responses from patients with both winter and summer SAD. Whereas the patients with winter SAD feel physically slowed down during depressions, those with summer SAD are often agitated. In addition, they express more suicidal ideas than their winter counterparts and may be at greater risk for harming themselves or taking their own lives. This is in keeping with studies that show that the peak time for suicide in the general population is the spring and early summer, not the winter.

Summer depressives frequently ascribe their symptoms to severe heat whereas winter depressives more often attribute their symptoms to a lack of light. Some winter depressives feel that the extreme cold of winter may also play a role in their symptoms, but this possibility has yet to be explored. Conversely, it is possible that some summer depressions may be triggered by the intense light, rather than the heat, of summer. One of my patients with summer SAD, a woman in her late thirties, experienced one of her typical "summer" depressions after a heavy snowstorm. Although temperatures were below freezing outside, we speculated that the bright light reflected off the snow might have triggered the unseasonable onset of her summer-type depression. Curiously, some patients report having both regular summer and winter depressions. For these people spring and fall are the only times when they feel good. Flora, for example, an editor in her mid-forties, recalls winter depressions since age sixteen, which last "from Thanksgiving until the daffodils begin to bloom in April." It's only in the last fifteen years that she has become aware of having summer depressions. Before then, she lived in upstate New York, where temperatures do not often go above eighty-five to ninety degrees—the point at which she has observed that she begins to feel "slowed down and stupid and for-getful and depressed." Her summer depressions usually last from the middle of June until the middle of September. She has become aware of this because, as a keen gardener, she has noticed that "I garden pretty seriously through June. Then I look up in September, and the garden is full of weeds." In her professional life, she is least proud of the editing she does in the summer.

Flora has noticed many similarities between her summer and win-ter depressions. She feels lethargic, needs more sleep, craves candy bars, and gains weight in both seasons. She has used light treatment for several winters but has not as yet been treated for her summer de-pressions. One difference between the two types of depression that Flora has noted is the rapidity and ease with which they can be re-versed. "During my summer depression, I feel better instantly if I go north. In the winter, on the other hand, if I am separated from my lights, it takes me several days to feel better again after I return to them."

The winter depressions tend to be longer and deeper for Flora. In the summer, she notes, "I never get so far from reality that I lose track of how it actually is. I can't always deal with it at that moment, but I don't think that I get really buffaloed, while in the winter I think I ac-tually lose touch with reality; I begin to get kind of paranoid."

One big problem for people with both summer and winter de-pressions is that they have to cram as much as possible into the spring and fall. Flora notes that because of her depressions, "I go through cy-cles of letting things slide, and then, when I feel better, I scurry around, pay my income taxes and bills, clean my basement and weed my garden, make new friends, and start a whole bunch of projects."

Gary is another person who has suffered both winter and summer depressions since he was ten years old. A tree surgeon in his early thir-ties, he loves outdoor activities, particularly rock climbing. In spring and fall he is lean and fit and strong, "like a horse let out of a starting gate." But when winter comes along, he gains up to thirty pounds and feels slowed down and sluggish. "I can't fight it. It's as if a switch has been thrown. Each time you think you've conquered the beast, the de-pression starts again." Summer sets him back in just the same way, de-railing his plans, frustrating the hopes that come with the spring. "You think, 'Look how far I've come since winter.' Friends come up and tell me how good my body is looking. And I can feel it. I'm stronger and fitter. Projecting the curve up, I think of how well I can do if it just keeps going that way. Unfortunately, that's usually exactly the time when I begin to get depressed again." Gary has responded very well to light therapy during the winter. In summer, his depressions have been prevented successfully by his taking Prozac. Because of his outdoor work, it is impossible for him to avoid the intense heat of a Washington summer.

Although most SAD patients retain the same "worst season" throughout their lives, some experience a shift in their seasonal problems and preferences over time.

Patients with regular spring depressions seem to be quite rare. One such person whom I have treated did not respond to light therapy but did well when given antidepressant medications. In people with spring depressions the potential role of pollen allergies should be borne in mind. Treatment with antihistamines or other anti-allergy medications may help.

Treatment of Summer Depressions

At this time, no specific physical treatments for summer depression have been developed properly. Researchers have considered trying to keep patients cool or to restrict their levels of environmental light. While some patients, like Marge, mentioned earlier, find that traveling to cooler climates, swimming in cool water, and staying in air-conditioned rooms have alleviated their symptoms, others find such measures to be either impractical or ineffective. One colleague has had success with recommending regular cool baths as opposed to showers, which he thinks cool people down more effectively. This is reminiscent of a nineteenth-century antidepressant method used in France called the *bain de surprise,* in which the patient was plunged unannounced into a tub of cold water. While lowering someone's temperature may help, I do not recommend startling anyone this way. Regular aerobic exercise can be helpful for summer SAD as for other types of recurrent depressions. The value of nonpharmacological approaches, administered either individually or in combination, has yet to be explored properly. Meanwhile, the mainstay of treatment remains antidepressant medications. My colleagues and I have had some success in treating summer-SAD patients with antidepressants. The trick is to treat early, at the first sign of symptoms, and to build up to adequate doses quickly. It seems easier to forestall depressions before they settle in than to reverse them after they are in full swing.

Here is an example of this strategy at work. Joan is a professional in her mid-forties, whose annual depressions typically last from March through September. So every February, we meet and I prescribe Prozac, an antidepressant that has been helpful to her in the past. In March, I increase the dosage of Prozac and we meet at regular intervals through the summer months so that I can monitor her progress and add in extra medications as needed. In October, I begin to taper Joan's medications, and by November, she is usually off all antidepressants. Using this strategy, Joan has been free of all symptoms of depression for the last three years without having to take antidepressants during the winter months, when she is not at risk for depression.

See Chapter 10 for more information about the use of medications in treating SAD. Also make sure that your physician checks your thyroid levels since reduced thyroid function can contribute to depressions of all sorts.

The Flip Side of Depression: Spring Fever

Although many people with SAD feel normally cheerful during the summer months, it is quite common for individuals to report feeling exceptionally energetic and creative at this time. Herb Kern, the first patient with SAD to be treated at the NIMH, was particularly productive scientifically during the summer—so much so that his boss was happy to let him cruise through his less productive winter months.

Such enhanced productivity is not universal for those who develop extra energy in the summer. In some people, this acceleration goes too far and may result in major problems—bank accounts overdrawn from excessive spending, difficulties getting along with friends and colleagues, and even trouble with the law. This state is referred to clinically as mania.

An exaggerated sex drive caused by a midsummer high resulted in problems for Marie, a housewife in her twenties, who was at home with her two young children. Although she was a faithful wife under ordinary circumstances, one summer she could not resist the attentions of a carpenter who was installing bookshelves for her husband. This dalliance caused her a considerable amount of guilt until she understood that her abnormal mood state had increased her libido while at the same time decreasing her inhibitions, thereby affecting her judgment.

Others may spend large sums of money that they can ill afford on items that at other times would seem extravagant. They may show poor judgment in their driving and speed along the highway, assured that their lightning reflexes make them invulnerable to accidents. Or they may suddenly and impetuously decide to undertake some long journey for reasons that to an outsider would seem frivolous.

The degree of acceleration does not have to reach manic proportions to be considered a problem by an individual or, more commonly, by the person's partner, friends, and colleagues. Others may frequently complain about not being able to get a word in edgewise or being interrupted repeatedly during a conversation. This condition, known as hypomania, often impairs efficiency. Although hypomanic people have a great deal of energy, they have so many ideas for projects that they find it difficult to focus on any single one. As a result, their energies are scattered, their attention darts from task to task, and, fueled by grandiosity, they are often left with several unfinished projects at the end of the summer.

Dr. Kay Redfield Jamison, in her book *Touched with Fire,* shows how artists and writers are most creative in spring and fall. Perhaps they are too slowed down in winter and too revved up in summer to do their best work.

Summer Highs: Scenes from a Marriage

Although Jack and Sylvia have some problems with each other when Sylvia is in her "low" winter state, her summer highs present the couple with more serious difficulties. Jack is an accountant in his middle years, and Sylvia is a housewife. The following excerpts from an interview with the two of them, conducted during the summer, illustrate some of these.

JACK: During her lows, Sylvia really gets down. She will say, "I don't know how anyone can love me" or "I'm so slow, I hate myself." And then in the summer, when she gets in the high, she'll say, "Aren't you fortunate to have somebody with my personality?" It's just a complete reversal. I'm amazed—sometimes the highs are more trying than the lows. A day can make a huge difference. In just one day she can come alive.

Most of our arguments come in the early spring, when she comes alive and wants to do all kinds of things. I remember going to Wolf Trap [an open-air amphitheater near Washington, DC] with some friends; she was so excited that everyone said, "Look at Sylvia, she's so high." She became the focal point of her friends because of her excessive energy. It is difficult for me because Sylvia gets after me to join in on her whirlwind of activities. Just the other day I said to her, "Look, I can't be as high as you unless I take cocaine, and I don't plan to take cocaine." At Wolf Trap she just bounced around—it was unreal. I thought she could fly, and I think Sylvia and all her friends thought she could, too!

Jack documents many incidents that have occurred during the summer as evidence of Sylvia's hypomanic state. She spends money on projects that he regards as unnecessary but that she feels are interesting or creative. For example, she bought an expensive video camera so that her sons could learn to make films. On another occasion, she bought a pet iguana, capable of growing to a length of eight feet. While Jack regarded the animal as a bizarre nuisance, Sylvia identified with its love for the sun. She remembers, "When he would get out of the house and I couldn't find him, I would wait for the sun to start going down and know that he would be in that one spot in the yard where the sun was still shining."

Although they have generally been able to resolve their financial difficulties amicably, Jack actually suggested taking Sylvia's credit cards away from her during the summer on one occasion. She became extremely angry and threatened to leave him, and he backed down.

They discuss their seasonal problems further:

SYLVIA: There's a kind of power struggle that goes on between us, because for six months you can just lead me anywhere, and then in the summer, I want to lead. And Jack is not the kind of person who likes a boss.

JACK: In the winter, Sylvia would be really down, and I'd feel really sorry for her and try to keep her spirits up. Then in the spring she'd almost turn on me. I almost got the feeling she didn't like the person she was in the winter, and the fact that I cared for that person in the winter was held against me in the spring. And I couldn't believe that. I think to myself, "I've done all kinds of things for you in the winter, driven you around, made excuses for you to your friends, but because you hate that Sylvia, you hate me, too."

SYLVIA: Jack's reactions to me have always worried me. I like myself in the spring and summer, but I don't think Jack really enjoys me then.

When asked how she feels about Jack's having helped her and taken care of her during the winter, Sylvia replies: "I don't like to think about it."

"Do you forget it, put it out of your mind?" I ask.

"I certainly do. I want to think about happy things," she replies.

Jack comments: "The heck with that! Next winter, I'm going to let her take care of herself."

Both Jack and Sylvia agree that she becomes short-tempered in the summer and is most likely to have run-ins with other people then. On one occasion, when Jack's mother came to visit during the month of May, she and Sylvia had an argument from which Jack says it took his mother two years to recover. As a result, Jack makes sure to keep the two women apart during the summer. Sylvia also has to stay away from meetings at her church then, because she is likely to monopolize them and antagonize some of the other church members with blunt and tactless remarks. She relates this with a certain amount of enjoyment and little evidence of regret.

Although Sylvia's high periods are a source of frustration for Jack, there are aspects of them—the humor, creativity, and liveliness—that he enjoys as much as she does. In the last year or two, however, Sylvia has become worn out from lack of sleep and excessive activity during her high periods. She has been reluctant to take any medications for this, and I have treated her by having her wear dark glasses during the summer days. This treatment has been quite successful, and at times she has even slept with eyeshades on to prevent herself from waking up with the first rays of dawn.

The couple has benefited greatly from marital therapy as well, which has helped them identify the symptoms of SAD, understand that biological processes are at work, and cope with these changes. Jack sums it up: "I think we're like ships passing in the night. We're very seldom at the same level. She's either below me or above, and only momentarily do we see eye to eye."

Although hypomanic individuals often feel euphoric, as in Sylvia's case, hypomania may also be an extremely unpleasant or dysphoric state. As with euphoric hypomanics, people with dysphoric hypomania also feel activated, experience racing thoughts, and speak in a pressured way. But unlike their euphoric counterparts, they feel uncomfortable both physically and emotionally and long for something to bring them down from their hypomanic state. To this end, they may resort to alcohol or cigarettes in an unavailing attempt to calm themselves down. They are irritable and snappy with those they come into contact with. As a consequence, friends and family often avoid them at such times, which may cause them to feel rejected and isolated. A few patients I have encountered with dysphoric hypomania in spring and summer have also complained of physical aches and pains.

The symptoms of hypomania may result from the impact of the rapidly increasing spring light levels on the oversensitive eyes and brain of individuals who have become accustomed to the low levels of environmental light typically found in winter. One young woman consulted me on a spring evening for her problems with dysphoric hypomania. Over the course of the consultation, she became increasingly agitated. I noticed that the lights in my office were very bright and suggested that we experiment by dimming them. Over the next half hour, her agitation subsided dramatically, so much so that I suggested she try treating herself with light restriction. She called me a week later in a state of elation and reported that she had become able to manage her hypomania without using the tranquilizers that she had previously needed, simply by going into a darkened room for a short period of time whenever she felt overexcited. This rapidly acting, nondrug treatment with which she was able to regulate herself not only relieved her symptoms but also gave her a sense of personal mastery over them. Other ways of restricting one's light exposure include wearing eyeshades while asleep to avoid exposure to early morning light, wearing wraparound dark glasses when outdoors, and avoiding brightly lit indoor environments in the evening. If these measures don't work, effective medications are available to lessen the uncomfortable and problematic aspects of this condition.

Although spring and summer hypomanias may cause problems, I should emphasize that for many people with SAD, hypomanias are joyful and creative times that do no harm and don't require treatment.

They need to be watched carefully, however, because they can progress to mania.

Mania

Mania, a more florid form of hypomania, is fortunately rather uncommon in SAD. In the many hundreds of people with SAD whom I have treated over the years, I have witnessed only a handful of manic episodes. But those episodes are not easily forgotten.

Symptoms of mania include extreme disruption of sleep, increased energy level, racing thoughts, pressured speech, enhanced sex drive, an exaggerated sense of one's own importance, excessive optimism, and grandiose ideas and schemes. People with mania often have little insight into their disturbed condition and experience others as being spoilsports and party-poopers who are throwing obstacles in their path because of envy or for other base motives.

At first mania can be great fun, and the affected person does not want the good feelings interrupted for any reason. Yet mania can be very disruptive to one's life and may result in reckless spending, sexual indiscretions, and other serious errors of judgment. One manic patient of mine was apprehended by state police as he walked down the median line on a busy highway, certain that he was invulnerable and that the cars would somehow magically miss him by whizzing by him on either side. On another occasion, while driving around the city in the early hours of the morning, he picked up a hitchhiker and generously gave him a ride into a very dangerous neighborhood, where he was stripped and robbed at gunpoint. Luckily, his life was spared, and he found his way through the bitterly cold winter air to a nearby police station.

Even without the occurrence of such hair-raising episodes, however, mania becomes exhausting. The lack of sleep, excessive activity, and rush of thoughts can become painful, and the feelings of elation become mixed with severe irritability and unhappiness.

The following points about mania are worth noting:

1. Mania is a clinical emergency that should be treated by a doctor without delay. We now have a number of medications with which to treat this condition, but they are most effective if administered earlier rather than later in the manic process.

2. Mania is often preceded by hypomania—so a hypomanic state

has to be watched carefully to make sure that it does not progress to mania.

3. If you are vulnerable to mania, as evidenced by a history of mania or hypomania:

- Be sure to get enough sleep; sleep deprivation fuels mania; even one or two nights of sleep loss should be flagged and brought to the attention of your doctor.
- Be sure not to get too much light; discontinue light therapy if you feel yourself getting manic and check in with your doctor.
- If you have been on lithium carbonate or some other mood stabilizer during the winter, do not stop it in the spring or summer. Doing so increases the likelihood of a manic episode.

4. Curiously, treating the depressive symptoms of SAD with light therapy in the winter seems to decrease the likelihood of developing mania the following spring or summer, perhaps by making certain brain receptors less sensitive to the sudden surge of light experienced as the days get rapidly longer and brighter in springtime.

The Heat and Violence Connection

> I pray thee, good Mercutio, let's retire.
> The day is hot, the Capulets abroad,
> And if we meet, we shall not scape a brawl,
> For now, these hot days, is the mad blood stirring.
> —SHAKESPEARE, *Romeo and Juliet*, III:1

Until recently, the idea that seasons or weather could fundamentally affect mood and behavior seemed absurd. Consider the relatively recent debate to explain the very well-documented association between the seasons and the incidence of sexual violence in the United States. Two leading researchers in the field, Drs. Richard Michael and Doris Zumpe, published a paper in the *American Journal of Psychiatry* in 1983 called "Sexual Violence in the United States and the Role of Season," in which they analyzed seasonal variations in over 50,000 rapes in sixteen locations in the United States. They found a seasonal variation, with peak occurrences in July and August. This corresponded closely to the seasonal variation in assaults, but not to that for robberies, which peaked in November and December, or for murders, which showed no specific pattern. The timing of the maximum incidence of rape closely paralleled that of the maximum temperature values. These researchers suggested that environmental temperature might influence this seasonal variation by its effect on the secretion of certain hormones. Indeed, the male sex hormone, testosterone, has been shown to have a seasonal rhythm in humans, with a peak in the summer months, and is known to influence aggressive behavior in both humans and animals.

An outcry followed. A strongly worded essay by Stephen Jay Gould in *Discover* magazine pointed out the hazards of confusing correlation and causation and suggested the "more obvious" association between hot days and the opportunity for violence when people are out and about. Two prominent psychiatrists wrote a letter to the editor, criticizing Michael and Zumpe for making "statements that appear to embody misperceptions of the experience of sexual violence and that look narrowly at an enormously complicated interaction between biological, psychosocial, and environmental determinants of human behavior." The researchers replied that they were not disputing the importance of all sorts of factors as determinants of rape, but simply drawing attention to the potential importance of temperature, "a factor that has been ignored by science for one hundred years." Indeed, the Italian scientist Morselli wrote about the influence of temperature on the seasonal variation of violent crime in the nineteenth century.

Michael and Zumpe, commenting on the outcry produced by their paper, suggested that this came from "all those who believe passionately that men and women should be in total control of their personal destinies and that, if they are not, then it is society that has perverted them." They addressed some of their critics in a follow-up study on domestic violence, a type of behavior where availability of the victim does not vary seasonally in the same way as in community violence. Once again, they found a peak incidence of crisis calls to shelters for battered women in the summer months, corresponding closely to the peak environmental temperatures. Besides the excellent work of these researchers, there is substantial scientific literature on the influence of temperature on irritability, which may in turn lead to anger, directed at someone who just happens to be in the way.

Full Moons, Air Ions, and Evil Winds

> Demoniac frenzy, moping melancholy,
> And moonstruck madness.
> —MILTON, *Paradise Lost*

> The wind's in the east. . . . I am always conscious of an uncomfortable sensation now and then when the wind is blowing in the east.
> —CHARLES DICKENS, *Bleak House*

So central is the influence of the moon in the mythology of madness that it would hardly be right to omit it from this book. The word *lunacy* derives from this belief. Yet the actual evidence of its influence on human behavior and emotions is rather slim. Dr. Arnold Lieber analyzed the patterns of homicides and aggravated assaults in Dade County, Florida, and showed that they tended to cluster around the time of the full moon. Others failed to replicate this work elsewhere in the country. Dr. Charles Mirabile analyzed medical records of psychiatric patients at the Institute of Living in Hartford, Connecticut, and found a small rise in paranoid behavior around the time of the full moon. The behavioral effects of the moon—if indeed they exist—may be due to its light or its gravitational effects on body fluids. I have occasionally come across individuals who say they are strongly influenced by the phases of the moon, but I have never seen this influence convincingly documented in any particular individual. Until someone is able to do so, the age-old beliefs in the powers of the moon over mankind will continue to lack a compelling scientific basis.

The weather has been held to have powerful effects on human functioning since the time of Hippocrates. In his famous works, he has an entire section, "On Airs, Waters, and Places," where he outlines his beliefs on the importance of our physical environment. He emphasizes the effects of good and bad winds. In a modern text, Dr. Felix Sulsman writes at length on the effects of weather on humans. He devotes an entire section to the "medical impact of evil winds." Prominent among these are warm winds that come down from the mountains—such as the Santa Ana in California, the *foehn* in Europe, and the Chinook in Canada. These winds blow vast amounts of positively charged air particles called *positive ions,* which have been shown experimentally to induce irritability in people. Curiously, these "ill winds" are reported to cause not only irritability but also restlessness, lethargy, depression, and general debility. The *foehn* has been associated with increased rates of crime, suicide, and traffic accidents. Later on in this book I will discuss the potential therapeutic value of negative ions and how you can use special machines called negative ion generators to treat the symptoms of SAD (see Chapter 8).

I have already discussed the important effects of heat on emotions and behavior, and since these mountain winds generally raise the environmental temperature abruptly by as much as fifteen to twenty degrees Celsius, it is possible that many of their effects may be due to heat alone.

Those who have studied the effects of weather changes on people observe that some individuals are particularly sensitive to these changes. Goethe wrote, "It is a pity that just the excellent personalities suffer most from the adverse effects of the atmosphere." He numbered himself among that unfortunate but privileged group. It does indeed seem as though different people react differently to various weather conditions. I have seen a few people who have reported marked feelings of depression or irritability when the weather changes, particularly when a storm is about to hit.

For Ahmed, a computer scientist in his early forties, the problem was serious enough to induce him to come from Saudi Arabia to Washington, DC, for a consultation on his problem. He noticed that just before clouds drifted across the sky, he began to feel weak and depressed. His stomach seemed bloated, and his head felt "blown up." When the weather was stable, he would feel even better than normal—exceedingly energetic and enthusiastic about life. Several members of his family reported almost identical weather-related symptoms. Unfortunately, he has never been able to pinpoint what elements in the atmosphere are responsible for his symptoms, nor has he had access to the technology that might help him reverse them. Medications have not helped his symptoms, and he continues to suffer from weather-related problems.

The effects of weather on vulnerable individuals have been a rather neglected area scientifically. Apart from the specific focus on SAD that I have already discussed, little systematic work has been done on other types of climatic influences. The literature is full of assumptions and old nostrums culled from the classics. It has been widely claimed that some people are able to predict the weather based on its effects on their minds and bodies. This phenomenon is also poorly understood, and we are little further along in our understanding of it than the author John Taylor (1580–1653), who wrote:

Some men 'gainst Raine doe carry in their backs
Prognosticating Aching Almanacks.
Some by painful elbow, hip or knee
Will shrewdly guesse what weathers like to be.

Recent research bears out Hippocrates' view that "Of natures, some are well- or ill-adapted for summer, and some for winter." Just as some people are affected adversely by the physical environment in winter—the darkness and cold—others have trouble with heat and humidity. Characteristic patterns of depression may result. The symptoms of winter SAD usually include decreased activity, overeating, oversleeping, and weight gain, whereas the symptoms of summer SAD often include loss of appetite and weight, insomnia, and agitation. It seems as though these two patterns represent extreme manifestations of physical changes seen in a large proportion of the population in these two seasons. Somehow, seasonally depressed people seem less well insulated against the effects of extreme changes in climate and are unable to function adequately in such conditions. The symptoms of depression result. Fortunately, there are many ways in which the depressed person can find relief from these symptoms. The second part of this book describes how this can be accomplished.

Feeling of Sadness When the Sun Goes Down

Some people report feeling sad at twilight when the sun goes down. One psychoanalyst recognized this symptom and called it "Hesperian depression" after the Greek goddess of the dusk, Hesperus. Some patients with SAD complain of this problem. For example, one woman observed that she could not keep working after the sunset. Another felt unable to make love to her husband except during the day, when the sun was shining.

It's a curious symptom because it suggests an immediate response to the light. This coincides with the experience of some patients using light therapy, in whom I have seen an increase in energy occur even within the first half hour of light treatment.

As we have seen, many people are markedly affected by the changing seasons and weather, and these effects can disrupt their lives. The chapters that follow describe in detail what can be done to alleviate these problems.

Part II
Treatments

Everybody talks about the weather; but nobody does anything about it.

—CHARLES DUDLEY WARNER

*A*lthough there may still be little that we can do about the weather itself—other than to escape from it—there are many things that we can do to alleviate the effects that the weather has on us.

Along with the initial description of SAD twenty years ago came the development of light therapy. In the last two decades light therapy has undergone many changes to make it as effective and practical as possible. Equally exciting, however, has been the development of other types of treatment, notably antidepressant medications and psychotherapy, which promise to make SAD more treatable than ever.

The detailed discussion of all these treatments in this section should enable you to evaluate what therapies might work best for you and how best to implement them. In my experience, knowledgeable individuals make the best patients. Nevertheless, there are limits to self-help. While you may be able to use light therapy (Chapter 7) and the measures described in Chapter 8 largely as self-help, you will of course need professional help if you choose to pursue psychotherapy or antidepressants (Chapters 9 and 10, respectively). Either way, a competent, empathic, and open-minded physician is an invaluable guide and companion for a depressed person. Depression is a serious condition that in its most extreme forms can actually rob a person of life. Therefore, *if your symptoms are causing you a great deal of pain, if they are disrupting your physical functioning, your work, or your personal life to more than a minor degree, and certainly if you have any ideas that life is not worth living, do seek the help of a qualified physician or therapist without delay.*

It is often easy to diagnose SAD on the basis of history, but other conditions can masquerade as SAD, such as underactivity of the thyroid, hypoglycemia, chronic viral illnesses, and chronic fatigue syndrome. These problems should be considered and ruled out before SAD is diagnosed. The first treatment you try may not be helpful. It is important not to despair, but to try other approaches as well. If a treatment fails, it is also possible that the treatment is not being implemented correctly. A professional may be able to detect this and make the necessary suggestions for correcting the problem. Side effects may develop, and an expert may be able to minimize these.

Even if you do have a physician or therapist, the information that follows may be useful in guiding you to recovery. I draw on many years of experience as a psychiatrist, researcher, and SAD sufferer. So read on to find out about the many things you can do to overcome SAD and feel well all year long. In addition, I have included a special chapter to provide guidance to friends and loved ones of people with SAD to help them through the dark winter months.

SEVEN

Light Therapy

"*Mehr licht*," exclaimed the famous German poet Goethe as he lay dying—"more light." With these words, Goethe summed up the chief principle involved in successful light therapy. Patients with SAD develop their symptoms during the short, dark days of winter or when they are deprived of light for any reason. The basic principle involved in light therapy is to replace the light that is missing and help a person with SAD feel more energetic and cheerful, more like the way he or she feels during the summer.

Before getting into the technical details of light therapy, here are a few important facts:

- Most people with SAD can benefit from light therapy.
- There are many tricks to making light therapy work best for you, as detailed in this chapter. If you are planning to embark on a course of light therapy, you would do well to read this chapter carefully. Otherwise, you could easily buy the wrong type of light fixture or use it in the wrong way so that you don't respond optimally. Then you might prematurely conclude that light therapy is no good for you, whereas in fact you just haven't been using it most effectively.
- Light therapy is usually only part of the solution (see Chapters 8–10 for other elements of treatment that can complement light therapy).

• For some people, light therapy is not the answer. Either they do not respond despite their best efforts, or it is too inconvenient. The good news for these people is that it is possible to treat SAD effectively without light therapy—for example, with medications or psychotherapy, as detailed in the chapters that follow.

• One way or another, most people with SAD can benefit substantially from available treatments.

There are many ways to bring more light into your life during the winter. You can make a point of going outdoors on a bright winter's day or bring more lamps into your house or work space—both useful strategies. In practice, however, the most effective and best-studied way of enhancing your environmental light is by means of a special light fixture or light box, the most commonly used method for administering light therapy. Other ways of administering light therapy include the portable, head-mounted light visor and various types of devices for simulating a summer dawn on a winter morning. In this chapter, I will discuss all of these, but since the light box has the longest and best-established track record for successfully treating SAD, it is a starting point for our discussion—and for most light therapy programs.

The Essentials of Light Therapy

After establishing that you need light therapy:

1. Obtain a suitable light box.
2. Set the light box up in a convenient place at home or at work, or both.
3. Sit in front of the light box for a certain amount of time (usually between twenty and ninety minutes each day).
4. Try to get as much of your light therapy as early in the morning as possible.
5. Be sure to sit in such a way that the correct amount of light falls on the eyes.
6. Repeat this procedure each day throughout the season of risk.

Although this remedy sounds simple, in practice many questions arise about the best use of light therapy. An enormous amount of research has been conducted on light therapy over the past twenty years:

about sixty controlled scientific studies by my latest count. A recent meta-analysis by Dr. Robert Golden, professor of psychiatry at the University of North Carolina, Chapel Hill, found that light therapy is as effective for SAD as antidepressants have been shown to be for nonseasonal depression in most published studies. Many light therapy studies explored important practical questions, such as the best time of day to administer treatment or how bright the light should be. In addition, many different devices are now available for administering light therapy. How can you make sense of these many studies and determine what type of device might be best for you? In the section that follows I will answer the most commonly asked questions about light therapy, referring to the research wherever possible. I will also draw on my own extensive experience with this form of treatment, personally and with hundreds of patients with SAD. I strongly recommend that you read through all the questions and answers to educate yourself fully about light therapy, but if you want a quick reference to specific questions, see Table 5.

TABLE 5
Frequently Asked Light Therapy Questions

(cont.)

TABLE 5 (cont.)

Questions Frequently Asked About Light Therapy

1. Should I involve a professional, or can I treat my symptoms on my own?

Ideally, anyone who undertakes light treatment for SAD should be supervised by a physician or other qualified therapist for several reasons. It is important that the diagnosis be confirmed by a qualified person, that a careful history be taken, and, if necessary, that a physical examination be performed. Professional input may also be very helpful in monitoring a person's mood and the side effects that may develop in the course of treatment. Light therapy may not work, and a professional can recommend or prescribe alternative or supplementary treatments. Above all, an informed perspective, encouragement, and support can be invaluable in guiding one through the ordeal of depression.

Practically speaking, though, a qualified professional is not always available, in which case someone with relatively mild symptoms could undertake a time-limited trial (no more than, say, two weeks) of light therapy to determine whether that will take care of the problem. If it does, treatment may be continued and no outside assistance may be needed. If problems persist, however, it is certainly worth bringing a professional into the picture sooner rather than later. Guidelines as to when it is really critical to involve a professional are provided on pages 58–60 and 111–112.

2. What is a suitable light box for light therapy?

A suitable light box is usually a metal fixture approximately two feet long and eighteen inches high, containing ordinary white fluorescent light bulbs set behind a plastic diffusing screen, which houses a film that filters out most of the ultraviolet (UV) rays from the fluorescent bulbs. These types of light fixtures have been used in almost all research studies that indicate the value of light therapy for SAD. The many smaller boxes on the market that have capitalized on the success of their larger counterparts are probably less effective. (See also question 5 below.)

Some of the most effective types of light fixtures are constructed so that they can be positioned toward the eye at an angle, so that the light source is tilted forward, permitting more light to enter the eyes. This angle also decreases the apparent brightness of the light, creating less glare and making it more comfortable to use. An upright type of light box, though perhaps not quite as effective for delivering therapy, is often more useful for illuminating an interior space because it projects light farther into the room. Some boxes are constructed so that they can be set up in either an upright or an angled position, thereby offering the user both choices. Three of the light fixtures that have been used extensively, both clinically and in research studies, are shown in Figure 3.

The amount of light (or intensity) that has been found to be therapeutic ranges between 2,500 and 10,000 lux (lux is a measurement of intensity). To give you an idea of how much light this is, the average room at night is illuminated at a level of 300 to 500 lux; offices are usually somewhat brighter—between 500 and 700 lux. The amount of light coming off the sky at sunrise, just before the sun crests the horizon on a cloudless day, is about 10,000 lux year round, whereas the amount of light coming off a summer sky is over 100,000 lux.

The initial studies of light therapy for SAD used light boxes that emitted 2,500 lux, which proved to be therapeutic. More recently, the higher levels of light intensity have been preferred because they are more effective and allow for shorter daily treatments.

Fluorescent bulbs are preferable to incandescent ones because they spread the light out over a wide surface area, which is safer and probably more effective. Incandescent lamps generate a great deal of light

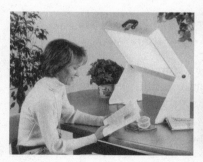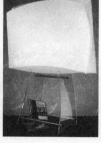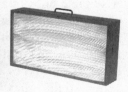

FIGURE 3. The SunRay II (left), DaylightXL (middle), and Brite Lite IV Oak (right). These three standard light boxes, manufactured by the SunBox Company, the Center for Environmental Therapeutics, and Apollo Health, respectively, have been used extensively and effectively both clinically and in research settings.

from small point sources. These can be dangerous to stare at directly, especially the intensely bright halogen lamps. Incandescent lights are fine to use as indirect lighting to enhance the general level of indoor illumination but are not generally suitable for formal light therapy.

The plastic diffuser adds extra protection to the light box by further spreading the light out over the surface of the fixture. A UV filter is a valuable addition because the UV rays that emanate from fluorescent light bulbs can be harmful to the eyes and the skin. By filtering out most of these rays, these potential harmful effects of light therapy are minimized.

Modern light fixtures contain special ballasts that remove the irritating flicker that can be associated with fluorescent lights, thus adding to the general comfort of using the light box.

Never stare directly at incandescent light bulbs, especially halogens.

3. Where can I obtain a suitable light fixture?

In general, light fixtures fall into two categories: desk or tabletop models such as those shown in Figure 3 and freestanding models such as those shown in Figure 4. In Part IV I list some of the established companies that sell light fixtures suitable for light therapy. All should offer thirty-day, money-back guarantees if you are not satisfied with their products. (Be sure to check on this before making a purchase.) All provide details about their products without charge and will ship the desired fixture to you.

4. How much does a light box cost?

Although prices vary, over the last several years most recommended light boxes have run between $250 and $350, an amount many people have found to be well worth the investment over time. Since most light box companies have a thirty-day return policy and since light therapy usually works within a few weeks—if it is going to work at all—you can make use of the return policy to test whether the investment is worth your while, without any cost to you.

5. What about smaller, cheaper light boxes?

Light boxes that are smaller and cheaper than those just described are widely advertised and appear to be quite popular. If you are suffering

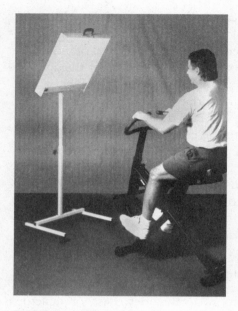

FIGURE 4. The Sun Square. This freestanding light box by the SunBox Company allows the user to receive light therapy in a variety of settings, including while exercising on a stationary bicycle or treadmill.

from depression as a result of insufficient environmental light, any light fixture that increases your exposure to light may be helpful. But these smaller boxes have not been researched in the same way as the larger boxes, and it is not known whether they are as effective. I suspect they are not, for two reasons. First, they do not give out as much light as the larger boxes. Second, the amount of light to which your eyes are exposed depends on the position of your head in relation to the light box, and with a very small light box, minor movements of the head will greatly decrease the amount of light to which you are exposed. Still, if a more expensive box is out of your reach, a smaller one is far better than nothing, and I have heard many favorable reports from people who have set such smaller boxes on their desks with beneficial results.

With the growing awareness of SAD and the beneficial effects of light, manufacturers are offering a greater variety of shapes, sizes, and designs, allowing consumers to choose those elements that best match their own needs.

6. Can I build my own light box?

Perhaps you can. The structure of a light box is not that complicated. When I first began recommending light therapy in the early 1980s, there were no commercial light box vendors. I told patients what sort of metal boxes to purchase, instructed them to be sure to wire the boxes properly so as to be electrically safe, and advised them as to what sort of light bulbs to obtain. Most found the process tedious and un-appealing and were very pleased when commercial light box providers arrived on the scene.

In addition, I was never sure a homemade box was giving off sufficient light, because different boxes have different physical properties. If the depression did not lift after a few weeks of therapy, it was never clear whether the box was unsatisfactory or the patient was not a good candidate for light therapy. Commercial fixtures have additional advantages over homemade products, such as a UV filter and special ballasts to decrease flicker. For a homemade version to be of comparable quality, these components would need to be included in the design. Before you go to all the trouble of making your own light box, consider all these factors. You might also want to check how much money you will save by doing so.

With all these caveats in mind, I have come across people who have set about building their own light boxes and seem pleased with the results. If you decide to build your own light fixture, be sure that:

- The amount of light emitted is between 2,500 and 10,000 lux.
- It is electrically safe.
- The UV light is filtered out as well as possible.
- The fluorescent bulbs are set behind a plastic diffusing screen; there should be no "hot spots."

One cautionary tale: A colleague of mine had a patient who built his own homemade light fixture, which consisted of fluorescent lamps without a plastic diffusing screen. The patient decided to treat himself with this device by staring at the unshielded light bulbs for extended periods and suffered a burn on his cornea as a consequence.

7. What effects might I hope for after starting light therapy?

The first sensations you may experience in response to light therapy may be physical—a sense of lightening of the body, calm, or increased energy. There may be a feeling of "butterflies in the stomach" or "pins and needles" in the hands. In the days that follow, people report that it feels as though some fundamental problem is being corrected; ideally, the symptoms of SAD disappear, one by one or all at once. In those people in whom this effect takes hold completely, the results may seem dramatic, almost a miracle. In others, the result is less complete, only partly helpful. In a small minority light treatment may not work at all. The good news is that over eighty percent of people with SAD or the winter blues may expect to benefit from light therapy, but you should not expect it to cure all your winter difficulties.

While on light therapy, people typically feel more energetic. Suddenly, chores and daily activities no longer feel like drudgery. Along with a physical sense of lightness, the burden of living, of carrying your body around from place to place, seems lighter, and the overwhelming need to sleep subsides. Suddenly, you feel less driven by cravings for sweets and starches. Cakes and candy bars become resistible. Even dieting seems possible again! Thinking becomes more efficient. No longer does your mind creak along like an old machine in need of oiling. Your computer is up and running again. Computations and calculations are possible, and new ideas spring readily to mind. You think of tackling problems in ways that hadn't occurred to you before. Exercise becomes less onerous—no longer does that trip to the gym, that walk, jog, aerobics class, or stationary bicycle seem like a mountainous obstacle. There is once again a wish to communicate: to call friends, write notes, arrange trips to the movies, a ball game, or the theater. Sex seems not only possible but desirable. In short, you feel human again.

If you wish to monitor your progress on light therapy, consult the Daily Mood Log at the end of the book (Appendix A, p. 348), which may help you measure your mood level on a daily basis.

8. How long does it take for light therapy to begin to work?

Although it varies from person to person, most feel the effects of light therapy within two to four days of starting treatment. Some experience a lift in mood and energy level after only one session of light therapy. Almost everyone who is going to respond to light therapy should feel the benefit within two weeks, though it may be worth persevering beyond that time.

Those who experience an immediate positive effect of bright light may be the ones who experience "light hunger" during the winter and have learned to seek out bright places. On the other hand, those who respond to light therapy more slowly, over days or weeks, may be the ones who have historically had difficulty connecting their feelings with the brightness of their environment. These people may seclude themselves when they feel depressed and rest in darkened rooms, thereby inadvertently making their symptoms worse.

When I think back to those who have experienced an immediate response to light therapy, the man who comes first to mind is a car salesman in his early thirties. He had suffered winter depressions for several years and had used cocaine in an attempt to increase his energy level and remain functional at his work during the difficult winter months. It is hard to imagine a job more difficult for a depressed person than that of a salesman, whose livelihood depends on being upbeat and persuasive. Although cocaine seemed to help in the short run, over time the drug made matters much worse. He became increasingly addicted and experienced many of the problems associated with this dangerous substance. He had quit cocaine a few years previously with great difficulty, but now, confronted once again with a severe winter depression and unable to function at work, he was considering restarting cocaine unless I could find something else to help his depression quickly.

As he began to tell me his story, he was so slowed down and listless that it was hard to imagine him capable of making any sales—or functioning at all for that matter. I wondered if he might feel better if I turned on the light box in my office and directed it toward him during the consultation. I did so, and within half an hour observed a marked difference. The pace of his speech picked up; life returned to his face and body gestures and enthusiasm to his voice. At that moment, I appreciated what a successful salesman he could be when he was feeling well. He used light successfully throughout the winter and did not even consider returning to cocaine.

I have since used the light box during treatment sessions with several patients with SAD, who have dragged themselves into my office at the beginning of the session and have left with smiles on their faces and a spring in their stride. On more than one occasion, the patients scheduled immediately after these rapid responders have turned to me and quoted that famous line from the movie *When Harry Met Sally*— "I'll have what she's having."

Such rapid responses are by no means universal, so don't be disappointed if you experience no immediate effects from the light. *You should not give up on light treatment until you have used it consistently for at least two weeks and reviewed the section on troubleshooting* (see p. 142).

Although most people who will benefit from light show some favorable response to treatment within the first week or two, there is evidence that the benefits may continue to grow over the weeks that follow. For this reason, I recommend that you continue treatment after an initial improvement, since your response to light may get even better over time.

9. Do I need to stare at the light box?

No. Studies show that it is not necessary to stare at the light box to derive its benefits. Just facing it with your eyes open is generally sufficient for obtaining a therapeutic effect. It is important, however, that your eyes be open. An early study by Dr. Thomas Wehr, myself, and others at the NIMH showed that the effects of light therapy, derived from typical light therapy fixtures, are mediated through the eyes rather than the skin. If you are using a properly made light box, it is quite safe to stare at the plastic diffusing screen for short periods (such as a few minutes). Because you are not obligated to stare at the light box, there are many things you can do while receiving treatment. (See question 12.)

10. Where is the light acting?

Evidence suggests that light therapy acts on the brain via connections from the eyes. (See Chapter 4 for more details.) That is why it is necessary to face the light box. One study showing that light exposure to the back of the knees could alter the timing of daily rhythms was never replicated. There is no basis for recommending that light be used in this way. The effects of standard light therapy fixtures are quite different from those of the lamps used in tanning salons, which I discuss in question 43.

11. How far do I need to be from the box for light therapy to be effective?

The answer differs for different light boxes and different people. Usually, the distance at which the light is active will vary between one and three feet and should be specified by the manufacturer. According to simple laws of physics, the intensity of light exposure falls off sharply with the distance from a light source. Studies of light therapy have shown a relationship between the intensity of light exposure and the strength of the antidepressant effect. If you are to obtain the maximum therapeutic effect in the minimum amount of time, it is important to stay within the recommended distance from the light box.

12. What can I do while I am receiving light therapy?

You can do anything you like while receiving light therapy, provided your eyes are open, you are facing the box, and you are at the proper distance. Some people use their light therapy sessions as an opportunity to catch up on chores, such as paperwork or returning business calls. For others, this makes light therapy itself feel more like a chore. I encourage these people to use their therapy time for enjoyable activities like reading a novel or catching up with a friend on the phone. Some people like to relax in front of their light boxes, others to exercise. It is possible to set up a light box in front of an exercise machine (as in Figure 4), and some of the distributors listed at the back of the book sell light boxes that are specially adapted for use in front of a treadmill or ski machine. I have a light box set up in front of a stationary bicycle and find the combination of light therapy and exercise to be particularly energizing. Research bears out the benefits of combining these two forms of treatment.

One common concern people have is how to find time for daily light therapy in the midst of a busy schedule. Analyze your daily activities and determine when you will be seated in one place for a period of time each day. For light therapy to work best, it should be incorporated naturally into your current daily activities so it does not become an extra burden when you already feel overburdened. Almost everyone has at least one daily sedentary period. If you can afford more than one light box, you can derive the benefits of light therapy by moving from one illuminated setting to another—say, from the kitchen at breakfast to your desk in the den—the way we do in summer, when many of us feel at our best.

13. What is the best time of day to receive light therapy?

This question has been researched extensively, and the answer is now in: For most people light treatments are most effective if administered early in the morning. According to researchers Michael and Jiuan Su

Terman, the earlier the better, especially if you are a person who generally functions best in the morning. These researchers have developed a formula that links how much of a morning or evening person you are with the best time for receiving light treatment. (See *www.cet.org* for further information about this.) The trouble with using light at the most effective time of day is that for many people the best times tend to be much earlier than is convenient, often intruding on their sleep time. According to the Termans' studies, however, response rate to light therapy can double, from forty to eighty percent, if treatments are shifted early enough, say from 8:00 A.M. to 6:00 A.M. In addition, using light therapy at an early hour of the day for several days tends to shift people's sleep schedules earlier, making it easier for them to fall asleep earlier in the evening and wake up earlier in the morning. This earlier schedule, however, doesn't work well for everyone.

Although most people can benefit from light therapy given at convenient times of the day, for some it may be critical to use light very early in the morning One of my patients, Hank, was just such a person. Unlike most people with SAD, who tend to become depressed in October or November, Hank would regularly become depressed toward the middle of August. Antidepressant medications combined with light therapy administered at conventional morning hours, such as 7:00 A.M., were unable to prevent the inevitable slide into sluggishness and misery at that time of year. It occurred to me that one event that occurs regularly around the middle of August is the arrival of dawn about half an hour later than at the summer solstice. Could it be, I wondered, that a mere half hour of light deprivation, occurring at this crucial time of day, was responsible for Hank's early symptoms? To test this theory, I asked Hank to start his light therapy at 5:30 A.M., the time of dawn at the summer solstice in our part of the world. Both Hank and I were pleasantly surprised at his powerful response, which endured throughout the winter. For Hank, the earlier timing of the light made all the difference. Most people, however, do not need to wake up as early as Hank to benefit from light therapy.

One regimen that I have found to be particularly effective is to place a light box a few feet away from one's bed and connect it to a timer that turns it on early in the morning. To avoid waking up with a jolt, it is best if the bright light follows an artificially simulated dawn, as described below (see question 36).

In practice, light therapy has been found to be helpful at all times of the day, including the evening hours. In addition, many derive benefit from light therapy administered more than once a day, often in the morning and the evening. If you are starting light therapy, try treatment first thing in the morning if your schedule permits. If you have been using light treatment in the morning with only minimal effect, try to shift sessions earlier in the morning. If you still see no improvement, switch to or add evening light therapy before concluding that you have obtained the maximum possible benefit.

14. How long do I need to sit in front of the light box?

This varies among individuals and even within the individual over the course of the year. A few people are exquisitely sensitive to light therapy, and five to ten minutes per day are as much as they can take. I often suggest such short treatments, at least initially, to those with a history of hypomania or mania, who may become overactivated by light therapy. Others may need to sit in front of their light boxes for hours. But most people end up using between thirty and ninety minutes (of 10,000 lux) per day, often divided into more than one light therapy session. This is either enough to achieve a complete remission of symptoms or about as much time as they are willing to invest, in which case additional types of treatment may be needed.

If you are starting light therapy at the beginning of the winter season just as you are experiencing your first winter symptoms, start with about twenty minutes in the morning for the first week or so. If that reverses most of your symptoms without any untoward effects, stay with that duration until your body tells you that you need either more or less treatment. If you are still feeling the symptoms of SAD markedly after the first week, increase your treatment to about forty-five minutes per day, either all in the morning or with no less than thirty minutes in the morning and the rest in the evening. Reevaluate your symptoms one week later and make adjustments again. You may find the chart at the end of this book of some help in evaluating your mood response (see Appendix A, p. 348). If you feel side effects related to light therapy, such as irritability, anxiety, insomnia, headache, or eyestrain (see the more complete list at question 22), you may want to scale back after the first week, to, for example, ten or fifteen minutes of therapy in the morning.

As the winter deepens, the degree of light deprivation increases and you may well need to increase your amount of daily light therapy. It is important to be aware of this ahead of time so that you don't despair that the treatment is no longer working for you. It is quite common, for example, to find that twenty minutes of light therapy per day is sufficient at the beginning of winter but that you need ninety minutes during January and February.

If you are already in the midst of your winter depression by the time you start light therapy, start with twenty minutes twice a day for a few days and then, after determining that there are no untoward effects, add an extra ten minutes twice a day until you have reached a total daily exposure of forty-five minutes twice a day. You should allow about two weeks at that dosage before deciding how effective the treatment is for you and whether any further steps need to be taken.

Remember, when the days begin to get longer and brighter in the spring, you will no longer need as much light therapy and will be able to taper off the duration of daily therapy accordingly. In fact, you may start to develop side effects in the spring, such as irritability and feeling "wired," indicating that you are receiving too much light therapy and need to cut back. After a while, you get good at recognizing whether you are receiving the right amount of light therapy per day. When the amount falls below a therapeutic threshold, you may begin to feel lethargic again, to start craving sweets and starches, or to feel unintelligent and unmotivated. Check the symptoms of SAD outlined in Chapter 2 if this occurs. Usually you will realize that you have slipped back into your winter doldrums again. When you are receiving too much light therapy, you may feel overenergized and overactivated, as though you have been drinking too much coffee. That is a sign to pull back. It is worth paying attention to how you feel each day and relating it to the amount of light you are receiving both from therapy and from the world outside. When it snows and the landscape dazzles, for example, you may be able to cut way back on your light therapy. Even old light therapy veterans would do well to focus on how they feel each day and relate it to the amount of light they're getting. At times, I find myself needing to remind some old friends of mine who have SAD that they may want to increase their light levels; if they observe me slipping, they don't hesitate to return the favor.

15. Is it important to use full-spectrum light?

Full-spectrum light is a type of white light, fluorescent or incandescent, that mimics the colors of sunlight more closely than ordinary fluorescent lamps or incandescent light bulbs. This type of light, sold under a variety of trade names such as Gro-Light or Vitalite, is often advertised as healthier than ordinary lighting, but there is no evidence in favor of these claims. Although many people prefer the color of full-spectrum fluorescent light, which appears a little more blue and a little less pink than ordinary fluorescents, you will probably do well with either type. One feature of some full-spectrum lights is that they include more of a certain type of UV light than ordinary fluorescents. Once again, there is no evidence that this feature confers any special advantage. On the contrary, it may present additional risks to the skin and eyes. This risk factor is largely offset, however, if a light fixture has a proper UV filter on its diffusing screen. The bottom line as far as full-spectrum lamps are concerned is "Suit yourself." Feel free to use them if you prefer the color and are using a box with a UV filter, but don't feel obligated to go to any special lengths or pay any premium for this type of lamp.

16. Is it true that blue light is better than white light for treating SAD?

If you have the impression that this is the case, you are not alone. Several companies have been marketing fixtures that emit blue light, advertising them as superior to regular white-light fixtures. Is this true, and if so, what is the science behind it? The bottom-line answer is, at this time stay with conventional white-light fixtures. We have decades of experience indicating that these are effective and safe. As of the writing of this book, there is not one published study on the effectiveness of blue light for treating SAD. Nor is there the long track record of safety. On the contrary, there is long-standing concern about potential toxicity of blue light to the eyes. The burden of proof as to whether blue light is safe and effective must fall on those who advocate this novel treatment. So far, in my opinion, this burden has not been met. For those interested in finding out more about the science behind this blue light approach, read on.

All physiological effects mediated by the eyes depend on specialized photopigment-containing receptors in the retina. Color vision, for example, depends on three different types of cone receptors that are especially sensitive at picking up certain wavelengths of light. Working together, these cones allow us to pick up different shades of color in the world around us. Another group of receptors, the rods, which use a different photopigment, are specialized for picking up light in dim surroundings. We depend on them for night vision.

In the past few decades scientists have discovered that light is capable of mediating many physical functions other than vision. It can suppress melatonin, shift circadian (daily) rhythms, make people more alert, and, yes, reverse the symptoms of depression in people with SAD. Researchers have attempted to tease out which receptors (or photopigments) are responsible for these nonvisual effects of light. One way to determine which pigment might be mediating a particular function is to expose that pigment to different wavelengths of light and develop a graph that describes the relationship between these different wavelengths and different degrees of absorption, a so-called absorption spectrum. The next step is to explore the effects of these different wavelengths of light on a physiological function, say melatonin suppression, and develop a similar graphic relationship, a so-called action spectrum. If the absorption spectrum of a photopigment or photoreceptor closely correlates with the action spectrum of a specific physiological function, the pigment in question might in fact be responsible for the action being observed.

Recently a novel photopigment called *melanopsin* was discovered in the retina, and its absorption spectrum indicates that it absorbs light most efficiently in the blue range. Dr. George Brainard from Jefferson Medical College in Philadelphia and colleagues from Dr. Charles Czeisler's group at the Brigham and Women's Hospital in Boston and from Dr. Anna Wirz-Justice's group in Basel, Switzerland, have set about to explore which colors are most active in mediating nonvisual effects of light. Blue light has emerged as the leading candidate, possibly exerting its effects through the photopigment melanopsin. These researchers have found blue light to be most effective at shifting the timing of circadian rhythms, at making people more alert, and at affecting body temperature rhythms and heart rate. The next step clearly will be to see whether blue light is more effective than white at reversing the symptoms of SAD.

Dr. Brainard and colleagues have conducted a small study of blue light therapy in SAD and have found that it is more effective than red light. They also found the blue light to be effective at levels far lower than those that have been traditionally used in therapy with white light. These data are quite preliminary, however, especially since the researchers did not have a white light therapy control.

In summary, this is an exciting new line of research that may hold out promise for developing more effective forms of light therapy in the future. From my point of view, however, a lot more testing is needed before we can conclude that blue light is safe and effective, let alone superior to white light. Remember, we now have over twenty years of experience with white light, which is both safe and effective. I there-fore recommend traditional white light—not blue light—for the treat-ment of SAD. This opinion may change depending on the results of research studies yet to be done.

17. Will light therapy still work if I take a break from it?

Yes. Short breaks in a light therapy session should not significantly de-crease the overall benefit.

18. If one light box is good, would two be better?

Even though this question has never been studied systematically, based on my personal experience, the answer is yes. I recently purchased two large light boxes (of the type shown in Figure 4) which I placed in my den, intending to give one as a gift. I put them in front of me, one slightly to the left and the other slightly to the right. To my astonish-ment, the effect was extremely intense, more powerful than from a sin-gle box. The second light box never left my den. As we know, a single example is no proof of anything, but I share my experience with you for what it's worth.

Dr. Teodor Postolache and others in my group at the NIMH found that patients with SAD don't generally feel as well in the winter following light therapy as they do in the summertime. Something about summer does more for their mood than a light box. Postolache has suggested that it may be the fragrances of summer and has actually shown that the smell of lemons boosts mood to a very small though significant degree in people with SAD. I have often wondered whether one therapeutic aspect of summer is that we receive light from the vast dome of the sky, which bathes a larger proportion of our retinas in light than is the case with a single light box. When two boxes are used, the resulting illumination may more closely resemble that of a summer sky, which may explain its greater effectiveness.

19. Can I simply replace all the lamps in my house with full-spectrum lights?

This is one of the most commonly asked questions that I encounter. Again, there is nothing special about full-spectrum lighting and no reason why such replacement of bulbs would be beneficial. But this question also reveals an underlying misunderstanding about what is special about light therapy fixtures—that they enable the user to receive high levels of light in a safe and standardized way, not that they contain light of a particular color range. On the other hand, there is no harm in putting full-spectrum light in your home, and if it makes the environment more cheerful or increases the overall amount of lighting, it may well do you some good.

I should mention that not everyone likes the color range of full-spectrum lighting. At one point, for example, the nurses on our research unit requested full-spectrum lighting, which they thought would create a more appealing environment for the night shift. To their surprise, they found the sharp, blue-white light unwelcome and soon voted to replace the full-spectrum lamps with the more usual "cool-white" fluorescents.

My personal preference is to use full-spectrum light for light therapy (I like the crystalline blue-white quality of the light) but to illuminate the rooms in my house with light of different colors, such as the sunny indirect light of halogen bulbs and the soft yellow of incandescents. Surface areas of different colors can also be used to create the desired atmosphere for each room.

20. Do I need to use light therapy every day? What happens if I skip a day or two? And when can I stop light therapy?

Once again, the answer varies from one person to the next and according to the season, the weather, and the amount of naturally occurring environmental light available. In the darkest depths of winter, most people with SAD need light on a daily or almost-daily basis. Some people manage quite well if they skip a day of therapy, but after skipping it for two days many feel some return of symptoms. One patient of mine recognized this trend and informed his wife that he could not undertake social activities (and skip his light therapy) two nights in a row during the winter.

Those who feel an immediate energizing effect of light therapy may be the first to miss this effect if they skip treatment for as little as a single day, whereas those who take longer to obtain a response may be able to hold on to the benefits for longer after withdrawal of light therapy. Just as low energy and difficulty waking up in the morning are often the earliest symptoms of SAD to appear at the approach of winter, so they may be the first to return when treatment is discontinued.

When spring arrives, it may be possible to skip more days of light therapy without experiencing a relapse. Similarly, if you can get out and about on a bright winter day you may get enough light to skip therapy that day. The principle here is simple. If you are getting enough light from some other source, it may be possible to skip your formal light therapy indefinitely without experiencing a relapse.

Another way to skip light therapy is to embrace one of the other treatment strategies, such as embarking on a vigorous program of daily exercise or starting an antidepressant medication, as described in later chapters. Otherwise, it is best not to skip more than one day of light therapy a week in order to feel well throughout the winter.

21. Is there an advantage to starting light therapy early in the winter?

In my experience, it is best to start light therapy as soon as the first symptoms of winter depression appear, before they progress to a full-blown picture of SAD. For some, this may be as early as August, while others may not begin to experience symptoms until January. Chapter 11, "A Step-by-Step Guide Through the Revolving Year," deals with this question in greater detail.

Some European researchers have suggested that treating SAD early, when the very first symptoms appear, for a relatively short period of time—say a few weeks—protects an individual from developing any further symptoms later in the winter without any further light therapy. Unfortunately these findings are not borne out by other research or by my own clinical experience. While early treatment often prevents the depression from becoming severe, treatment almost always needs to be continued throughout the season of risk to prevent a relapse.

22. What are the side effects of light therapy?

Light therapy is generally very well tolerated; side effects, when they occur, are usually mild. It is the rare individual who is unable to use light therapy altogether because of side effects. When they occur, the most common side effects of light therapy are:

- Headaches
- Eyestrain
- Irritability or anxiety

- Overactivity
- Insomnia
- Nausea
- Fatigue
- Dryness of the eyes
- Dryness of nasal passages and sinuses
- Sunburn-type reaction of the skin

You can deal with these side effects as follows:

- *Headaches and eyestrain.* These can usually be managed by decreasing the duration of treatment—for example, to fifteen minutes per day—and then building it up gradually over a week or two to the more usual exposure durations. Alternatively, sit slightly farther away from the light source until symptoms subside. It is generally possible to move closer to the light box again after several days without experiencing a recurrence of these side effects.
- *Irritability, anxiety, and overactivity.* People who become irritable during light therapy often compare those feelings to how they typically feel during the summer. This side effect generally responds well to decreased exposure (either by shortening the duration of therapy or increasing the distance from the light source). Such irritability (together with insomnia, increased energy, racing thoughts, and pressured speech) is among the symptoms of hypomania and mania. If you experience these symptoms, I recommend that you review the features of these conditions on pages 101–106. Usually, reducing the amount of light treatment (or discontinuing it) is sufficient to bring these side effects under control within a few days. If these measures fail to do so within this time frame, consult your doctor without delay.

Although light therapy generally decreases the anxiety associated with SAD, in some people—usually the same ones who tend to become irritable or hypomanic—light therapy may cause anxiety, panic, and a feeling of overstimulation. One of my patients who developed these feelings on light therapy experienced stomach discomfort as part of her anxiety state, and at certain times of the year it was necessary to decrease the duration of light therapy—at times to as little as five minutes per day—to prevent these side effects. At other times of the year she was able to tolerate longer durations of treatment and, despite the anxiety, found light therapy to be very helpful overall.

- *Insomnia.* Insomnia is most apt to occur when the lights are used late at night. Some people complain that the lights make them feel too energized or "wired" to go to sleep. The best remedy is to shift the treatment to an earlier time of day; if not morning, then afternoon or even earlier in the evening may be fine.

- *Nausea.* According to Michael and Jiuan Su Terman, nausea is the one side effect that tends to go along with a favorable response to light therapy. As with some of the other side effects, the best remedy is to decrease the exposure until the nausea subsides and then gradually increase duration of treatment.

- *Fatigue.* Fatigue may occur after several days of light therapy, especially if the amount or timing of sleep has been changed to accommodate treatment. If feelings of fatigue persist, the best remedy is to try to get to bed earlier at night. Alternatively, it may be necessary to move treatment to a later hour in the morning, a less desirable choice as it may prove less effective at that time.

- *Dryness of eyes, nasal passages, or sinuses.* This problem may be due to the heat generated by the light box, which can dry out the surrounding air. In contact lens wearers, dry eyes may be more than just an irritant and may actually result in abrasions of the cornea. Artificial tears may help to overcome this problem, as may a humidifier placed in the vicinity of the light box. Dryness of the nasal passages and sinuses may also be relieved by a humidifier, as well as by drinking hot beverages while undergoing treatment. An added advantage to keeping the air humid is that humidity promotes a higher concentration of negative ions (charged particles) in the air, which may boost your mood (see pp. 183–185 for more information about this).

- *Reddening of the skin.* This problem, similar to a mild case of sunburn, may occur, especially in those with fair, sun-sensitive skin or in those taking certain medications that sensitize the skin to light. Such reddening is evidence that despite all attempts at removing ultraviolet rays, some of them are getting through the screen and reaching the skin. If this is a problem, consider using sunblocking creams.

Suicidal attempts or ideas have been reported, in very rare instances, within two weeks of starting light therapy. There is also one documented case of suicide after five days of light therapy. Dr. Raymond Lam and colleagues analyzed their clinic experience with 191 patients with SAD and found a significant decrease in suicidal tendencies in forty-five percent following light treatment, with only three percent showing worsening in these tendencies. Since suicidal ideas and tendencies are part of mood disorders in general (and SAD is no exception here), it is reasonable to assume that they fluctuate to some degree as a result of fluctuations in the severity of the illness. It is therefore possible that the increases in suicidal ideas or tendencies seen in a small percentage of patients with SAD might have been unrelated to the light therapy. On the other hand, it is well known that increased activation in depressed people can sometimes bring out suicidal tendencies, as may also occur rarely following antidepressant treatment. In any event, the bottom-line message is: *If you experience any suicidal ideas before, during, or after light therapy, do yourself and everyone who cares about you a favor and report it to a health care professional without delay.*

23. Is light therapy harmful to the eyes?

This question has raised concern, especially in those who use light therapy year after year. The good news is that no problems of this type have arisen to my knowledge over the last twenty-five years, when light therapy has been used as recommended and under proper supervision. The one isolated cautionary tale mentioned on page 121—the only one known to me where light therapy was clearly associated with an eye injury—occurred in someone who used a homemade light fixture in an unsupervised setting.

Two follow-up studies—one by Dr. Paul Schwartz and colleagues at the NIMH and the other by Dr. Chris Gorman and colleagues in Calgary, Canada—revealed no evidence of eye damage in fifty-nine and seventy-one patients, treated for an average duration of nine years and five years, respectively. All these data are based on people whose eye functioning was normal before treatment was initiated. They may not necessarily apply to people with abnormalities of visual functioning.

If you have any history of visual difficulties (apart from the need for ordinary corrective lenses), be sure to consult your eye doctor before undertaking light therapy. Certain retinal problems, such as macular degeneration and retinitis pigmentosa, can be made worse by exposure to bright light. These conditions may first appear as visual difficulties. Medications that sensitize the skin to sunlight (a property generally noted on the medication bottle) may also sensitize the retina to bright light. This may or may not be subjectively apparent to the person using both the medication and the light. Although the concomitant use of these medications has not generally been considered a reason to avoid light therapy, it does warrant extra caution. Be sure to draw your doctor's attention to the possible interaction and proceed more cautiously, for example, by increasing the duration of light therapy more gradually than is generally recommended or sitting a little farther away from the light box. It is possible that if you are taking a medication that sensitizes your tissues to light, you may derive benefit from lower doses of light than are generally needed.

The absence to date of any reported cases of eye problems related to light therapy is encouraging and is in keeping with our expectations, given the amount of light used in standard treatments. Even the highest-intensity (10,000-lux) light boxes give out no more light than you would receive if you looked at the horizon just after sunrise.

In fairness, I should note that some researchers have sounded a precautionary note about possible long-term consequences—as yet undiscovered—of long-term light therapy. To minimize this possibility, it is important that manufacturers of light boxes screen out as much UV light as possible. They should make available the transmission spectra of their light fixtures (the graphs of all wavelengths of light transmitted) so that consumers can make informed choices. At this time, such information is not generally available, and so far there are no Food and Drug Administration (FDA) guidelines for how much UV light transmission from therapeutic fixtures is acceptable.

The good news is that a growing number of researchers and clinicians are treating ever-increasing numbers of patients for extended periods with no evidence of any eye problems so far. Of course, should you develop any eye-related symptoms while on light therapy, such as visual changes, irritation, or increased light sensitivity, it would be prudent to take these problems to your doctor promptly.

In summary, there is no evidence to date that standard light therapy, when administered properly to individuals with normal visual functioning, is harmful to the eyes.

24. Should everyone have an eye examination before starting light therapy?

In practice, most clinicians and researchers do not routinely give eye examinations to people with normal visual functioning. If you have any problems with your eyes, however, check with your doctor before starting light therapy.

Eye exams should be given before initiating light therapy to any-

one with a history of eye problems (over and above the need for corrective lenses) or anyone in whom visual difficulties or eye-related
symptoms develop during the course of ongoing light therapy. Absent
these special circumstances, however, it is not standard practice to administer eye exams before initiating light therapy.

25. Is it safe for me to receive light therapy if I have sensitive skin?

As already mentioned, some UV rays get through the diffusing screen,
and while these cause no problem for most people, they may lead to
problems in those with sun-sensitive skin—people with a history of
skin cancers, those on medications that sensitize the skin to sunlight,
and those with conditions, such as systemic lupus erythematosus,
where there is enhanced sensitivity to sunlight.

For such light-sensitive individuals, I encourage the use of sunblocking creams on the face, though even the most powerful of these
do not appear to screen out all the potentially damaging UV rays. If
you have a history of skin cancer, check with your doctor before starting light therapy and have your skin monitored for possible recur-
rences at regular intervals. To put things in perspective, you will probably be exposed to far less UV light from your light box than from
going outdoors. Even so, the UV rays coming from the light box may
increase your chances of a recurrence of skin cancer. For this reason
you and your physician should do a cost–benefit analysis of the potential benefits of light therapy to your mood versus the potential harm to
your skin. If you are considering the relative merits of antidepressant
medications versus light therapy, remember that many antidepressants
sensitize the skin to environmental light and may also represent a risk
factor for people with sensitive skin.

On a reassuring note, I have come across several patients with a
history of both lupus and SAD who have benefited from light therapy
without suffering any skin problems.

26. How can I tell how likely I am to respond to light therapy?

Although it is not possible to predict exactly who is most likely to respond to treatment with bright light, the following factors predict a
more favorable outcome:

- A history of mood improvement in the winter when you have been exposed to more light in a natural context, such as when you have traveled south or spent time in brighter indoor environments, or when you lived closer to the equator.
- Certain symptoms of winter depression, including fatigue, oversleeping, overeating, carbohydrate craving, weight gain, and social withdrawal.

In contrast, severely depressed people who lose sleep, eat less, and lose weight during their winter depressions tend to do less well with light therapy. But even if you do have these particular symptoms, light therapy is still worth a try if you have a clear-cut pattern of winter depressions, especially if your mood has been responsive to the amount of light in your environment.

One further predictor: if you feel a beneficial effect after one hour of light exposure, the chances are that you will continue to benefit over time.

27. What can I do if I dislike fluorescent lights?

Fluorescent lights make some people feel anxious, irritable, or "wired." Such people are understandably concerned when fluorescent light fixtures are recommended as a treatment. In my experience, patients with SAD rarely object to the quality of the light emanating from standard light-treatment fixtures; on the contrary, they generally find them relieving, soothing, or invigorating. Modern light fixtures contain special devices that minimize the irritating flicker that many associate with fluorescent lights.

People with seizure disorders, who have been told to avoid strobe lights, have wondered at times whether there is any reason to avoid light therapy. They have no reason to be concerned, since there is no evidence that standard light therapy fixtures pose any risk for seizures.

28. Is it safe to use light therapy while I am pregnant?

All evidence suggests that light therapy is safe for pregnant women, and I have known several pregnant women whose winter depressions have been treated successfully in this way and who have subsequently given birth to normal, healthy babies. Besides having psychological problems, depressed people also experience physical difficulties, such as sleep disruption, that might potentially have an adverse effect on the developing baby. For the sake of both mother and baby, it makes sense to treat the physical and psychological symptoms of SAD, and it would seem far better to do so, if possible, without introducing any chemicals, such as antidepressant medications, into the system. After twenty-five years of prescribing and studying light therapy, I have not encountered a single report of any ill effects to a baby whose mother used light therapy during pregnancy.

29. Can I use light therapy while nursing my baby?

Yes, but only if the infant's face is turned away from the light box. The eyes are much more sensitive in infants than in adults and could potentially be harmed by the intense light from a standard light fixture. So, if you decide to use light therapy while you are breast feeding, be sure to shield the baby's face from the direct rays from the box.

30. Is it all right if older children are around the light box while I am being treated?

It is quite common for parents who are using light treatment to have children around, whether they are toddlers jumping on the parent's lap or older children with questions to ask or opinions to offer. There is no reason to think that the casual light exposure involved in such activities will harm the child in any way. If the child has SAD, it might actually be beneficial to spend some time in front of the light box, and the companionship and identification with the parent that come from the shared experience can be very reassuring to a child or adolescent.

31. Will the bright light be harmful to pets?

Many people have commented that their pets seem to react favorably to the lights. Cats in particular seem drawn to the light and sit mesmerized in front of it. The best pet story I have heard concerned a cat and a parakeet that was able to open his own cage. Ordinarily, when the cat encountered the bird, he would give chase and the parakeet would make a dash for his cage and slam the door shut behind himself. However, when the bright lights were turned on, the parakeet emerged from his cage and strutted in front of the light box, despite the dangerous proximity of the cat. The cat, for his part, appeared so entranced by the lights that he showed none of his usual interest in pursuing the parakeet. In summary, there is no reason to believe that any harm will come to your pet from sitting in front of your light box.

32. How can I handle other people's reactions to my light box?

Some people are embarrassed to have friends or colleagues see the light box. You may worry that they will speculate about what is wrong with you, make judgments about your competency or mental health, or ask embarrassing questions. It may also feel like an invasion of your privacy to have people speculating in this way.

Bringing a large box that emits intense light into an indoor environment is certain to have an impact on those around you. Those who use the light in work or home settings observe that some people are drawn to it and find it pleasant, while others dislike it and find it irritating.

The concern that bringing a light into the workplace will label you as disturbed or peculiar in some way is understandable and may in some instances be well founded. Generally, you will have the best sense of how accepting the people at work will be and whether it is advisable to use the lights in that setting or not. The reactions of colleagues will clearly vary from one work setting to another. Colleagues and supervisors at a graphic design company or a mental health center, for example, may be more understanding and accepting of lights than senior officers at the CIA or the Pentagon, settings where it might not be prudent to bring the box in to work. Most people, however, have been pleasantly surprised at how accepting their colleagues are of the light box and the underlying condition that its presence implies. Perhaps it is because most people understand that seasons can affect behavior in animals, and the majority of the population experiences some seasonal changes, albeit to a milder degree. In fact, my patients have often told me how friends and colleagues tend to congregate around their light boxes on dreary days.

Questions about the lights are generally best handled in a matter-of-fact way, though one college student I know chose humor instead. When asked by his roommates why he used the lights, he replied that experiments had shown that bright light kept rats in a state of constant sexual arousal. That put an end to the questioning.

33. What should I do if light therapy doesn't start working within a week?

The one-week mark is generally an excellent time to take stock of how your light therapy is working. If light therapy has not yet begun to work after one week, the following are a few points to consider:

- Make sure you are using the equipment correctly.
- Do you have the right sort of box? Is it large enough? (Remember, research studies have used light boxes about one foot high by eighteen inches across.)
- Have you placed the box at eye level?
- Are you sitting at the right distance from the fixture?
- Have you been using the lights for long enough each day? Some people need at least forty-five minutes in both the morning and the afternoon.
- It may be helpful to shift the treatment to a different time of day (usually earlier in the morning, but sometimes to the afternoon or evening).

If the therapy is not helping at all after one week or is only partially helpful after two weeks, check in with your doctor or therapist if someone is monitoring your treatment. *Above all, don't give up too soon, since significant improvements may take at least two weeks to occur.*

34. What can I do if light therapy is helpful for a while but becomes less effective over time?

Although this problem may occur, it is rarely because the benefit of the light has been lost. A mood decline after an initial response may occur because of:

- A change in your life circumstances
- Decreased environmental light
- Inconsistent light treatment
- Loss of intensity of the fluorescent lamps

Consider each of these possibilities and ask yourself:

- Has my life become more stressful in any way? For example, has anything changed at work or in my relationships? If so, it is important to attend to the underlying stresses in your life so you can alleviate their effects on your mood.

• Has it become darker outside? Light treatment that is completely effective in November and December may become only partially effective in the darker days of January and February. In those months, the days are getting longer, but they are also often cloudier, so less light is available. To combat this climatic change, you may need to increase the amount of light or add some other type of treatment.

• Have I been using the lights consistently, or have I slacked off, skipped days, or cut my treatments short? Am I using the lights properly? For example, am I sitting at the right angle, so that my eyes are exposed to sufficient light?

• How old are the fluorescent lamps in my fixture? After one or two seasons of use, the amount of light given off by the lamps may decrease enough to diminish their effectiveness. If you feel you are responding less well to treatment than you were previously, and the lamps in your fixture are more than one year old, consider replacing them.

35. Do insurance companies cover light boxes?

Some people have successfully filed for insurance reimbursement for their light fixtures, but many people suffering from SAD have had their claims denied, usually because light therapy is labeled "experimental" by the insurance company. The real reason is that the insurance company is trying to save money. The best strategy for obtaining reimbursement for your light fixture is to send the invoice for the light box to your insurance company along with a letter from your doctor. A sample of the sort of letter that I have sent for my patients is shown on page 144.

Two developments would greatly enhance the extent to which light therapy units are reimbursed by insurance companies: lobbying by patient advocacy groups and approval of light fixtures as effective medical devices by the FDA. Unfortunately, patients with SAD have been less successful than those with other conditions at developing a support group. Such support groups typically have a variety of constructive agendas, which may include dealing with insurance companies. Insurance companies often look to the FDA to legitimize a medical device. This has not occurred with light boxes so far, despite discussions about doing so for over a decade. One reason for this delay is that getting approval of drugs and medical devices by the FDA is

SAMPLE LETTER FOR INSURANCE REIMBURSEMENT

To Whom It May Concern:

This is to certify that Ms. Jane Smith has been a patient of mine since _____. I have treated her for recurrent major depressions (DSM-IV-TR 296.3), with a seasonal pattern. This condition, also known as seasonal affective disorder (SAD), has been shown in many studies in the United States and elsewhere in the world to respond to treatment with bright environmental light (light therapy). Light therapy is no longer considered experimental but is a mainstream type of psychiatric treatment, as evidenced by its inclusion in the authoritative *Treatments of Psychiatric Disorders, Third Edition,* a publication of American Psychiatric Publishing.[1] The effectiveness of light therapy was further confirmed in a recent meta-analysis published in the prestigious *American Journal of Psychiatry.*[2] To administer light therapy adequately, a light box, such as the one described on the attached invoice, is required.

Although a light box is an expensive piece of equipment, the experience of clinicians who have used it for many patients indicates that it saves a great deal of money over time by reducing the number of doctors' visits and the costs of medications and laboratory investigations of persistent symptoms, as well as the indirect costs of lost productivity. I maintain that in Ms. Smith's case, the use of such a light fixture should be regarded not only as a medical necessity, to be used in preference to, or in addition to, other forms of treatment, but also as a means of reducing her overall medical costs.

[1]Oren, D. A., & Rosenthal, N. E. (2001). Light therapy. In G. O. Gabbard (Ed.), *Treatments of psychiatric disorders* (3rd ed., Vol. 2, pp. 1295–1306). Washington, DC: American Psychiatric Publishing.
[2]Golden, R. N., Gaynes, B. N., Ekstrom, R. D., et al. (2005). The efficacy of light therapy in the treatment of mood disorders: A review and meta-analysis of the evidence. *American Journal of Psychiatry, 162*(4), 656–662.

very expensive. The costs for obtaining such approval are usually borne by large pharmaceutical companies, which bankroll the process. Even the largest manufacturers of the type of fixtures used for light therapy are only small businesses, and none has found it feasible as yet to spearhead such an effort. One can only hope that the FDA will address this problem as soon as possible and approve light boxes for the treatment of SAD, a step which, in my opinion, is long overdue.

36. Can I get my light therapy while I am asleep?

Surprisingly, you can get some benefit from light while you're sleeping. Researchers have found that simulating the light of a summer dawn helps patients with SAD wake up in the morning and feel better during the day. This should make sense to many people (and not only those with SAD) who are aware that on a sunny day they wake up in the morning and jump out of bed even before they realize what type of day it is outside. In contrast, on a dreary, cloudy day it may be difficult to pull yourself out from under the covers even before looking out of the window and recognizing that the reason for the problem is the bank of cumulus clouds blocking out the sunlight. Presumably, in the final hours of sleep, the eyes are registering the quality of the light in the environment and signaling to the brain whether to jump out of bed or linger under the covers.

For many years, I have recommended that patients attach a bedside lamp to a timer, which is set to turn the lamp on about an hour or two before the person intends to rise. New research by Drs. Michael and Jiuan Su Terman at Columbia Psychiatric Institute supports the value of having light turned on rapidly (in their case, over a thirteen-minute interval) before wake-up time. But you can simulate a more naturalistic type of summer dawn thanks to devices called *dawn simulators*. The Termans originally suggested the use of such dawn simulators, which were later tested extensively by Dr. David Avery and colleagues at the University of Washington in Seattle.

One such dawn simulator, the SunUp, shown in Figure 5, a small electronic gadget that fits into the palm of one's hand, can be plugged into an ordinary bedside lamp. Advantages of the SunUp are (1) its compact size, which is perfect for travelers—I don't leave home during winter without mine; (2) the fact that you can plug it into any incandescent lamp (though fluorescent lamps don't work with this device); (3) its flexible programming capacity,

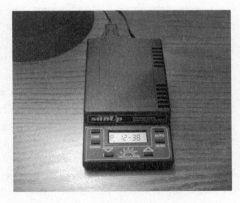

FIGURE 5. The SunUp dawn simulator.

which enables the user to regulate the duration of the artificial dawn—the interval between complete darkness and the maximum intensity of the light source; and (4) substantial research demonstrating its effectiveness in reversing the symptoms of SAD.

I recommend attaching the dawn simulator to a lamp containing a light bulb of no more than a sixty- to one-hundred-watt intensity and programming it to create an artificial dawn lasting between one and one and a half hours. The eyes appear to be very sensitive to light in the early morning hours, and a bedside lamp that is too bright may disrupt sleep and cause unpleasant feelings of irritability and over-activation. If this occurs after you have started to use a dawn simulator, decrease the intensity of the light source, increase the distance of the lamp from your pillow, or shorten the duration of the artificial dawn.

It is curious that dawn simulation works while the user is asleep, given our understanding that the antidepressant effects of light therapy are probably mediated via the eyes. It is also paradoxical that this effective treatment involves light that is no brighter than that emitted by an ordinary bedside lamp, many times less bright than a light therapy box. Our best understanding of the demonstrated benefits of dawn simulation is that the eyes are probably so sensitive during the pre-dawn hours that they are capable of responding to even the very small amounts of light transmitted through the sleeper's closed eyelids.

Several other dawn simulators are now available and can be located by checking the merchandise of light companies listed in Part IV. Some of these have the light source embedded in the device, in which case the light might be too dim or set at too low an angle in relation to the user's eyes to be fully effective. Do check on these elements before purchasing such a device, to make sure that you obtain the best results.

One stylish alternative type of dawn simulator device is the SunRise clock (Figure 6). The SunRise clock combines a pleasant light source, which resembles the sun, with an alarm clock and a mechanism geared to producing an artificial dawn lasting thirty minutes. The advantages of this device are its stylish design, its all-in-one quality, and its price. As of the time of writing, the

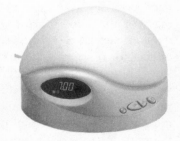

FIGURE 6.
The SunRise clock.

SunRise clock retails for about $120 versus about $200 for the SunUp. Its disadvantages are its relatively dim light source, which, under ordinary circumstances, would be at or below the level of a sleeping person. Ideally the light should come from above, as is the case with a natural dawn, coming through the windows on a summer day.

Interestingly, the very first alarm clock ever invented incorporated both sound and light in its mechanism. It was the first profitable invention of Jean Eugene Robert Houdin (1805–1871), who created a gadget containing a bell that would ring to wake the sleeper and a lighted candle that came out of a box.

37. If I had to choose one light treatment device, should I go with the light box or the dawn simulator?

Studies suggest that light therapy, administered in a standard way with an appropriate light fixture, is more effective than dawn simulation. So if you have to choose one of the two, the light box is probably the better choice. But the two devices work very well together, the dawn simulator helping you to wake up and get your day going and the light box continuing to provide a summer light signal to help reverse your SAD symptoms. Therefore, although it is an additional expense, the combination is highly recommended. Remember, if you cannot afford a dawn simulator or SunRise clock, you can still create an artificial dawn—albeit a rather abrupt one—by plugging your bedside lamp into an ordinary timer, which costs only a few dollars. Although you will not get the gradual increase in light that the more expensive devices generate, you may well find the less expensive solution to be perfectly satisfactory. As yet, no research studies have shown any advantage of the more expensive devices over this cheaper solution.

38. What about creating an artificial dusk? Is there any advantage to that?

Both the dawn simulator and the SunRise clock permit the user to generate an artificial dusk by turning the light source off gradually until the bedroom is completely dark. Although there is no evidence that the dusk feature confers any benefit to the treatment of SAD, I have found it to be helpful in people with insomnia or disturbances of their daily rhythms. Some parents have also commented that it has been helpful to their children, who are afraid to go to sleep in a darkened room but have difficulty falling asleep with the light on. In some cases, an artificial dusk has resolved this difficulty.

One useful feature of the dawn simulator is that it permits a person to gradually increase or decrease the intensity of the bedside lamp without disrupting the programming of dawn or dusk. This feature is helpful at night if one person in a couple comes to bed later than the other. The dawn simulator allows you to turn the bedside lamp on very gradually at night so as not to disturb your partner. It also allows you to turn the light off gradually when you want to go to sleep. Gradually decreasing the intensity of the light in the bedroom can help slow down your thoughts and ease the transition between the day's activities and the night's rest.

39. How about receiving light therapy by means of a head-mounted light device?

The head-mounted light device, also known as the light visor, received national attention when it was featured on an episode of the television series *Northern Exposure*. In this episode, Walt, an elderly gentleman, develops SAD and is given a light visor to wear on a daily basis. The device not only reverses his symptoms, but it drives him manic in the process. He is overenergized, interrupts people, and undergoes a personality transformation, as manics often appear to do. His friends recognize that these changes are probably due to the light visor, to which Walt has now become addicted, and they devise an intervention where they confront him and persuade him to give up the visor. The last scene shows Walt going to the clinic, where the nurse rations out a prescribed fifteen minutes of daily therapy with the visor.

In this case fiction was stranger than truth. I have never encountered anyone who has become manic as a result of using the light visor, though it certainly could happen. Nor have I encountered light addiction of such magnitude that an intervention has been necessary to persuade the user to relinquish the treatment device. Implausible as the story might have been, the episode was useful in bringing the problem of SAD and the powerful effects of light therapy to the attention of the general public.

The biggest debate about the light visor, a version of which is shown in Figure 7, is whether it works at all. In several multicenter studies, in which visors of different intensities were used, researchers were unable to show a relationship between intensity and effectiveness. This relationship has been used as one of the tests of whether a light therapy device is specifically active and not just a placebo. Despite the equivocal results of these studies, in my opinion, the light visor works. Duration of recommended daily usage is similar to that for the light box.

The major advantage of the light visor is its portability, a useful feature both for travelers and for those who want to move around while receiving treatment. Just as with the dawn simu-

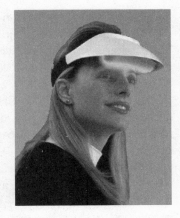

FIGURE 7. The light visor.

lator, if you have to choose between a light box and a light visor, the box is probably the better choice unless it is very important for you to be able to move around while receiving light therapy. The light visor works very well in conjunction with the light box, and one small study found that SAD patients who had responded to therapy with the light box maintained their responses when they switched to the light visor for a week. This finding is relevant for travelers, who may be able to maintain their response to the light box by using the far more portable light visor while away from home.

In summary, although the light visor is far more portable than the light box, this advantage must be offset against research data that are less clear-cut in demonstrating the visor's effectiveness. In addition, remember that even though the light visor permits you to move around while receiving light therapy, some activities, such as driving, operating machinery, and walking up or down stairs or in hazardous areas, are not recommended during therapy with this device. Despite these limitations, the light visor is a useful addition to the anti-SAD arsenal.

40. Could I get my light therapy by making a whole room in my house bright enough?

The answer is yes, but it would take some doing. This is how light therapy is administered in Sweden, where, when last I checked, there were approximately eighty such light therapy rooms distributed in

clinics across the country. I had the good fortune of sitting in one such
room when I visited St. Gjöran's Hospital in Stockholm, a center for
light therapy research in Sweden. All the lighting in the room was indirect—emanating from recessed fluorescent tubes reflected off the
ceiling and the walls, all of which were white. To increase the amount
of light reflected off the surfaces in the room, the overstuffed chairs
and sofas were all draped with white sheeting and everyone in the
room was given white hospital clothes to cover his or her street
clothes.

The atmosphere in the room was otherworldly. It was October
when I visited Stockholm, and there was a definite wintry feeling in
the air. The sun, slung low on the horizon, offered me a chilly welcome, and despite the warm and friendly reception I received from
friends and colleagues, I could feel the juice ebbing out of me. That
changed after thirty minutes in the light room. The immediate effect
was extremely pleasant, both calming and energizing. Sitting there, I
felt my energy return to me just in time to be appropriately animated
for my presentation.

The goal of the Swedish light therapy rooms is to emit light of
about 2,500-lux intensity to anyone in the room, regardless of the direction in which the person is looking. If you want to replicate this effect in a room in your house, you might try to incorporate the same elements used by the Swedes, namely:

- Indirect lighting—although the Swedes used fluorescents, you
  can use incandescent lights as well, as long as you don't stare di-
  rectly at them.
- White walls
- Light carpeting and furniture
- White robes for everyone sitting inside the room

Of course, it is not necessary to go to these lengths to create a
bright and cheerful room, which can be very therapeutic even if it falls
short of these stringent standards.

If you want to check how much light there is in the room, you can
purchase a light meter from a photographic store and take measure-
ments when the device is pointed in different directions.

One of my patients with SAD, a physician himself, spent a lot of
time in his kitchen and decided that if he was to get as much light as
possible, that was the best room to modify. He went to the trouble of

actually installing lights in the cabinetry. Such radical remodeling is rarely necessary. Modifying your home to increase indoor light levels may be as simple as washing windows, trimming hedges around them, or removing low-lying branches of trees near the house, or as elaborate as constructing skylights. One useful product, the Sunlight Pipe, is a shiny aluminum tube extending from the outside of the roof to just below the ceiling. Like a skylight, it transmits natural light into the house. Not only is the extra indoor light welcome, but there is the added advantage of feeling connected to the passage of the sun across the sky and even to the moonlight when the moon is full (see Part IV for suppliers of this device). Many of my patients with SAD who have a decorative flair have found attractive ways of using bright colors and surfaces to good effect. Dark wood paneling can be replaced with light-colored wallpaper. Splashes of yellow and orange on curtains and cushions seem to work well, as do white or off-white carpeting and furnishings. Before buying a new home, people with SAD should pay attention to the size of the windows and the directions that the rooms face.

41. If there is more light outdoors on a winter's day than I get from my light box, why not just go for a walk instead of doing light therapy?

It is true that if you stare at the sky (never directly at the sun!) on a bright winter day, you will be exposed to more light than you get from a light box. But the same would not apply for a cloudy day, of which there may be many during the course of a winter, depending on where you live. In other words, winter days are unreliable. In addition, they can be cold and unpleasant, and when you are depressed, you may be disinclined to walk outdoors regularly. A light box in a cozy room is generally a more practical proposition. Even if there is a lot of light coming off the sky, you may not benefit much from it as most people do not gaze upward when they walk. They are more likely to focus on the landscape, and the amount of light coming off the ground and winter vegetation is often minimal and certainly variable. When the landscape is covered with snow, there may be more than enough light around; you may even need to wear sunglasses. On the other hand, a dreary winter landscape reflects very little light and is unlikely to provide much cheer.

In one study, Dr. Anna Wirz-Justice and colleagues in Basel, Switzerland, found that walking outdoors for thirty minutes each morning was very therapeutic for their patients with SAD. But the winter weather where you are may not be as conducive to good spirits as that in Switzerland, and you may find it difficult to muster up the same degree of discipline as the Swiss subjects in Dr. Wirz-Justice's study. While walking outdoors is an excellent way to supplement your light therapy program, it is probably impractical for most people to rely on this alone. To enjoy their outdoor walks, some of my patients have chosen to work the evening shift so that they can capture as much outdoor sunshine as possible during the day. Surprisingly, even in sunny places it may be important to go outdoors during the day. According to one psychiatrist, his patients with SAD develop symptoms even in sunny Hawaii because they don't venture out into the sunlight. He has found that simply encouraging them to do so can provide them with sufficient light to control their depressive symptoms.

42. Is it possible to combine light therapy with antidepressant medications?

It is commonplace to use these different types of treatment together. Light therapy can be used in conjunction with any antidepressant and often allows for lower dosages of antidepressants to be used, resulting in fewer undesirable side effects.

43. Will it help to go to a tanning salon?

Although research shows that light therapy fixtures work via the eyes and not the skin, some of my patients have reported immediate mood improvement following visits to tanning salons. A recent scientific study by Dr. Steven R. Feldman and colleagues at Wake Forest University Baptist Medical Center in Winston-Salem, North Carolina, lends credence to my patients' reports. These researchers exposed volunteers to tanning beds with or without ultraviolet filters for two days. On the third day subjects were allowed to choose which tanning bed to use, and eleven out of twelve chose the bed with the UV rays. Other research shows that UV light can cause certain skin cells to release the substance beta-endorphin, an opium-like substance that may account for UV light's euphoriant effect. Although UV light on the skin may improve mood, I recommend against such tanning sessions because of the known potential for these rays to cause skin cancers, including potentially deadly melanomas.

44. How does light therapy stack up against antidepressant medications?

Two studies have examined this question, comparing light therapy to Prozac. Essentially, both found the two treatments to be roughly equivalent, though light therapy kicked in quicker. Although the particulars of the two studies do not allow for a general answer to the question of which treatment is better, these results reinforce my clinical impressions that a person with SAD has more than one viable option for effective treatment. I emphasize once again, though, that these treatments are by no means mutually exclusive. On the contrary, they often work particularly well together, especially when part of a good collaboration between an observant patient and a skillful clinician.

Creating a Light Therapy Program That Works for You

As you can see, there are many different ways of enhancing your environmental light. Different strategies work best for different people, but most people benefit from combining strategies in a way that maximizes the overall amount of light exposure day after day through the months of risk. Remember, SAD symptoms can develop at unexpected times if the weather becomes cloudy. So be ready to use light therapy out of season if necessary. Ideally, a comprehensive light therapy program involves moving seamlessly from one light-enhanced environment to another at different times of day. Perhaps the best example I can offer of how this can be accomplished is to share with you my own light treatment program. As you will see, I do combine other nonmedical types of treatment, about which I have much more to say in the chapter that follows.

My Personal Winter Routine

When people ask me whether I suffer from SAD myself, I know the answer is "yes," though it has been years since I have experienced the

symptoms of the condition in a sustained way to any significant degree. The reason for this is that for many years I have taken a series of
measures to keep these symptoms at bay. I suspect that without all
these preventive actions I might not do too well, especially since my
work as a clinician and SAD researcher means that winter has been my
busiest and most stressful season.

My typical winter day begins at 5:30 A.M., when my dawn simulator is set to turn on my bedside lamp. Although I am still asleep at that
time, I can imagine the lampshade gradually becoming brighter as the
light enters the pupils of my eyes through my closed eyelids. At 7:00
A.M. my first alarm clock begins to ring, and the process of turning it
off ensures that my head comes out from under the covers and my eyelids open wide enough to let in a fair amount of light. By this time, my
bedside lamp has reached its maximum intensity, and all of a sudden, a
light box, set on a timer three or four feet from my head, goes on and
my eyes are exposed to about 2,500 lux of light. Believe it or not, I
continue to doze as I stir, aware that the end of the night is rapidly approaching. It takes the second alarm clock, set for 7:30 A.M., to bring
that message finally home to me, and I am able to get out of bed fairly
easily. This stands in sharp contrast to those days when, for whatever
reason, the lights do not come on, and I feel that I have to drag myself
out of a coma to get up.

I walk outdoors in the morning in all sorts of weather and reserve
a stationary bicycle in front of a light box only for days when there is
ice on the ground. I often walk with a friend and find that unless I
make a commitment to meet someone at a set time, the temptation to
play hooky is very great. Working out first thing in the morning seems
to energize me for the rest of the day.

After my workout I eat breakfast and read the newspaper in front
of a light box before starting my work. At other times, I repair to
other brightly illuminated parts of the house. I also have a light box in
my office, where I see patients. Depending on the amount of light to
which I have been exposed during the course of the day and the needs
of the individual patient, we may elect to turn the light box on during
one of our sessions.

By now I rarely have to calculate how much light exposure I have
had on a given day and how much more I need. It has become quite
instinctive. When I am feeling sluggish and lethargic, I can tell that I
need more light. On the other hand, when I have had too much light,
I feel a sort of edginess, as though I have drunk too much coffee. It is

important to develop this ability to gauge one's own light require-
ments, since they vary over the course of the winter and no single regimen will work all the time. For this reason, I encourage you to focus
your attention inward to evaluate whether you have had the right
amount of light and to adjust your light exposure schedule accordingly.

Luckily for me, these steps—together with planned winter retreats
to sunny places—have been sufficient to keep me on an even keel
through the winter. In fact, I now look forward to winter as a season
with its own pleasures and challenges (see Chapter 18 for more information).

I recently had my eyes checked, and I was pleased that the oph-
thalmologist found no problems even though I have used light therapy
for the last twenty-five years.

The way in which I have structured my winter days works for me,
and I offer it as a detailed example of how one person has succeeded in
preventing the symptoms of SAD. But remember, everyone is different; strategies that work for me may not work for you. It has taken me
some time to learn all these tricks for making my life easier during the
difficult winter months. In a similar way, you can be creative in finding
those strategies that work best for you or someone you care about.

Another example of someone who has successfully developed her
own light therapy program comes from a reader who wrote me from
Albuquerque, New Mexico:

> I would like to see [you discuss] how important it is to work
> with the lights in order to fine-tune them to one's own needs
> (which can be very unique). Thanks to light therapy, in 1993
> I had my first depression-free winter in ten years. *But*—the
> light box did not work by itself!! It *did* work in the early fall,
> when the sun was still coming up pretty early. But when the
> mornings were dark, the box ceased working—no matter
> how long I used it or at what time. I carefully read all the var-
> ious books—to no avail.
>
> Almost hopeless, I asked *myself* what was wrong and real-
> ized that what I craved was to be submerged in light—like I
> was sitting on a beach. Sitting in relative darkness, with regu-
> lar home lighting, focusing on a single strong light source
> (the light box) didn't feel "right" to me. I followed my in-
> stincts, set up my light box in my bedroom, along with all my
> old homemade light boxes—a total of eight four-foot-long

fluorescents, which had worked moderately well in past winters (if I used them for four hours a day!). I submerged myself in light in the mornings—and that's what turned the
switch on again. And it stayed on consistently through the
winter. How do I know I have gotten my dose? My hands
tingle! It's like the circuit is connected.

She adds the following comments about doctors who have been
dismissive of her symptoms or have given her casual advice that has
not gone far enough in addressing the seriousness of her winter problems:

Soon I hope the doctors in this area will stop saying, "You
can't have SAD in Albuquerque—it's sunny here." Don't they
read? . . . Beware of doctors who claim that "going out for
an hour a day," adding more light bulbs in home fixtures,
etc., is all you need. This is what I was told by various psychiatrists—of course, it didn't work, and I discovered what I
need to do only through my own reading and my depression
support group.

This reader has discovered the critical importance of using her in-
ventiveness, taking some responsibility for her own treatment, cus-
tomizing it to her needs, and not relying entirely on her doctors. I encourage you to do the same.

Other Therapeutic Applications
of Light Therapy

Following the success of light therapy for SAD, researchers and clinicians have looked for other potential applications of this novel form of
treatment. These applications fall into two categories: (1) attempts to
influence circadian (daily) rhythms and the body clock and (2) the
treatment of other psychiatric disorders.

Influencing the Body's Clock

There are several circumstances where the body's clock is out of sync
with the outside world and its rhythm of day and night. In some cases,

this maladjustment may be temporary, such as when people fly across several time zones and develop jet lag or when they work changing shifts. In others, however, it may be a permanent state resulting from some internal abnormality of the body clock. This category includes people who are extreme "night owls," who cannot fall asleep until very late at night and cannot wake up easily at conventional hours—a condition known as *delayed sleep phase syndrome* (DSPS). On the other end of the sleep–wake spectrum are those with *advanced sleep phase syndrome* (ASPS), who tend to fall asleep early in the evening and wake up early in the morning. Many elderly people fall into this category.

All the circadian rhythm disturbances mentioned have two things in common. First, they all result in discomfort and difficulties if the individuals concerned are expected to adhere to a schedule that is at odds with their body clock and are not free to sleep and wake when they choose. Second, they can all be helped by appropriate modifications in exposure to light and dark.

Understanding how exposure to light and dark can affect the timing of the body's clock requires some appreciation of what is known as the phase response curve (or PRC). All creatures studied to date, from single-celled organisms to human beings, have been found to exhibit a PRC to light. This curve describes the relationship between the time of an animal's twenty-four-hour day when it is exposed to light and the resulting effect on the animal's circadian rhythm on subsequent days. For example, in the case of human beings, light exposure late at night tends to push the person's circadian rhythms later on subsequent days. On the other hand, light exposure in the early hours of the morning, say at 6:00 A.M., tends to push the person's circadian rhythms earlier on subsequent days. I should point out that keeping people away from light, in other words, in the dark, has an effect on their circadian rhythms that is approximately opposite to the effect of exposing them to bright light at that same time of day.

Delayed and Advanced Sleep Phase Disorder

Our knowledge of the human PRC leads to direct applications in the treatment of those whose daily rhythms deviate from the norm in one way or another. For example, my colleagues and I at the NIMH found that bright light exposure in the morning, together with avoidance of bright light in the evening, helped extreme "night owls" to readjust their sleep–wake schedules to more conventional hours.

For people with late-night jobs, such as actors or bartenders, a delayed sleep pattern may fit in well with their lifestyle. Clearly, one way to deal with a circadian rhythm pattern that is out of the ordinary is to adapt your lifestyle to fit in with your rhythms. Unfortunately that is not possible for everyone. When extreme "night owls" choose—or are required—to live on a 9:00 to 5:00 schedule, they are likely to encounter problems. I have seen businessmen, stockbrokers, and accountants who are unable to succeed at their jobs because they can't get in to work on time and therefore miss out on the crucial early morning hours. DSPS is not uncommon among adolescents and young adults, who may struggle—at times unsuccessfully—to get to their early morning classes and have school difficulties as a consequence. Many of these teenagers find that even when they can get their bodies into class, their minds really want to stay in bed, and they find it impossible to concentrate during the morning hours. For all those who cannot easily adapt their lives to their sleep schedules, the good news is that much can be done to readjust their sleep–wake schedules to more conventional times.

ASPS, a condition found most frequently among the elderly, responds to a pattern of light exposure opposite to that required for treating DSPS. Bright light exposure should be administered in the evening hours, and subjects should be kept in darkness in the early morning hours.

Jet Lag

Jet lag is a condition in which the rhythms of the body clock are temporarily out of sync with those of the external world as a result of traveling across several time zones. The condition can persist for up to ten days, depending on the number of time zones crossed and the individual's capacity for shifting circadian rhythms. In its milder forms, jet lag can be a nuisance, causing people to wake up when they want to sleep and doze off when they should be awake. Imagine how annoying it would be to travel thousands of miles to see some legendary tourist attraction, only to find yourself standing in front of it, unable to keep your eyes open. But jet lag can be more than an annoyance, as the resulting disorientation can cause errors of performance or judgment. Consider, for example, the difficulties a businesswoman would encounter trying to negotiate a deal at a time that would be 4:00 A.M. in her hometown. Even though it may be midafternoon at her destination, to her it feels like 4:00 A.M., and her body is telling her it's time to sleep, just when she is supposed to be at her sharpest.

An understanding of the PRC can allow a person to treat his or her own jet lag. Appropriately timed exposures to bright light and darkness can greatly diminish the length of time necessary to shift a person's rhythms into sync with local time. For example, instead of a week of jet lag following a transatlantic trip, proper treatment with light and dark may shorten the adjustment time to one or two days. Understanding exactly when to administer bright light and dark to overcome jet lag is more complicated than treating DSPS or ASPS. In these two conditions, we know that light exposure in the early morning hours will shift circadian rhythms earlier and that light exposure in the evening hours will shift rhythms later, because we have a good idea where the phase response curve is in relation to the hour of the day.

When people travel across time zones, however, their internal body rhythms (including their PRC) remain in the same position as they were at the point of departure for several days after they arrive at their destination, until they have shifted into the new time zone. This makes it much more complicated to calculate when someone should be exposed to light or to dark in order to shift his or her circadian rhythms in the right direction to speed up adjustment. Such knowledge is crucial, since exposing someone to light or dark at the *wrong* time on the phase response curve may actually shift rhythms in the *wrong* direction, *delay* adjustment to the new time zone, and *increase* the duration of jet lag. Exactly how to calculate when someone should be exposed to light or dark after traveling across several time zones is beyond the scope of this book.

Shift Work

Just as those suffering from jet lag experience distress as a result of being fatigued when they are supposed to be alert, and suffer sleep difficulties, so do shift workers, who can be considered to be chronically "jet-lagged" as a result of their shifting work schedules and the resulting disruption of their sleep times. The circadian problems of shift workers can induce not only discomfort—or even physical illness—in the worker, but also sleepiness on the job, and errors in judgment can result in serious industrial accidents. It has been pointed out, for example, that the nuclear accidents at Chernobyl and Three Mile Island both occurred in the early hours of the morning, and researchers have speculated to what degree worker error resulting from fatigue and circadian disruption might have been responsible.

Just as properly timed exposure to bright light and dark can be used to help those suffering from jet lag, it can also be used to help shift workers adjust to the demands of changing shifts. One well-publicized instance of successful use of this strategy is with astronauts. The astronauts on the shuttle, for example, may need to take off at night, when they would normally be going to sleep. Proper adjustment of their circadian rhythms in the days leading up to the takeoff can result in their being wide awake and ready to go at midnight. Once up in space, astronauts generally work in shifts that require them to be asleep and awake at times different from their usual sleep–wake schedules. Once again, judiciously timed light and dark exposures in the days before takeoff can enable them to do so comfortably and effectively.

As with jet lag, it is complicated to work out exactly when shift workers should be exposed to light and dark to speed up their adjustment. There is no easy formula that can readily be applied and, to date, no good manual for shift workers to consult. One of the leading researchers in this particular area, Dr. Charmane Eastman, warns against simple remedies, such as "Try thirty minutes of bright light each morning." She points out that light, if administered at the wrong time, can sometimes delay adjustment to the new shift. Environmental influences, such as sleeping and waking at certain times, can help the shift worker adjust to a new schedule. Unless light and dark signals work in the same direction as these social time cues, the resulting competition between external influences may delay adjustment.

Dr. Eastman's advice to night shift workers is to wear dark sunglasses on the way home from work and go to sleep as soon as possible in a dark room. On days off, adopt as late a sleep schedule as possible, for example from 4 A.M. to noon. Get as much bright light as possible during the night shift, especially before about 5:00 to 6:00 A.M. These techniques can reset the circadian clock later and make you better adapted to working the night shift and to sleeping during the day. For those working rapidly rotating shifts there is no way to adjust your body clock fast enough, so expect to feel very sleepy during the night shift and early morning shift and to have difficulty sleeping during the day.

Insomnia

Patterns of light and dark are capable of influencing circadian rhythms with respect not only to their timing but also to their amplitude (or strength). If you think of circadian rhythms (of alertness or body temperature, for example) as waves—with the peak of the wave being the highest temperature or level of alertness and the trough being the lowest level—then the strength or amplitude of the rhythm is the difference between these two extremes. There is evidence that when people have circadian rhythms of low amplitude, they may have difficulty falling or staying asleep. This happens, for example, in extreme northern countries during the weeks of continuous winter darkness. The artificial indoor lighting may be inadequate to provide sufficient contrast between daytime and nighttime light levels. The result is midwinter insomnia—a condition of disrupted sleep that afflicts many people living at very high latitudes during the winter. There is some evidence that even for those insomniacs who do not live in the far north, light therapy may have some value in improving the quality of their sleep.

Dr. Scott Campbell and colleagues at Cornell University in White Plains, New York, successfully treated elderly patients who have difficulty staying asleep with bright light exposure for two hours in the evening. Following treatments, patients woke up less during the night and showed an overall increase in sleep even though they did not spend more time in bed. In other words, their sleep efficiency increased. This type of treatment can be as effective as sleeping medications—without the side effects. Light treatment for insomnia is certainly worth further research to evaluate its scope and limitations in the management of this common and distressing condition.

Light Therapy for Other Psychiatric Disorders

Just as seasonal variation in its symptoms was a clue that SAD might respond to changes in environmental light, so researchers have wondered whether any other seasonally varying conditions might prove similarly responsive. Our group and others have found that subgroups of patients with eating disorders (both bulimia and anorexia), obsessive–compulsive disorder, panic disorder, and schizoaffective disorder show a degree of seasonal variation, with symptoms worsening during the winter. It would be reasonable to consider light therapy for individuals suffering from any of these conditions. The best studied of these to date is bulimia.

A Woman Who Couldn't Stop Bingeing: Light Therapy for Bulimia

Phyllis is a twenty-four-year-old travel agent who presented to my colleague, Dr. Raymond Lam, Associate Professor of Psychiatry at the University of British Columbia in Vancouver, with a history of bulimia going back at least ten years. "I lose control of myself," she told him as she described her typical binges—two boxes of crackers or a dozen cookies within an hour, followed by self-induced vomiting. Afterward she would feel awful—guilty and angry at herself. She was preoccupied with her weight and unhappy with the shape of her body. At 5'4", she weighed 130 pounds, 10 pounds of which she had gained during the previous winter, and believed that she should weigh no more than 110 pounds. In the past, she had abused laxatives and exercised excessively in an attempt to achieve her desired weight. In addition to her bingeing, Phyllis had been quite depressed in the two months before seeing Dr. Lam. She had frequent crying spells, a low energy level, and difficulty getting to sleep, and once sleep came, it was fitful and unrefreshing. Her concentration was poor, and she had to take sick leave because she was unable to perform her usual duties at work. She reported that her bingeing had been worse during the winter months but that during the previous summer she had managed to keep her binges to no more than one or two per week.

Dr. Lam treated Phyllis with light therapy, 10,000 lux for thirty minutes per day in the early morning. After two weeks of this treatment, her mood brightened and her energy and concentration improved. So did the bingeing, which settled down to its summer pattern after a month of treatment. She then entered a cognitive-behavioral group psychotherapy program, which helped her stop bingeing entirely. She continues to use light treatment during the winter and feels that "I've gained back the lost winter months."

There are by now several studies by Dr. Lam and other researchers that show benefits of light therapy for patients with bulimia, even when they do not also suffer from SAD. Those bulimics whose binges increase during the winter, however, may be the most promising candidates.

A Teacher with PMS: Treating the Monthly Blues

Joan was a thirty-three-year-old sixth-grade schoolteacher who entered a research program run by Dr. Barbara Parry, Professor of Psychiatry at the University of California in San Diego. Her premenstrual symptoms had begun some five years earlier, after the birth of her first child. Initially these symptoms lasted only two to three days, but they worsened over time to occupy about two weeks of every menstrual cycle, from shortly after ovulation until two or three days after the start of her menstrual period. During these days a sense of "doom and gloom" settled over her. She felt inadequate as a wife, mother, teacher, and woman. All she wanted to do was to "hibernate"—to sit on the sofa and eat "bon-bons." She slept poorly, woke frequently during the night, and felt tired the following day. She avoided social engagements, found herself more irritable with the kids and her husband, had no motivation, and easily broke down in tears. She had a desire to "get away from it all" and on one occasion even thought of admitting herself to a hospital.

Joan entered Dr. Parry's light treatment study because she didn't want to take drugs and get "all those bothersome side effects." She had tried treating her symptoms with vitamin B_6, a common treatment for PMS, without success. She improved after three to four days of light treatment (10,000 lux for thirty minutes) and preferred receiving light therapy in the evening rather than the morning, when it made her feel as though she had drunk too many cups of coffee. The evening light also allowed her to stay up later and spend more quality time with her husband. After the study she continued to use lights on a monthly basis, starting a week before her period was due. Light therapy remained just as effective over time as it had been during her participation in the research study. When she was asked to stop the light therapy for one month for research purposes, her symptoms returned right away and in full force. In the many months since that time, Joan has remained free of her monthly symptoms as a result of her continued, diligent use of light therapy.

Dr. Parry has now conducted several controlled studies of light therapy for PMS. More recently, Dr. Raymond Lam and colleagues at the University of British Columbia in Vancouver replicated Dr. Parry's studies and found bright light administered in the afternoon to be superior to a dim light control in reversing the symptoms of PMS. It is especially appealing because the mainstream alternative treatment, medication, generally needs to be taken all month long to be effective. Many women consider the presence of side effects all month to be too high a price to pay for treating a condition in which the symptoms last for only one or two weeks per month. I would expect the popularity of light therapy for PMS to increase, given the low level of side effects and the ease of administration.

It is not clear whether most women would benefit more from light therapy in the evening, as Joan did, than in the morning, which tends to be better for people with SAD. Dr. Parry suggests that those people who wake up and go to sleep early might benefit more from evening light therapy, whereas those who go to sleep and wake up later may benefit more from morning treatments. According to Dr. Parry, light therapy may be beneficial even for women whose PMS symptoms do not seem to vary seasonally. She speculates that light therapy may work for women with PMS by helping synchronize their rhythms to the environment. It is also possible that light, acting via the eyes and the hypothalamus, may exert a favorable influence on the secretion of female reproductive hormones.

Additional conditions for which light therapy has been tried with greater or lesser success include the following:

• *Stabilizing menstrual periods in women with irregular period length.* As early as 1967, Edmund Dewan reported that such irregular cycles could be stabilized by the light from the hundred-watt bulb of a bedside lamp left on overnight. This work was more recently picked up by Dr. Daniel F. Kripke, Professor of Psychiatry at the University of California in San Diego, who has demonstrated such stabilization in a controlled study.

• *Treating nonseasonal depression.* Dr. Daniel Kripke began his work on the use of light therapy for nonseasonal depression at about the same time as my colleagues and I began to study SAD at the NIMH. Since then, there have been numerous studies of light therapy for SAD, which have yielded mixed results. Perhaps the best use of light therapy for nonseasonally depressed patients will turn out to be in combination with antidepressants. In one of the most interesting examples of the value of light therapy used in this way, Dr. Siegfried Kasper and colleagues added morning light treatment for a group of nonseasonally depressed patients who had failed to respond to Prozac. Within three to four weeks, patients showed a remarkable improvement in mood compared with a control group that received dim light control treatment in conjunction with Prozac. It is worth considering the addition of light therapy if you are depressed and have not responded fully to other treatments, but it is important to wait for several weeks, longer than the time frame for a response to light therapy in SAD patients, before judging the outcome of such a trial. A recent panel commissioned by the American Psychiatric Association to investigate the value of different forms of treatment concluded that light therapy is effective for nonseasonal depression, based on data from research studies.

• *Other conditions.* There have been a few studies suggesting that exposure to bright light during a period of withdrawal from alcohol may ease the feelings of anxiety, irritability, and mood instability that are commonly experienced in such circumstances. Small pilot studies have tried light therapy for other conditions, but it is premature to draw any firm conclusions from them.

Conclusions

• Light therapy has been highly successful for the treatment of SAD.

• I have summarized the many tricks involved in making the most out of light therapy. Read them carefully because, with light therapy, the devil is often in the details.

• Although there is much that you can do on your own, if you are markedly depressed, *especially if you have any suicidal ideas*, do be sure to involve a professional in your care.

• Light therapy works very well along with other treatments for SAD, such as psychotherapy, antidepressant medications, and a variety of self-help techniques outlined in the next chapter.

• Light therapy may also be helpful for conditions other than SAD, most notably disturbances of sleep rhythms such as DSPS and ASPS, jet lag, shift work, premenstrual syndrome, bulimia, and nonseasonal depression.

EIGHT

Beyond Light Therapy
Other Ways to Help Yourself

Live in rooms full of light
Avoid heavy food
Be moderate in the drinking of wine
Take massage, baths, exercise, and gymnastics
Fight insomnia with gentle rocking or the sound
of running water
Change surroundings and take long journeys
Strictly avoid frightening ideas
Indulge in cheerful conversation and amusements
Listen to music
—A. CORNELIUS CELSUS, physician, first century A.D.

Although most people with SAD can benefit from light therapy (as well as or in addition to antidepressants or psychotherapy, described in the next two chapters), many still don't feel as well in the winter as they do in the summer. Light therapy studies find that most patients with SAD are still left with some symptoms after treatment. In fact, in most light therapy studies, more than one-third of patients fail to respond completely to active light therapy. Luckily, there are many other ways in which people with SAD can help themselves to overcome winter depression—or, indeed, depression at any time of the year. In this chapter I will discuss things that you can do yourself to make winter a more cheerful season.

Understanding SAD: The First Step

One of the most useful things about diagnosing SAD is that it provides you with a new way of understanding your difficulties. Even two decades after we first described SAD, however, the condition remains underdiagnosed and undertreated. Recent large-scale studies found that fewer than fifty percent of patients with SAD had been treated for their condition, even though they had suffered through an average of thirteen winter depressions. Diagnosis is the key to proper treatment. In addition, it is important to appreciate just how much the symptoms of SAD can rob you of your ability to function and enjoy yourself during the precious winter months.

It is one thing to understand intellectually that you have SAD, but another to acknowledge the degree to which it is interfering with your capacity to enjoy yourself or to be productive. I have seen many patients suffer unnecessarily for several winters after being diagnosed with SAD simply because they have had trouble accepting the severity of their condition and its impact on their lives. One woman, for example, who had a tendency to neglect her own well-being, did not sit in front of her lights on a regular basis for two winters until she came to accept, as part of her ongoing psychotherapy, that she had trouble attending to her medical needs. After she came to terms with her condition and its impact on her life, she had her best winter ever.

Sometimes taking SAD seriously means making significant life changes to ease the difficulties of everyday living during the winter. One of my patients with SAD had to spend many hours in her car each day commuting and carpooling her children, which added enormously to the daily stresses of her life and prevented her from being able to exercise regularly and get sufficient light exposure. By taking her problem seriously, she managed to persuade her husband to put their much-loved home on the market and move. This life change undoubtedly will pay off richly for the patient and her family in the coming winters.

Changing the Environment

More Light

The benefit of increasing environmental light can be obtained not only from formal therapy in front of a light box but also whenever your environment is brighter. Some people have several light boxes in the house, from which they can get lots of light without feeling trapped in one location. Extra light need not come only from special boxes but can be obtained by installing more lights on the ceiling or placing more lamps in the room. Once you pay attention to the amount and quality of your environmental light, you will come up with all kinds of ways to enhance it, which will help you feel more comfortable and cheerful. For more information on modifying your environment to bring more light into your life, see pages 150–151.

Winter Vacations

Many of my patients have learned that if they have a choice, it's better to take vacations in winter than in summer. Two weeks in a sunny climate in January can effectively interrupt the worst stretch of the winter. I am reminded of a television commercial in which a somber-looking man stands on the beach in Jamaica on day one of his vacation, looks a little more cheerful on day two, and is positively blissful by day three. For the SAD sufferer, this is truth in advertising! People seem to feel better in this natural sunlight than they do up north, even with light therapy. As an alternative to popular seaside resorts, some of my patients have undertaken adventurous trips—to Antarctica (where the days are very long when it's winter in the northern hemisphere) or the Galapagos Islands, for example, with similarly beneficial results.

Unfortunately, the beneficial results of winter vacations are usually short-lived, and after you return from a vacation, the regimen of light therapy usually must be resumed. In some instances, patients have reported feeling worse in the days after they return from a sunny climate than they did before they left the dreary weather to go on vacation. The likelihood of this happening can be reduced by restarting light therapy promptly after you return from your trip. Should depression return in full force, be sure to consult your doctor and actively step up the various elements of your self-care program. Another cautionary note applies to those people who can feel overstimulated by sudden exposure to intense sunlight in the middle of winter, as they often feel in summer. If this applies to you, be sure to watch out for the signs of overstimulation, such as loss of sleep, racing thoughts, and excessive exuberance, and decrease your exposure to sunlight should this occur.

It should not really come as a surprise that a Caribbean vacation may be more uplifting than a light box perched atop a desk on a dreary New England day, but there is also a small, growing body of evidence suggesting that sunlight might affect mood via the skin as well as the eyes. One recent study described in Chapter 7 showed that tanning beds, which emit UV light, may have a euphoriant effect. Subjects in the experiment were exposed on different occasions to such a tanning bed or a control tanning bed that looked exactly the same but emitted no UV rays. Later on, when asked to choose between these two tanning beds, the vast majority preferred the one with the UV rays. Other research has shown that UV rays can stimulate cells in the skin to secrete the chemical beta-endorphin, which produces opiate-like euphoriant effects and may explain the UV phenomenon.

Even though tanning, whether on the beach or in tanning salons, may make you cheerful, I can hardly recommend it, given its potential to cause skin cancers including the sometimes-fatal melanoma. By all means enjoy winter vacations in sunny places, but do be careful to limit direct sun exposure to the skin with sunblock and appropriate clothing (including a hat or cap).

Relocation

Several of my patients have chosen the dramatic solution of moving permanently to a place with a sunnier climate. Generally, patients who have relocated feel more energetic and their energy level is more evenly distributed year round. There are, of course, many factors other than climate that have to be taken into account in a decision to relocate. Besides the potential impact of lifestyle, consider the following:

- How well can the SAD symptoms be controlled by light therapy and other means?
- Will you really feel better during the winter in the new climate? One way to test this is to visit the place during the winter before making a commitment to move.
- What are the exact weather conditions in the place in question? For example, even though a place may be located in the South,

local weather conditions may cause clouds to obscure the sun for much of the winter. You can order a booklet summarizing comparative climatic data for the United States from the National Oceanic and Atmospheric Administration in Asheville, North Carolina [phone: (828) 271-4800].

• What is the summer like in the new place, and how do you respond to heat and humidity? Be careful that a move doesn't result in exchanging one climatic problem for another.

Diet and Exercise

Diet and exercise are important considerations for SAD sufferers, not only because they can have a valuable effect on mood control but also because of their beneficial physical effects. Patients with SAD often put on weight during the winter, as a result of a combination of overeating and inactivity. Although it is easier to lose weight during the summer, there is a tendency to retain pounds with each cycle of the seasons, which over the years can result in obesity. Researchers have shown that obesity resulting from cyclical increases and decreases in body weight can be particularly bad for one's physical health. Light therapy, in my experience, for all its benefits, often proves disappointing to those who hope that they will automatically shed their excess weight as they begin to feel better. Diet and exercise should therefore be part of the overall health maintenance plan of patients with SAD.

Exercise

There is growing evidence that regular aerobic exercise has a beneficial effect on mood control in those who suffer from depression in general. Not surprisingly, research shows that exercise is helpful for people with SAD as well—as helpful as light therapy, according to one study. Researchers Arcady Putilov and colleagues in Siberia compared two different types of treatment in two small groups of patients with SAD: light therapy (2,500 lux for two hours in the afternoon) and exercise (one hour of pedaling on a stationary bicycle at roughly the same time of day). They were equally effective. It is only fair, however, to point out that the light used in their study (2,500 lux) is not as bright as that now generally used for therapy in the United States (10,000 lux). Also, we know that the afternoon hours are a less favorable time for light therapy than the morning. So, the researchers did not test light therapy at its best. But for all we know, exercise might also be more effective as an antidepressant in the morning; to my knowledge, that has not yet been studied.

The Siberian researchers added an interesting angle to their study. They tested the rate of oxygen consumption (also known as the metabolic rate) in people with SAD and in healthy volunteers. They found that people with SAD had abnormally low levels of oxygen consumption at baseline. This is compatible with the theory that SAD may have evolved as an adaptive mechanism to deal with the lack of energy supplies (in the form of food) during the winter in harsh environments. These results are also compatible with the observed weight gain that occurs in people with SAD during the winter. Putilov and colleagues found that a week of both light therapy and exercise increased oxygen consumption in patients with SAD (and also in healthy controls). Their findings are completely in agreement with my own experience that regular exercise plays a vital role in both mood and weight control in people with SAD. The researchers did not include a group that used both light and exercise, but I would wager dollars to donuts that such a group would do better than those treated with either lights or exercise alone.

In practice, of course, it is easy to exercise and increase your light exposure at the same time, thereby enhancing the antidepressant effect. It is simple to do so, for example, by walking briskly or jogging outdoors on a bright winter day or working out in front of a light box. Typically, people with SAD who rely on exercise alone to prevent their winter symptoms have trouble mustering up the willpower to continue it through the winter months. The light therapy may help keep you motivated to exercise. Exercise, of course, has the added virtue of reducing weight or, at least, preventing the much-dreaded winter weight gain.

Most patients with SAD can derive some benefit from exercise. The most important factor in finding the best regimen for you is to choose something you enjoy. This could be brisk walking, swimming, jogging, cycling (moving or stationary), cross-country skiing, or aerobic dancing. If you enjoy it, you are much more likely to stick with it. If you choose the exercise on the basis of its aerobic properties or therapeutic value and don't enjoy it, it's unlikely to work out over the long haul. Finding a friend who also wants to exercise can be a valuable support, and you can bolster one another's motivation during the dark days. Some people find it easiest to exercise as part of a group. I frequently see a group of neighborhood women out for their regular brisk morning walk—they always seem to be having a good time. Likewise, I know several men who enjoy working out together at the gym before heading in to their jobs. If you can afford it, hiring a personal trainer may be one way to ensure that you stick to your exercise program.

A key to losing weight is raising your metabolic rate—the rate at which you burn calories. One way to accomplish this is through vigorous exercise, especially when carried out for a sustained period, for example, twenty minutes or more. An added benefit of this "fat-burning" exercise is that you continue to burn off more calories than usual for some time after you have stopped exercising, since it takes a while for your metabolic rate to settle back down to resting levels. Another way that exercise can increase your metabolic rate is by losing fat by building muscle, which occurs, for example, with regular weight lifting. Since muscle cells have a higher metabolic rate than fat cells, you can think of your muscles as calorie-burning factories. By increasing your muscle mass, you are also increasing the rate at which you burn calories, even at rest.

But it is not necessary to engage in vigorous exercise or weight lifting to derive some benefit from exercise. Walking briskly or even slowly also helps burn calories and can improve your overall mood. The bottom line is *do whatever it takes to resist the very strong temptation to be a couch potato when you have SAD and do something—anything—to keep your body active through the winter months.*

Diet and SAD

People with SAD often have a voracious appetite for foods rich in carbohydrates, such as cookies, donuts, pastries, chowders, and stews, often reporting that such foods comfort them, energize them, or otherwise make them feel good when nothing else seems to do the trick. One of the problems with regulating your mood and energy with food is that the resulting satisfaction is very short-lived. Within an hour or two, the carbohydrate craver is hungry, lethargic, or irritable once more and sets out to treat these uncomfortable feelings with another dose of carbohydrates.

I once believed that little could be done about these cravings. I had read that there is a set point for weight somewhere in the brain and that your body will cause you to eat more or less to ensure that you remain at that set point. Diets don't work, I was informed. Biology is destiny. I was more impressed by this theory each time I stood on my bathroom scale and found my weight more or less unchanged, despite the variability in my eating and exercise from day to day.

This was the dietary philosophy that informed my own eating patterns during the difficult winter months. I kept the fat content in my diet relatively low, the fiber content relatively high, and exercised as much as possible. That, I reasoned, was about as much as I could do—and it didn't work.

Now millions of people have begun to realize that you can influence your weight by the *types* of food you choose to eat. There has been a nationwide shift away from carbohydrate-rich diets as a means of weight loss. Instead, diets such as the Atkins diet emphasize the benefit of limiting carbohydrates. The popular South Beach diet echoes the same theme while extolling the value of certain types of carbohydrates over others. In my experience, different diets work for different people. But most patients with SAD need to limit their carbohydrate intake if they hope to avoid gaining weight during the winter. It is particularly important to avoid carbohydrates that consist of "empty calories"—foods that don't contain useful nutrients, such as sugar and white flour. While entire books are written about diets, let me simply outline a way of eating that has worked for me and many other carbohydrate cravers with or without SAD. In addition, in Part IV, I provide a week's worth of menus and recipes that give you an idea of how you can prevent winter weight gain while still eating well. These were created by Bette Flax, a nutrition counselor with whom I have collaborated successfully in helping patients keep their cravings and weight gain in check. Remember, everybody is different when it comes to diet and weight regulation. What will work for some will not work for others. For example, some people may need to limit their carbohydrate intake more drastically than others. In the diets provided, some recipes are more carbohydrate restricted than others, letting you choose the proportions that are right for you. I would also caution against extreme diets (for example, almost no carbohydrates at all). We just don't know what their potential long-term ill effects may be. We certainly don't want to exchange one health problem for another, as yet to be determined.

"Are You a Carb Craver?"

Most people with SAD crave carbohydrates in the winter and sometimes year round. As a consequence, they gain too much weight. To find out whether you are a carb craver, answer the following questions:

1. Do you struggle to keep your weight within acceptable limits? Yes No

2. Do you crave carbohydrate-rich foods like bread, cake, cookies, cereal, desserts, pretzels, sweetened sodas, fruit, or fruit juice, between meals? Yes No

3. When you are eating carbohydrate-rich foods, do you have the next handful, spoonful, or forkful ready before you have finished swallowing the previous one? Yes No

4. If you have had a carbohydrate-rich breakfast, do you feel hungrier in mid- to late morning than you would have had you skipped breakfast altogether or just drunk a cup of coffee that morning? Yes No

5. Do you find yourself snacking on carbohydrate-rich foods between meals or after dinner at least four times per week? Yes No

If you answered yes to question 1 and to at least two of the four other questions, you are probably a carb craver. This is even more likely if you answered yes to more of the questions.

Profiles of Carb Craving

I was recently at a business meeting that took place in the middle of the afternoon. Several of my colleagues sat around a conference table discussing the issues of the moment. The woman who had called the meeting graciously put a large bowl of popcorn in the middle of the table, and its wonderful aroma filled the room, evoking a movie theater atmosphere. I was careful to avoid the popcorn, which was really no effort since I had no craving for it, despite the pleasant associations it brought to mind. Across the table from me, a slender, attractive woman, an accomplished athlete who participates in triathlons, reached out for a handful or two that she put on her plate. During the meeting, she picked away at the popcorn with a take-it-or-leave-it air, and indeed, at the end of the meeting, some was left behind on her plate.

At the end of the table sat another colleague, who is clearly overweight. He reached out for some of the popcorn as soon as it arrived and piled several handfuls on his plate. He then proceeded to tuck in ravenously as though he could barely pack the calories in quickly enough. Before he was able to swallow one mouthful, he had the next one waiting in his hand so as not to interrupt the flow of his binge. His eyes glazed over, and a dreamy expression crossed his face, like an opium addict lost in the pleasures of contemplation of some distant place, far from the meeting room and the dreary subject matter being discussed. Recognizing the profile of a carbohydrate craver, even without asking him any questions, was not difficult—especially for me. Before I went on a reduced-carbohydrate diet, I might easily have gobbled the popcorn in exactly the same way he did.

Although I hope I would have restrained myself from overeating in public, my carb gorging began with breakfast. I would pour myself a full bowl of low-fat, carbohydrate-rich cereal and fill the bowl with skim milk. It was delicious. I would finish off the cereal before the skim milk, which I would then "top up" with more cereal. Now the mix was too dry, so I poured in more skim milk. And so it would go. By the time breakfast was over, distracted by the morning paper, comforting myself all along with the idea that the food in front of me was low-fat, I might easily have packed in 1,000 calories.

By lunchtime, I was starving and could barely hold out until noon before eating. Often, carbohydrate-rich foods were part of the midday meal. In the depths of winter, I would crave cookies in the middle of the afternoon. Sometimes I would yield to the craving, while at other times I would "white-knuckle" it until the craving passed. Dinner was a replica of lunch. But the eating day was not over. Late at night the cravings would hit me once again, and I would spoon out some frozen yogurt (low-fat, of course) straight from the carton. Given the number of calories I was consuming, it was no wonder that I was gaining weight progressively. Yet I was so driven by the cravings, it was inconceivable to me that I could eat any differently or do anything other than yield to them and accept the fate dictated to me by my so-called weight set point. All this changed when I went on a reduced-carbohydrate diet.

Some Practical Suggestions

The idea behind all carbohydrate-restricted diets is very simple: limit the amount of carbohydrate-rich foods. When you do eat carbohydrates, avoid foods that contain pure sugar, as well as white flour. That means minimizing white bread and pasta. For good measure, also minimize potatoes and white rice. What follows is a broad outline of how such a diet may play out over the course of the day. Be sure also to check out Part IV for detailed menus and delicious recipes that will allow you to lose weight without eliminating the joy of eating.

1. Start with breakfast. For carb cravers, starting the day with the standard cereal, toast, or orange juice is a surefire way of getting your cravings going all day long. Instead, consider protein-rich alternatives.

- Eggs or egg substitutes. There are many ways to be creative with eggs so that they don't become boring. See Part IV for some of these ideas.
- Fish. This could be steamed shrimp, which takes no time at all if you use the frozen type, canned tuna, or salmon. One good thing about canned salmon is that most of it is wild and free of some of the pollutants recently discovered in farm-raised salmon. Canned sardines are also good. Because they are lower on the food chain than larger fish, they are less likely to contain mercury and other pollutants.
- If you add in carbohydrates, do so sparingly. Whole wheat tortillas, a good complement to the protein elements, are readily available at whole-food markets, and are ideal for a quick meal.

2. An excellent lunch is a green salad with chicken or fish. Caesar dressing is low in carbohydrates and therefore good for those whose cravings get triggered by even small amounts of carbohydrate such as you will find in sugary vinaigrettes and other sweet dressings. For

those wanting to minimize unhealthy fats and carbohydrates, pure olive oil and regular vinegar works well. In addition, nowadays entire aisles in supermarkets are devoted to low-carbohydrate products. If you want to add small amounts of healthful carbohydrates to your salad, you can do so by sprinkling a few walnuts or low-sodium whole wheat crackers over it.

3. Dinner should be a well-balanced meal containing protein, green vegetables, and fruits. Different people can get away with different amounts of carbohydrates, but, once again, try to avoid items containing white flour. Whole wheat breads are preferred.

4. Snacks between meals are encouraged. Sticks of part-skim mozzarella or a handful of unsalted walnuts or almonds work well. These nuts contain omega-3 fatty acids, believed to be good for the heart and perhaps for mood as well.

Since I have been adhering to this type of diet, I have lost weight, gained energy, and no longer have to anticipate with horror that regular winter ritual of stepping into my winter trousers and finding that they no longer fit. Best of all, the cravings have gone and I no longer feel as though I am constantly deprived. Many of my patients have had similar good luck, so I pass these observations on to you in the hope that you too will find them useful.

Remember, no diet is right for everybody. There are many different kinds of diets out there, and if a diet described in this book doesn't work for you, be sure to consider other approaches. If you have special needs, such as those posed by diabetes, you would do well to consult with a dietitian or your doctor to be sure that the diet you choose is right for you.

Weigh Yourself Every Day

It seems as though people are divided into two types: those who like to weigh themselves and those who don't. I fall into the first group. Any scientist knows that in order to find out the results of an experiment, you have to measure something, and in the case of a diet that measurement is weight. For people with SAD, the pounds can sneak on relentlessly throughout the winter unless you keep an eye on the scale, and increases in weight invariably lead to drops in mood. To get the best handle on your mood and weight, I recommend that you weigh yourself daily. That way, you can establish a baseline and find out what factors influence your own weight fluctuations. Then when you start a diet, you can discriminate the effects of the diet from the ordinary weight fluctuations that occur, for example, with the menstrual period. You can set realistic goals for yourself and see where you are in relation to them.

How Does Limiting Carbohydrates Work for Patients with SAD?

Drs. Kurt Krauchi, Anna Wirz-Justice, and colleagues in Switzerland have shown that patients with SAD secrete more insulin in response to a glucose load than nonseasonal controls. When you consume sugar or other carbohydrates, your pancreas secretes insulin, which causes sugar to pass from the blood into the tissues, resulting in lower blood sugar levels hours after the glucose is consumed. If patients with SAD have exaggerated insulin responses to carbohydrate-rich meals, resulting in lower than normal blood sugar levels, this could trigger cravings for more carbohydrates and on and on. Ultimately all the calories consumed are converted into fat and the unwelcome weight gain seen in patients with SAD. By limiting carbohydrate-rich foods, you can minimize this cycle, reduce cravings, and contain your weight. The Swiss researchers have found that light therapy reverses the tendency to oversecrete insulin in response to a glucose load, which may explain why light therapy reduces carbohydrate cravings.

Fiber

Low-carbohydrate diets tend to be rather constipating. Salads, vegetables, and fruits tend to minimize this, but many people have to supplement these diets with fiber such as psyllium. Watch out for some fiber-containing supplements, which are quite caloric in their own right. If you're going to consume calories, you may as well enjoy it with high-fiber foods rather than bulk-forming laxatives. I recommend psyllium in capsule form with no starch or sugar added.

Herbs, Vitamins, and Supplements

You need look no further than your daily papers to find advertisements for herbs, vitamins, and supplements for all sorts of ailments, including SAD. It is important to sort out fact from fiction as these supplements can be expensive and are not necessarily harmless. So, what can truthfully be said in favor of supplements for SAD? Most of the data come from studies in nonseasonal depression, which may be valid for people with seasonally occurring depressions as well, just as antidepressant medications that work in nonseasonal depression also appear to be effective for SAD. In this section I will summarize what we know about these herbs and supplements.

St. John's Wort

This ancient herbal remedy, extracted from the leaves and flowers of *Hypericum perforatum,* has a reputation as an antidepressant going back 375 years. The physician Angelo Sala recommended extracts of hypericum for melancholia (depression), claiming "I effected cures which you can achieve neither with all the rest of your Apothecary." In recent years, numerous studies in nonseasonal depression suggest that Sala was right. To date, only one study, by Dr. Siegfried Kasper and colleagues in Vienna, has tested the value of St. John's wort for SAD. The patients in their study did well, but since there was no placebo condition, it is not possible to conclude with certainty that St. John's wort is effective for SAD.

Typically St. John's wort has been given in dosages of 300 milligrams three times per day, though lower or higher dosages can be used, based on individual response patterns. Although this is an herbal remedy, since it is an active substance, if you are thinking of using the herb, you should consider involving a doctor in your care. One problem with St. John's wort and all herbal remedies is that you cannot be sure that the amount specified on the bottle is correct since there is a great deal of variability from one brand to another and even between different batches in a given brand.

As with other antidepressants, St. John's wort generally takes a few weeks to exert its antidepressant effects. Like most active drugs, it also has side effects, most commonly headaches, nervousness, nausea, abdominal pains, and increased sensitivity to light. This last side effect is of particular concern to those using light therapy in conjunction with St. John's wort. In an open-label study conducted by the SAD Association of Great Britain, several patients who were using both St. John's wort and light therapy complained of an unpleasantly increased sensitivity to light and painful eyes. For this reason, I do not currently recommend that people use light therapy and St. John's wort together—a reversal of the position I took in my 1998 book *St. John's Wort: The Herbal Way to Feeling Good*.

Vitamins

Leaving aside the larger question as to whether vitamin supplements are necessary or beneficial to those eating a well-balanced diet, what can one usefully say about the benefits of taking vitamins specifically for SAD? Not much, it turns out. A few studies have examined the potential benefits of vitamin D for SAD. There's a sort of logic to these studies in that sunlight is responsible for vitamin D production in the skin. The numbers of subjects involved were small, and even though the authors concluded that the vitamin had an antidepressant effect, the data are certainly too weak to warrant any recommendations.

The most compelling case for the role of vitamins in treating depression in general involves vitamin B_1 (thiamine): four separate controlled studies found a mood-elevating effect for 50 milligrams per day. I outline the case for vitamins in treating depression in general in my 2002 book *The Emotional Revolution: How the New Science of Feelings can Transform Your Life*.

Fish Oil Extracts

There has been considerable excitement about the possibility that omega-3 fatty acids, contained in fish oil extracts, walnuts, and almonds, may be beneficial for depression. The data on its value for alleviating depression in general is mixed. No specific studies have examined its value for SAD in particular. Fish oil extracts may be beneficial for the heart as well as your mood, so there may be an all-around value in taking a modest amount of this supplement, for example, 1 gram per day.

Watch Out for Alcohol and Marijuana

As A. Cornelius Celsus advised two thousand years ago, "Be moderate in the drinking of wine." I thoroughly agree. Alcohol tends to make depressed people even more depressed. True, you may get an initial buzz that may even carry you through an evening, but in many cases depressed people will pay dearly for this in the form of lowered mood and energy over the next few days. This warning applies even more strongly against marijuana, which can increase depression and sap you of much-needed motivation, and is notorious for causing "the munchies."

Stress Management

If you are a seasonal person, you have the advantage of being able to predict that at some times of the year your energy level will be low and you may find it difficult to accomplish certain tasks, whereas at other times of the year it will be high and you may be able to tackle all sorts of things. You can use this information to regulate your stress level throughout the year. Some stresses are unpredictable and cannot be planned for, but many can be anticipated. These include purchasing a new house, moving, starting a new job, beginning a major undertaking, and many other projects that we impose on ourselves. Beware of setting spring deadlines and delivery dates on projects. A common trap when you are riding high during the summer is to promise to complete a project within nine months, which may seem ample, only to find yourself having to struggle to meet your overoptimistic projection when your energy level is at its lowest winter ebb.

Many people use the summer months for the creative aspects of their work and the winter months to consolidate and work on more humdrum tasks. Our original seasonal patient, Herb Kern, adopted this pattern. An engineer at a large laboratory, he conceived his best ideas and conducted his most exciting experiments in the summer, then wrote up his data—a more routine task—in the winter months. There is evidence that some famous composers, most notably Handel and Mahler, were seasonal and did most of their composing in the summer months.

In Chapter 11, "A Step-by-Step Guide Through the Revolving Year," I help you look over your year in its entirety and plan accordingly.

One way to reduce stress in winter is to pay for help and services. You can use some of that money you are not spending for the type of socializing and shopping you do in the summer to pay others to help you with difficult chores such as taking your clothes to the laundry, hiring a cleaning service, and buying takeout dinners. Mothers can have a particularly hard time meeting the demands of small children when they are feeling depressed, and paying for extra child or home care can provide a great deal of relief. If you have some money to spare, think of ways to solve a problem by hiring someone else to do chores, such as grocery shopping and housekeeping. You may find yourself coming up with some rather creative solutions.

Sometimes feelings of guilt can be an obstacle to getting the help you need. In that case, remind yourself that you are not being lazy, neglectful, and all the other negative adjectives that depressed people are so good at using on themselves. Reduced levels of energy and motivation and inability to cope are key symptoms of depression. Even though you may be doing many things to reduce these symptoms, these measures may not be completely effective. It is therefore very important to reduce your stresses and commitments, and if paying others to help out is financially possible, it is worth it for your mental health. Remember, too, that paying someone to take care of certain chores may give you more time and energy to devote to your job, and it is false economy to skimp on help with chores if your job is at stake.

A major problem for depressed people is concentrating and remembering. Many seasonal people have developed methods of coping with these difficulties. One woman I know has developed some tricks to help her remember things in the winter. For example, she records everything on her calendar and doesn't assume that she will remember things that she would recall easily in the summertime. She cross-indexes the people she relies on for help of various kinds under a section labeled "H" for "Help." This section includes addresses and phone numbers of plumbers, workmen, and even her doctors, whose names she often forgets in the winter. She leaves notes for herself on the back door, where she will see them as she goes out of the house, and writes notes to herself late at night about what she needs to do the following morning. She also writes down other information, such as friends' birthdays and directions to people's homes.

For many older patients with SAD, retirement offers a particular type of relief from stress. One such gentleman who had worked for many years as an architect said, "I have been free of all SAD symptoms for the past three years since I retired, and I recommend it to everyone." Retirement, like relocation, is a major life decision that involves many considerations, including the loss of a meaningful job, reduced income, and having to structure the days that were previously filled up with work. The dilemma was articulated by a couple who consulted me about how best to manage the wife's SAD symptoms. She had been a head nurse on a busy unit for many years and was finding it increasingly difficult to function effectively during the winter. Her husband, also a professional and very supportive of his wife, was concerned that she would feel even worse if she lost the daily structure that her work afforded her. When I suggested that the work appeared to be more of a stressor than a comfort, his wife expressed great relief at the idea of either quitting her job or giving up the head nurse position and working part time in a way that gave her more control over her hours. When he saw her relief, her husband pointed out that they would have more than enough money to enable her to stop working and supported her decision.

As far as stress management is concerned, the bottom line is *nurture your resources and use your creativity to find shortcuts and ways to conserve your energy to help keep you going through the down season.*

Negative Ions

As I mentioned earlier in the book, positively charged particles in the air, also known as *positive ions,* have long been regarded as mentally disturbing to those in their path. These positive ions are swept along at high density by "ill winds," such as the hot Santa Ana winds in California, which, as writer Raymond Chandler so aptly put it, sent housewives reaching for their kitchen knives while eyeing the backs of their husbands' necks. An old, patchy literature suggested a remedy for the unsettling effects of such ill winds: exposure to negatively charged particles, also known as *negative ions.* A negative ion generator would shift the balance of ambient negative to positive ions in a favorable direction. As you may recall, negative ions occur in nature near waterfalls, the pounding surf, or after a rainstorm. Until recently there was no good evidence in support of the therapeutic value of negative ions. In just the last few years, however, that has changed, with new studies offering an entirely new approach to the treatment of SAD and even nonseasonal depression.

Drs. Michael and Jiuan Su Terman at Columbia Psychiatric Institute rigorously tested the effects of negative ions on patients with SAD. They found that sitting in front of a machine that puts out a flow of negative ions at a high rate (a negative ion generator) for thirty minutes each morning for a week produces as powerful an antidepressant effect as sitting in front of a 10,000-lux light box for the same duration. The high-flow-rate ion generator maintains a high density of

ions in the room. A control negative ion generator calibrated for only
a low flow rate of negative ions (low-density ion generator) was vastly
inferior, no better than a placebo. The results of the Termans' first
study were exciting but preliminary. Scientists always like to see results
replicated before getting really excited. Well, the Termans have just
replicated their original findings, but with a slight twist. This time
they administered the negative ions to patients with SAD during the
last forty-five to ninety minutes of sleep. To ensure that the ions really
went to the patients and not to the radiator and other grounded struc-
tures in the room, the Termans connected the ion generator to a
grounded sheet on which their subjects slept. Once again, the high-
density ion generator turned out to be roughly as effective as light
therapy (thirty minutes at 10,000 lux) and vastly superior to a low-
density control generator. So far, no side effects have emerged; nor is
there any theoretical reason to expect side effects since we routinely encounter high densities of negative ions under natural circumstances.
So, I have felt comfortable recommending the high-density ion generator, used as noted above, to my own patients. I also plan to try it out
myself.

Jack, one of my patients, a physician in his mid-forties, has used a
high-density ion generator with good results. Jack has a long history
of severe SAD, for which I have treated him in several different ways.
As with Sara, the nurse I mention later in this book (see p. 221), I had
to throw the kitchen sink at him. While living in Maryland, despite being on hefty doses of antidepressants, he could not stay free of depression during the winter unless he spent almost all day in front of his
light box. Adding in a high-density ion generator made a big difference, freeing up some precious hours, which he needed to spend away
from his lights. In the end, like Sara, Jack chose to relocate, in this instance to Arizona. But his ion generator continues to be a valuable
part of his overall treatment plan. I have used the term *high-density* deliberately because, as you can tell from the Termans' studies, the density of charged particles really does make a difference. Therefore, if you
decide to use a negative ion generator, I suggest you use the version
shown in Figure 8 and mentioned in Part IV. This version is similar to
the ones used by the Termans in their studies. It features a wire that
connects the ion generator to a bracelet around the person's wrist,
which helps guide the ions to the person and not to other grounded
objects in the room. Another way to help keep negative ions in the air
rather than having them whizzing off to grounded objects (other than

yourself) is to increase the humidity in the room with a humidifier. The Termans caution against using a light box and an ion generator simultaneously as the ion flow could be diverted to the grounded light box.

The Termans have now extended their work to nonseasonal depression as well, where they report favorable results in a small controlled study.

How do negative ions work? Nobody knows. As we have learned with light therapy, it takes years to obtain a consensus among scientists that a treatment works at all. Figuring out how it works is always a more difficult

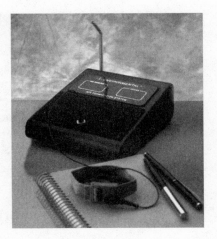

FIGURE 8. The negative ion generator available from the Center for Environmental Therapeutics. Photo by Gary Regester.

problem. Michael Terman muses that the ions may work via a sensitive structure in the nose. But right now, he acknowledges, that is pure speculation.

No medications, no effort, no side effects! It sounds too good to be true. But that is what the data suggest. So, expect to see a lot more about negative ions in the years to come. Meanwhile, you can try this novel treatment for yourself simply by purchasing and plugging in the ion generator shown in Figure 8 and listed in Part IV and switching it on and off next to your bed with a standard silent electronic timer.

Sleep Restriction

One surprising way to handle the sluggishness associated with SAD may be to sleep less. This may seem odd, since we usually think of sleep as refreshing and providing extra energy, but it may actually increase depression. Robert Burton, in his classic *Anatomy of Melancholy*, noted that

> sleep . . . may do more harm than good in that phlegmatick, swinish, cold, and sluggish melancholy. . . . It dulls the spirits, if overmuch, and

... fills the head full of gross humours, causeth distillations, rheums, great stores of excrements in the brain and in all other parts.

Some modern researchers agree with Burton's sentiments and have shown that sleep deprivation can have antidepressant effects. Forcing yourself to wake up at seven or eight in the morning instead of ten or eleven may have a salutary effect on your mood and energy level. A dawn simulator (see Chapter 7) will help you wake up earlier and enjoy more light, less sleep, and more energy. Likewise, successful light therapy often reduces the need for excessive sleep.

Support Groups

Just as patients with numerous other conditions have found support and comfort in associating with others who are similarly affected, some patients with SAD have been helped by associations that deal with mood disorders. Several of these organizations are listed in Part IV. Patients who have been involved with these organizations report many benefits, including having access to the latest information about the condition and its treatments, the support and friendship of fellow sufferers, and devices and strategies that others have found useful in coping with the problem. One important concrete goal of a support group for SAD sufferers would be to work toward universal reimbursement for light fixtures by insurance companies and HMOs.

Unfortunately, I know of no fully functional nationwide support group specifically for SAD in the United States at this time. In contrast, the highly successful Seasonal Affective Disorder Association of Great Britain (SADA) answers around a thousand queries about SAD every week, has regular annual meetings, and raises money for research into the condition. This group, which has done an enormous amount of good for people with SAD in the United Kingdom, has relied heavily on a small core of dedicated volunteers. In addition, its existence would not have been possible without the indefatigable perseverance of its founder, Jennifer Eastwood.

Certainly there is a need for the same services in this country. Millions of people are suffering from the condition, relevant new scientific and technical advances are being made every year, and the public has a tremendous need for support and up-to-date information about SAD and its treatment. It is hard to believe that a country as vast and resourceful as the United States cannot maintain our own support group for SAD. With a relatively small core of effective volunteers, it is surely possible to found and maintain a vibrant SAD support group. Along with a fine group of people, I tried several years ago to establish the group NOSAD, National Organization for Seasonal Affective Disorder. It still has a website (*www.nosad.org*), but as of this time it is a group awaiting leadership, membership, and inspiration. I point this out in the hope that one or more of the readers of this book might find the idea an appealing challenge and act on it.

One problem that a SAD support group faces is that all its members tend to be at their lowest ebb at the same time—during the winter—just when there is the greatest need for information and support. For this reason, it would be a good idea to hire an unaffected person or recruit friends and relatives of those with SAD, who could keep a support group running during the winter. In the meanwhile, you may wish to look into existing support groups for those suffering from depression in general, which are listed in Part IV and may be of value to patients with SAD.

Acceptance

Sometimes, even with the best therapy, mood control is not perfect. As long as the lows are not too low or too long, a measure of acceptance can sometimes be very therapeutic. Many of us expect to function happily and at peak levels at all times. By expecting this, we often place unreasonable demands on ourselves, which require machinelike efficiency. A great measure of contentment can be attained by accepting as inevitable some degree of fluctuation in energy, mood, and ability to function as part of the ordinary ebb and flow of life. This concept is more in keeping with Eastern than Western thinking. For example, the ancient Chinese medical guide, the *Nei Ching,* advises people to behave in certain specific ways during each season, recommending, for example, that during winter people should go to bed early and arise late. The message is to yield to the physical and emotional changes that come with the changing seasons, rather than to oppose them. After you have done all you can to reverse the unpleasant and disabling symptoms of SAD, that is not bad advice.

I counsel acceptance only after every reasonable means to counteract depressive symptoms has been tried. For example, I have one patient whose moods have not been controlled successfully, despite all manner of treatments. Bright light helps her, but only to a modest degree. We meet at intervals, discuss possible approaches, and evaluate new ideas for treatment as they come up. But she has reached a degree of acceptance of her condition and is not willing to try new approaches that appear to hold little advantage over those she has tried before. I support her acceptance while we both search for a better long-term solution.

Acceptance often comes slowly, bit by bit, rather than all at once. There is a great temptation each year, as spring arrives, to think that the problem is over, only to have it reappear again the following fall. I have seen many reactions to this familiar experience. For example, one woman with a fifteen-year history of SAD has been treated with light therapy, antidepressant medications, and psychotherapy with considerable success. Her depressions no longer disable her as they once did, but she is still less energetic, enthusiastic, and effective in the winter than in the summer. Last winter, for the first time, she felt enraged at the limitations the condition imposes on her, the way her life seems to flip-flop between feeling good and feeling depressed every six months. This anger is one more phase in her slow journey toward acceptance.

To summarize, there are many different approaches you can take to help yourself cope with winter depression and turn a previously dreaded season into a time of joy. A first step requires the recognition that the difficulties associated with depression—low energy level, pessimism, lack of motivation, low self-esteem, and withdrawal, to name just a few—are symptoms of an illness, not flaws in your character. They require understanding rather than judgment and condemnation, serious attention rather than denial and minimization, and the first person who needs to understand them and take them seriously is the depressed person. This is helpful in itself. In addition, for seasonal depressives, changing the environment may be quite beneficial. Brighten your living and work areas, travel to sunny places in the winter, or, if all else fails, relocate permanently to a better climate.

Exercise moderately and regularly in a way you find enjoyable. Find a companion to join you, and help each other stick to your routine. Diet sensibly and consider a low-carbohydrate diet. Limit stresses. Don't make commitments during your summer highs that you are unable to keep in the winter. Anticipate predictable chores and use your creativity to figure out solutions to them ahead of time. Stay informed. New treatments and devices, such as negative ion generators, are being discovered all the time—and yesterday's insoluble problem may have a solution today. If you're the kind of person who derives comfort from others who are in a situation similar to yours, join a support group of fellow sufferers—or establish your own! Finally, *accept* that which you cannot change. Life has its ups and downs, and no one understands that better than the SAD sufferer. But before resigning yourself to your problems, be sure that you have explored all the treatments outlined in this book, including psychotherapy and antidepressant medications, which I discuss in the next two chapters.

NINE

Psychotherapy and SAD

For many people with seasonal difficulties psychotherapy may be helpful, but it is by no means universally necessary. How do you decide when to seek therapy?

Having made the decision to enter therapy, what sort should you seek? There are various types of therapy. Which is likely to work best? And how do you find and choose a therapist—someone in whom you can put your trust? You generally tell your therapist your deepest and most private thoughts. How do you know whether you can trust him or her to treat these precious thoughts and feelings with respect? How do you know whether he or she is competent, will understand your problem, and know the appropriate thing to say or do about it?

Once in therapy, how do you manage to integrate psychotherapy with light therapy or antidepressant medications? How do you know whether the therapy is working? All these are difficult questions, yet they are often foremost in the minds of those in search of psychological help.

When Should You Consider Entering Therapy?

Suppose you suffer from winter depressions. You seek out a therapist qualified to treat you with light therapy or antidepressant medications

190

and find that this takes care of many, if not all, of your symptoms. In addition, you take steps to embrace a positive lifestyle as outlined elsewhere in this book. You now have an explanation for your seasonal difficulties and, moreover, a way to treat and control them. This frees you to get on with your life, to love and to work, as Freud would say, and also to enjoy yourself. Do you need psychotherapy? Of course not.

Now imagine a different scenario. Your seasonal symptoms have responded to treatment. You no longer sink to the depths of depression familiar to you for so many years. All should be well, but it is not. Something is amiss. Perhaps you feel stuck where you are in life. You have been following certain routines and activities that once were fulfilling but now are not. Some change is necessary, but nothing suggests itself to you. Persisting in the same course gets you nowhere in this mission. Or perhaps you feel trapped in certain gloomy ways of viewing yourself or the world around you. At this point, psychotherapy can be beneficial. It can help you define the problem and search within yourself for solutions that may be very difficult to find on your own.

I am reminded of a fly, trying to escape from a room by banging against a window. He does not realize that the door behind him is open. He can see the world he longs for stretched out in front of him, but his limited perspective dooms him to bang his head repeatedly against the windowpane. Fruitless, repetitive behavior of this kind is commonly found in people, too, but it can be modified by psychotherapy. The example of a woman who gets into a series of relationships with men who mistreat her has become almost a cliché in recent years. However, like all clichés, this one is grounded in reality, and the pattern is all too familiar. So is the situation of the man (or woman) who repeatedly fails just when success appears to be within reach. It has often been said that people with neuroses do not remember, they repeat; and most clinicians have seen this pattern many times.

Freud provided insights into the compulsion to repeat damaging behavior, tracing it back to childhood events. An image that comes to us from our age of computers is that some bug has been incorporated into the software that causes a program to make the same error again and again. Following this analogy a little further, insight-oriented psychotherapy can be seen as an attempt to track down the problem in the software and reprogram it to succeed rather than fail. Returning to the vignette of the fly and the windowpane, we can compare the process of psychotherapy to showing the fly that there is another way out of the room—through the open door. A wonderful, therapeutic sense of free-dom accompanies a new way of seeing a problem and new strategies for dealing with it.

One type of programming error that is often responsible for unhap-piness involves self-esteem. In growing up, you may have incorporated incorrect or derogatory images and opinions of yourself into the soft-ware of your brain, and these may continue to haunt you into adult life. Apart from your upbringing and early childhood experiences, other in-fluences from both the outside world and your own internal experiences can shape self-esteem. For example, suffering from repeated depres-sions—long stretches of time when you are unable to function prop-erly—can have long-term detrimental effects on self-esteem and self-image. Even after these depressions are treated, self-esteem problems may persist and may require psychotherapy to be resolved properly.

Melissa, an artist in her early forties, is a case in point. Intelligent, talented, attractive, and with a charming personality, she nonetheless grew up believing that she should aspire to be an empty-headed blonde. According to the voices of her upbringing, women were sup-posed to be pretty but vacuous and always available to support the men in their lives. Signs of burgeoning talent were viewed as danger signals that might scare off eligible men. Women were meant to con-ceal their talent and intelligence and to draw men out. After graduat-ing from high school, Melissa went on to get a degree in counseling, choosing this "appropriate" profession over the artistic areas that were her real love. Two unhappy marriages followed.

After entering the seasonal program at the NIMH and having her winter depression treated with light therapy, Melissa embarked on a course of psychotherapy. Through this process she was able to under-stand how she had been programmed to believe she had to become someone at odds with the person she really wanted to be. Therefore, no matter what she did, or how successful she was, it didn't feel right to her. She was not fulfilling those early programs and her parents' ex-pectations. Although she was a fine mother, a talented artist, a good friend to many, and a delightful person, none of this felt good enough. Once she understood the origins of her feelings of failure, she was able to alter her expectations of herself and recognize that these new expec-tations—her own—were both legitimate and compatible with what she truly wanted to do with her life. Psychotherapy was a liberating ex-perience for her. Whereas light therapy reversed the symptoms of her winter depression, psychotherapy helped her understand and come to terms with problems from her past—something that light therapy by itself would never have been able to accomplish.

I have seen many people besides Melissa reap successful and liberating effects from good psychotherapy. I have also seen psychotherapy and other forms of treatment work well together, as they did for Melissa. If you have significant problems like Melissa's that persist after treatment with light therapy or medications, you should certainly consider psychotherapy.

Cognitive-Behavioral Therapy for Seasonal Affective Disorder

Of all types of psychotherapy for SAD, cognitive-behavioral therapy (CBT) has the most going for it. Not only does a recent study provide evidence for its effectiveness specifically for SAD, but these results are buttressed by a huge literature showing that CBT is effective for depression in general. For people who do not choose to use light therapy or antidepressants, CBT alone may be sufficient for successfully treating SAD. What does this amazing treatment consist of and how can you incorporate its principles into your daily life to combat the symptoms of depression even without a therapist? For answers to these questions, read on.

The mind, like ancient Gaul, can be divided into three parts: what we think, what we feel, and what we do—or, in psychological terms, cognition, emotion, and behavior. All problems of the psyche result from disturbances in one or more of these domains or in some disconnect between them. All efforts to treat these disturbances involve tinkering with either one or more of these domains or with the connection between them.

Freud's influence led therapists and patients alike to believe that, to solve their problems, they had to probe for some hidden sorrow, uncover it, and, in so doing, resolve it. There may still be a role for such an approach in certain situations. But the proponents of CBT take a completely different tack. They deal with what is readily apparent in cognition, emotion, and behavior. They examine the content of these three domains and their relationships to one another and seek to alter or correct these apparent disturbances. In the words of Dr. Aaron Beck, one of the pioneers of CBT, there is more to the surface than meets the eye.

To their immense credit, CBT researchers have developed standardized ways of conceptualizing problems of cognition, emotion, and behavior and standardized methods to help fix them. These methods can be explained in terms readily understandable to the depressed person and can be implemented in therapy. Although you may be able to derive some benefit from CBT by reading about it and implementing its principles in your own life, it is far better to work with a therapist with expertise in this form of treatment. But even those undergoing CBT under the guidance of such a therapist are urged to do homework between sessions. This emphasis on homework is soundly based on both behavioral observations and basic brain science.

Both the Beck Institute for Cognitive Therapy and the Academy of Cognitive Therapy maintain websites where you can locate a certified cognitive therapist in your area (see Part IV).

Practice, Practice, Practice

It is a commonplace that practice makes perfect, but true nonetheless. That golf swing, video game, or piano fugue you are trying to master, the new language you would love to speak, your bridge, Scrabble, or chess game will improve by only one means: practice. So it is with all skills. To improve, you have to practice them. CBT therapists typically assign written homework in which they ask patients to record their feelings, thoughts, and actions. In depression these all typically take on a gloomy turn. The therapist teaches the patient to question these downers and turn them into uppers instead. An old song exhorted the listener to accentuate the positive and eliminate the negative. It sounded simplistic. Amazingly, though, it works, but only through continuous repetition.

Brain imaging techniques show that practice expands that portion of the brain involved in carrying out the task in question. Violinists, for example, who use their left hands to form the notes that make their music show expansion in parts of the brain responsible for orchestrating the movements of the left hand. In contrast, those parts that govern the right hand, which violinists use to move their bows up and down, a far simpler task, show no such expansion. London cab drivers, who are required to learn the location of all of London's many streets to get their licenses, grow that part of their brain responsible for spatial memory.

Although it may take a violinist years to master her art, it is not necessary for practice to occur over such a long period for it to change the brain. On the contrary, humans and other primates taught simple skills over the course of days undergo changes in those parts of the brain responsible for the skills. New connections between nerve cells are forged, and the brain regions involved actually grow. It is a wonder to contemplate the brain, this intricate mass of mortal coils, actually growing and changing throughout adult life. For this change to be purposeful, however, practice needs to be guided. We need a teacher, coach, or mentor to show us what we are doing wrong and how to fix it. We need to learn new methods, implement them, and practice, practice, practice. That is how CBT therapists approach the treatment of depression, and they have evidence to back up their recommendations.

Using brain imaging techniques, Helen Mayberg, a senior scientist at the Rotman Research Institute in Toronto, and colleagues have shown brain changes in depressed patients following a course of CBT. Specifically, certain cortical areas that may contribute to the chatter of negative thoughts quiet down after CBT, while core parts of the emotional brain become more active after therapy. These results suggest that CBT made changes in those brain regions involved in attention and memory and that those changes drove the antidepressant response. These findings are consistent with the idea that CBT involves "top down" processing whereby patients learn to short-circuit their negative thinking patterns, as measured by decreased activity in their cortical or "top" regions, and that this boosts mood, as measured by increased activity in the emotional or "bottom" regions.

CBT versus Light Therapy

There are by now so many studies showing the benefits of light therapy for SAD that it seems like a given that light is an effective treatment for this condition. Yet it took fourteen years from our first controlled study of light therapy for the field as a whole to definitively accept this treatment, and, for all I know, there may still be some diehard skeptics out there. In contrast, to date there has been only one small study of CBT for SAD. Preliminary results are so encouraging, however, that they are definitely worth a good look, especially since they lead to specific steps that people with SAD can take to alleviate their suffering.

The study in question was the brainchild of Dr. Kelly Rohan, an assistant professor of medical and clinical psychology at the Uniformed Services University of the Health Sciences in Bethesda, Maryland. Dr. Rohan compared three different forms of treatment for patients with SAD: conventional light therapy, CBT, and a combination of the two treatments. In a study of twenty-three patients with SAD, she found all three treatments to be equally effective, but perhaps her most interesting findings emerged the following winter. Rohan found that significantly more patients who had been treated exclusively with light therapy relapsed as compared with those patients who had received CBT as part or all of their treatment.

As best I can understand, the likely explanation for this distinction is that with light treatment alone the researchers encouraged patients to focus only on the light and not at all on their lives. With CBT, on the other hand, they encouraged patients to work hard to change their thoughts and behavior during the winter and thereby to improve the quality of their lives. I have long encouraged the latter approach, as you can tell from the contents of this book. An active, even aggressive, attitude toward your SAD symptoms and the winter is best. Many elements in this book echo those in Dr. Rohan's program: pursuing positive thoughts and activities and avoiding negative ones, keeping active, and interacting with people who lift your spirits. But in addition to these recommendations, Dr. Rohan's program borrows from classical CBT teachings to include specific elements that are part of what CBT is all about. Let us first examine the essentials of Dr. Rohan's program, which is based on the teachings of leading CBT practitioners. After that, let's explore some of the specific techniques of CBT.

Dr. Rohan's Anti-SAD CBT Program

Dr. Rohan conducted her program in a group setting over six weeks, offering two sessions each week. Here are the key elements of a CBT program such as hers that you can try out for yourself.

1. Educate yourself about SAD.
2. Consider how your activities contribute to your SAD symptoms.
3. Seek out pleasant activities.
4. Consider how your thoughts contribute to your SAD symptoms.
5. Correct erroneous thought patterns (cognitive distortions).

6. Identify themes in your negative thinking.
7. Challenge your core negative beliefs about yourself.
8. Maintain your gains and work to prevent relapse.

Self-Education: SAD as a Vicious Cycle

The more you know about SAD, the better equipped you will be to deal with and overcome it. You will find in the pages of this book much of what you need to know to do so. One important aspect of SAD that Dr. Rohan stresses in her work is how SAD can be a vicious cycle. Some of the behaviors that typically occur in patients with SAD can actually make SAD symptoms worse, which in turn aggravates those very same behaviors. A key example of this is sleeping late, which prevents you from being exposed to light in the early morning, which makes your SAD (and oversleeping) worse. Likewise people with SAD often avoid social engagements, which further isolates and depresses them.

Think of the behaviors that contribute to your SAD symptoms and write them down in a special homework log.

Seeking Out Pleasant Activities

Pleasant activities by definition elevate your mood. Make a list of those activities that give your mood a boost and push yourself to do them even if they don't come easily to you. Plan ahead by making an appointment with yourself to do a specific activity, even scheduling it into your daily planner for a specific day and at a specific time, to increase the chance that you will follow through. That way you will be less likely to back out of an activity that may improve your mood.

Remember, these activities can be pursued either indoors or outdoors. Most people can find something that will propel them out of hibernation mode. Think hard and find your own mood-boosting activities. In my own case, that means pushing myself to go walking first thing in the morning (with the help of a friend if necessary) and throwing myself into the whirl of holiday socializing even if I don't always relish the prospect. My reward: more energy during the day and an enjoyable sense of being connected with congenial people.

Dr. Rohan urges her study participants to make a commitment to pursuing pleasant activities. Analyze what is preventing you from having fun and remove all obstacles. You can do this, for example, by being sure you put enjoyable pursuits high on your priority list. Plan ahead to ensure that you get work and chores done to allow you time for joyful or spiritual activities.

Once again, make a list, keep a log of what works, and practice doing it, even if it is only for ten minutes a day. Remember, what you practice repeatedly changes the structure and function of your brain and shapes the quality of your life. In the words of the writer Annie Dillard, "How we spend our days is of course how we spend our lives."

Understanding How Your Thoughts Affect Your Mood

One of Aaron Beck's great insights was the recognition that our thoughts affect our moods. By changing your thoughts you can change your mood with positive results.

This profound insight may seem obvious now, but it was by no means so several decades ago when I was training to become a psychiatrist. Although psychiatrists recognized that depressed people had gloomy thoughts, many concluded that these were an irreducible part of the clinical picture that would resist any reasoned attempts to alter them. By their research studies, Beck and his colleagues disproved that notion. They observed that in depressed people negative thoughts flow automatically and these automatic negative thoughts (or ANTs, as they are often called) can be identified and altered. The acronym "ANTs" calls to mind ants crawling all over one's brain—not a pleasant image but one that might readily conjure up a counterimage of oneself as exterminator, systematically getting rid of them.

CBT therapists talk of the A-B-C model, in which A stands for *antecedent event*, B for the *belief* (or ANT) that this event produces, and C for the *consequence* of the event, or the emotion it produces. In depressed people, things often happen to make them feel worse. What CBT encourages you to do is to catch the intervening thought, between the event and the feeling, and work on changing that thought. Many research studies have shown that disputing depressed thinking, or ANTs, can elevate mood. So, D for *dispute* is added to the A-B-C mnemonic to suggest the therapeutic remedy for this toxic sequence of thoughts and feelings.

How does the A-B-C model play out in practice? Consider the example of Jack, who is turned down by a young lady when he calls her up for a date. That knocks him into a tailspin. He believes he is unattractive and undesirable to women, and that he will never find a soulmate. These unbidden gloomy thoughts (ANTs) flood his mind and plunge him into a profound state of morbid pessimism and despair. Jack is an excellent candidate for CBT, as the sections that follow reveal. He should keep a log of his negative thoughts each day and try to understand what triggers them and how they affect his mood. He should be encouraged to act as a researcher, to investigate the workings of his own mind as a basis for addressing his problems.

Here is the type of dialogue that a CBT therapist might encourage Jack to practice both in therapy sessions and on his own.

THERAPIST: What evidence is there that she finds you unattractive and undesirable?

JACK: She turned down my invitation.

THERAPIST: Other than finding you unattractive and undesirable, why might she have declined your invitation?

[It is important to acknowledge that the ANT is one possible explanation for the woman's behavior, but to explore plausible alternative explanations.]

THERAPIST: Let's assume that this one woman really does find you unattractive and undesirable. So what? Could you live with that?

JACK: It will hurt, but probably I could.

THERAPIST: Have there been any past instances when other women behaved as though they found you desirable or attractive?

[Jack must now collect evidence against his beliefs that all women will find him unattractive and undesirable and reject him.]

THERAPIST: What qualities do you look for in a partner?

[This is an important question because it emphasizes that everyone has qualities that they look for in a mate, himself included. It also helps him question whether he has been seeking out the right kind of woman for himself. After all, the right kind of mate is one who likes *you*.]

THERAPIST: Have you ever declined an invitation for a date?

JACK: Well, yes, I have on a few occasions.

THERAPIST: Why was that?

JACK: I just didn't find the one woman appealing, and the other one was loud and unkind. I saw her shouting at her little sister in the mall.

THERAPIST: It seems as though those women didn't feel like good matches for you. Obviously, matches are a two-way street and they have to feel right for both parties.

JACK: I guess you're right.

THERAPIST: What qualities do you think women are looking for in a partner?

JACK: Good looks, kindness, the ability to earn a decent income.

THERAPIST: How do you feel you stack up on those qualities?

JACK: Well, I'm not a bad-looking guy, and I'm a nice guy, but I don't have much money.

THERAPIST: Can you imagine some woman out there being interested in someone who is good-looking and kind even if he doesn't have that much money right now?

JACK: I guess.

THERAPIST: What's the worst thing that could happen with your love life?

JACK: That nobody will ever want to date me again.

THERAPIST: That is an important ANT for you to think about because if you hold on to it too firmly, it could become a self-fulfilling prophecy. It's an ideal type of ANT for us to work on. What's the best thing you can imagine happening in your love life?

JACK: Finding Ms. Right tomorrow and living happily ever after.

THERAPIST: Okay, let's look at the likelihood of these two different extreme scenarios. Rate the likelihood that each will happen on a scale of zero to 100.

[Sometimes it is useful to look at extremes to recognize that the most likely scenario lies somewhere in the middle. It's a way of bringing home the fact that in the dating game—and in life in general—there are hits and misses but that perseverance pays off in finding a compatible partner with whom to lead a good life.]

THERAPIST: What else would you like to achieve in your life, other than finding a soulmate? How are you doing in each of these areas?

[This sort of question is very useful as it broadens one's thinking about what is important in life and how you define your worth in your own mind. It is important also to point out that romantic love is only one kind of love and that the love of family and friends is also important and can bring feelings of closeness and satisfaction.]

As you can see, it really helps to have a trained therapist asking the right questions and keeping you on task. But whether or not you have such a therapist, consider keeping a daily log of your thoughts and feelings and see if you can identify which thoughts lead to negative beliefs that lower your mood. Nail down the A-B-C sequence in your own life as a necessary prelude to D, disputing and challenging this sequence and thereby improving your spirits.

Recognizing Different Types of Cognitive Distortions

CBT therapists have ingeniously categorized cognitive distortions in a very helpful way. The young man in the example above displays three types of cognitive distortions: *overgeneralization, magnification (catastrophizing)*, and *fortunetelling*. He blows the episode out of proportion and, generalizing from this single event, concludes that he is universally undesirable. Then he looks into his crystal ball and predicts that he will live out a life of lonely isolation. He considers these thoughts to be the only possible way of viewing that one event, being turned down by the young lady. He doesn't consider any other explanations for her behavior or other possible future scenarios for himself. She may be involved with another man or woman. Her cat might have died the previous day. Or she may not be interested in him, but another woman might find him irresistible.

The CBT therapist would teach him to diagnose the nature of his cognitive distortions and help him dispute them and ask "What other reasons may there be for her rejection?" and "What other outcomes can you envision other than a life of unremitting misery and loneliness?" That might then result in new behaviors that would help correct the cognitive distortion and glum forecasting, such as asking another woman out on a date (or another ten women, if necessary). After all, the young man in question is seeking only one fine lady. So what difference does it make if he finds her on the first try or on the tenth?

Let us now consider other types of distortions. Janet receives a

B+ on a term paper in an important course. When she sees the grade on the paper, her heart sinks. She believes that it represents a shockingly bad performance and that her professor, for whom she has the highest regard, must despise her for it. She had worked hard to maintain an A average throughout the semester and now regards herself as a failure who will bring shame on her parents, who have scrimped and saved to put her through school. "I must do better next time," she tells herself. "I just have to, or I will be doomed to be a failure for the rest of my life."

Janet is engaging in several types of cognitive distortions: *black-or-white thinking, magnification (catastrophizing), minimization, mindreading, fortunetelling, labeling,* and *"should" statements*. She sees her performance in black-or-white terms: either as wonderful or terrible. She doesn't consider that a B grade on the paper might be quite good when assigned by a strict professor. She magnifies the importance of the grade out of all proportion and minimizes her performance on other elements in the course. Perhaps the paper counts for only a percentage of the final grade, and even if it pulls her grade down to a B, that might be very respectable. And that one class may count for very little when viewed as part of her larger transcript. A skillful CBT therapist will encourage Janet to ask the right questions: "Do I have to see this single event in black-or-white terms? Am I making a mountain out of a molehill? Am I minimizing other aspects of my performance? How else might I view this development?"

Furthermore, Janet is engaging in *mindreading* when she jumps to the conclusion that her professor must think poorly of her. She might ask instead, "How else might he view me?" and "Even if he does not regard this particular effort as stellar, how much difference will that make in the long run (or even short run)?" Janet is also engaging in *fortunetelling* (that she will bring shame on her parents) and *personalization* (the idea that she is personally responsible for her parents' emotional well-being on top of their impoverished state, which she believes she has caused by siphoning money from the family coffers for her higher education). Finally, she engages in *"should" statements*, berating herself with thoughts that she must do better in the future and flagellating herself with the imagined consequences of failing to do so. See if you can take each of Janet's cognitive distortions and act as her CBT therapist, finding the questions that will help lead her lead to less morbid conclusions and improve her mood. Then skip to Table 6 and look at some of the questions that a skillful CBT therapist might ask her.

TABLE 6
Questions That a Skillful CBT Therapist Might Ask Janet

- What is the evidence that your professor despises you?
- What have your past interactions with this professor been like?
- What kind of feedback did he give you on this paper?
- What about on other assignments?
- How do you think the professor regards the students who got an A on this assignment?
- What about the students who got a C ... or an F?

[These questions are geared toward disputing mind reading and black-or-white thinking based on empirical evidence.]

- What written or verbal feedback have you received on your past performance from professors in other courses?

[Look for evidence that some professors hold her in high regard.]

- Let's assume this one professor truly thinks you are a dunce. So what? Could you live with that? How would you regard a professor who forms judgments of students on the basis of a single paper grade?
- What is the evidence that a B is a poor grade on this particular paper? What was the class average and the grade distribution?
- What does this single B mean for your overall grade in this particular course?
- How much is your final grade determined by this paper?
- How are you doing in the other areas that will factor into your grade?

[If possible, mathematically work out what it would take to earn an A through an F and the estimated likelihood of each outcome.]

- What would it mean to you if you ended up with an A, B, C ... F in this course?

[This explores and challenges the personal significance of this course in Janet's life. Once again, it confronts her all-or-none thinking, showing her that there are degrees of excellence and keeping her away from gravitating toward the extremes.]

- How would your cumulative GPA or overall academic standing be affected?
- What is the evidence that your parents are actually ashamed of you?
- What have they said to you about your academic performance?
- You say that your parents have made sacrifices to send you to school. What would they say if they were here now?

[The degree of sacrifice involved may not be as great as Janet makes it out to be, and they may be happy to do it.]

(cont.)

TABLE 6 (cont.)

- What do your parents actually expect from you in return for their financial support? [It's probably not straight As.]
- Given this grade, what is the worst thing you can imagine happening in terms of your academic performance?
- What is the best thing that could happen?
- What is the likelihood of each outcome, from 0 to 100?
- What is actually the most realistic outcome?

[You may recognize we used the same favorite techniques for Jack. They are widely applicable and extremely helpful.]

- What makes for a successful and fulfilling life?
- What other ways do you have for measuring success in your life?
- How much does your performance in this course realistically contribute to future successes in each of these important areas?

Identifying Your Core Negative Beliefs

Once you begin to log your negative thoughts regularly, you may find that they cluster around certain themes that come up again and again, sometimes with maddening regularity, especially during your depressions. These themes or patterns are called *core beliefs*, and they often seem to drive the negative thoughts. Melissa, the artist discussed earlier, believed that unless she chose a career path that pleased her parents, she would not be living a valuable and worthwhile life. That was a core belief, which filled her with self-doubts and made her very unhappy. Although the therapy she received was not strictly CBT, identifying that core belief and correcting it proved key to her recovery.

Peggy, another patient with SAD whom I treated, had a core belief that she was stupid and incompetent, based no doubt on messages she had received as a child. Even though she had tested very well in school and had all sorts of academic laurels to her credit, whenever winter rolled around, she would feel like the dunce of the class. At those times she believed she was a fraud and teachers had given her good grades because they liked her, not because she had earned them. Although Peggy's feelings of incompetence were no doubt fueled in part by the concentration difficulties so common in winter depressions, her repeated tendency to minimize her accomplishments and generalize her winter difficulties to encompass her entire life reached the level of a core belief.

Some core beliefs, like Peggy's, revolve around your concept of yourself: for example, a belief that you are defective, inadequate, vulnerable, or a failure. Other core beliefs pertain to your view of the world: for example, that you will be abandoned, disliked, or will or should be punished. Just as it can be very helpful to challenge your distorted cognitive thinking, it is useful to challenge your core beliefs, which is the next step in this program.

As you can see, a trained CBT therapist will energetically press the patient to challenge her ANTs and, in doing so, help the patient challenge them on her own. It is not quick or easy–but neither is straightening out your golf swing or your bridge game. Both Janet and Jack could benefit from extensive CBT work. On reading their brief vignettes, Dr. Kelly Rohan commented, "Both could take sessions of hammering away at the ANTs to make progress, and both are screaming of underlying core beliefs that complicate things. For Jack, it's 'I'm unlovable and unattractive,' while for Janet it's 'I'm incompetent and I must be perfect.' "

Challenging Your Core Negative Beliefs

You might already be able to guess the elements of this next step. Log your core beliefs, dispute them, and, as always, practice this activity regularly. Dr. Judith Beck, director of the Beck Intitute for Cognitive Therapy and Research, has actually constructed a Core Belief Worksheet, which is very useful for this task (see Appendix B). Here's how you can use the worksheet. On the top of the sheet, write down the core belief that you wish to change. For example, Janet, the student who obtained a B+ grade on her paper, might jot down "I am inadequate and will never amount to anything." Assign a percentage to the most and the least that you ever hold the core belief, for example, eighty percent and forty percent, respectively. On the lefthand side of the page, write those points of evidence that support your core belief, on the right, write those points that are against the belief. Follow each negative statement with a "BUT" and a rebuttal. For example, Janet might jot down "I earned a B on a paper in a very important course" but might immediately follow that with "BUT it could have been a lot worse" or "BUT many people would be pleased with that grade." Then, on the righthand side of the vertical line she would list evidence against her core belief; for example, "I have maintained an A average all semester." After sorting out the pros and cons very thoroughly, the next task is to come up with a new, more realistic core belief, which would be written on the bottom of the paper. In Janet's case that might be "I'm a good student with a very promising future, and though I'm not always perfect, nobody is." Then ask yourself "How much do I believe this new core belief?" and "How much do I believe the original core belief?" Assign percentages to answer these two questions and see how the new percentages compare with the initial ones.

Maintaining Gains and Preventing Relapse

As I mentioned, those patients in Dr. Rohan's study who had been treated with CBT the previous year were less likely to relapse the following winter than those treated with light therapy alone. Studies of patients with nonseasonal forms of depression have also found that both cognitive and behavioral techniques can help prevent relapse. So, watch out for the return of the ANTs and be ready to exterminate them at first sight, using the techniques outlined in this chapter. Likewise, guard against the tendency to retreat from enjoyable activities. Entire books have been written on CBT, and Part IV provides a guide to those seeking to pursue these strategies further.

Other Forms of Therapy

Most skillful therapists combine different forms of therapy to achieve the best results. *Insight-oriented therapy* refers to a process of exploring the basis of various symptoms as a way of providing the patient with understanding and relief. For example, one woman with SAD who was in her mid-forties went into psychotherapy to help resolve the guilt she felt at having been the only healthy child out of six siblings. A middle-aged man with SAD struggled for years on his PhD thesis but was unable to complete it, not because of any intellectual limitation but because it raised anxiety in him about competing with his father, who had been much less successful than he was.

Other forms of therapy have been developed to deal with the long-term consequences of traumas, which can arise from a wide variety of situations such as combat stress, rape, or child sexual abuse. The scope of these various therapies goes beyond the present book, but my book *The Emotional Revolution* (see Part IV) has a more extensive discussion of the topic. It may also be useful to bring a patient's family or partner into the treatment process at certain times.

Like all effective treatments, however, psychotherapy is not without hazards. Probing a person's past and stirring up buried secrets, while very helpful in some cases, is not universally so. Psychotherapy can actually amplify feelings of depression and anxiety and should be performed only by a skilled and properly trained therapist. That person should also be familiar with the biological treatments of depression so that the patient is not allowed to spin his or her wheels discussing childhood conflicts while a raging depression goes untreated.

Choosing a Psychotherapist

It is extremely important that you choose your therapist carefully. It is surprising to think that the same person who might take several days researching a car purchase—consulting consumer reports and friends, visiting several dealerships, and test-driving cars—might head straight for the Yellow Pages to find a therapist. A therapist is someone with whom you need to be able to share your most important personal thoughts and feelings. That person's judgment, training, and suitability for *you* should be the primary basis for your choice. How do you find such a person?

I believe that recommendations from other professionals are the best guide. Start with a health professional whom you respect and who has some knowledge of you as a person—a medical doctor, psychologist, or social worker. Briefly explain to this person the type of problem you are dealing with. Then ask his or her opinion as to who might be suitable for you. If possible, ask more than one professional, to see whether the same name appears on more than one list. Once you have obtained one or two names, set up an appointment to interview the prospective therapist. He or she should, of course, ask you questions about your problem. Consider whether the questions are on target. Does the therapist appear to be exploring the problem thoroughly, asking about it from different angles? Does he or she seem to understand what you are saying—not just intellectually but also emotionally? Does he or she appear empathic—on the same wavelength as you? These early impressions are important and should be taken into consideration in making your decision.

Remember, although medical doctors, psychologists, and social workers may all be able to provide psychotherapy, only medical doctors can prescribe antidepressant medications. If you need both medications and psychotherapy, it is possible to obtain both types of help from a psychiatrist or to obtain medications from a doctor and therapy from someone else. I have worked with patients in both of these formats, and either situation can be successful. If two professionals are involved, both should be competent, and they should work well as a team. The patient's responsibility is to keep each professional informed in general terms of what the other is doing.

You are certainly entitled to ask questions of the prospective therapist. What is his or her background and training? Does he or she subscribe to any particular school of therapy? If these questions are asked in an ordinary, matter-of-fact manner, they should be met with ordinary, matter-of-fact replies. Any defensiveness about the replies, questions in response to your questions (such as "Why do you want to know?") or interpretations (such as "It seems as though you suspect my competency") might reasonably raise suspicion about insecurity on the part of the therapist.

At the end of the initial consultation, the therapist should provide a formulation of the problem—a diagnosis and some clarification of the issues—as well as specific recommendations about treatment. Sometimes, however, if the situation appears to be complicated, more than one meeting might be necessary before the therapist is ready to provide a formulation and recommendations. It's important for you to consider this formulation and these recommendations as just *one* way to see the problem. There may be other ways to see it as well, and you may wish to seek other opinions before making up your mind about which therapist is right for you.

TEN

Antidepressant Medications

By now it is common wisdom that antidepressant medications have revolutionized the treatment of depression. In this chapter I will present the evidence for the value of antidepressants in treating SAD. How much is it reasonable to expect from these medications? What are their side effects and liabilities? What are the differences between available antidepressants and what is the best choice for any given person with SAD? And finally, how do these drugs work? These are particularly important questions because light therapy is not right for everybody. Some people do not respond to light therapy, many respond only partially, and others find it too cumbersome or inconvenient.

To date, dozens of studies have been undertaken to examine the value of medications in the treatment of SAD. The problem with most of these studies is that they involved small numbers of patients and were poorly designed. As a consequence, the results, though generally positive, are not compelling enough to allow for solid medical recommendations. But a reasonable bottom-line conclusion for practical purposes is that antidepressants in general work for SAD just as they do for other types of depression.

Typically the way in which a drug gets approval for use with a particular condition begins with at least two very large studies. If these studies show the medication to be reasonably safe and effective, the drug manufacturer petitions the FDA for permission to make a claim for its drug for the condition in question. If the data show the medication to be safe and effective, the FDA will generally grant the claim. That is when you see advertisements popping up on TV and in the print media directing you to ask your doctor whether a certain medication might be helpful for a condition that might be ailing you. These direct appeals to the consumer have become a powerful force in educating the public about specific conditions. Accompanying education of medical and mental health professionals has also served to direct attention to the condition in question, stimulating research in that area and the medical help that comes with increased awareness. Until recently few such efforts have been applied to the treatment of SAD.

It has been of concern to me that the power of the pharmaceutical industry has not been of benefit to those suffering from SAD, a condition near and dear to my heart. Until now, that is. I wondered why this might be. In part it seemed that the success of light therapy had perhaps discouraged interest by pharmaceutical companies. As a long-standing practitioner and consumer of light therapy, however, I was all too acutely aware of its limitations and realized the need for alternative and supplementary treatments. Another problem may be that SAD has not been given a category of its own in the DSM-IV-TR, the standard lexicon of psychiatric illnesses. Rather, it is relegated to an adjectival modifier of recurrent depression, "with seasonal pattern." Arguably, companies might be more hesitant to invest millions of dollars in an adjective as opposed to a noun.

These thoughts were preoccupying me when I received an unexpected call from a renowned psychiatrist and scientist, Dr. Jack Modell, at GlaxoSmithKline, a large pharmaceutical company. He was contemplating undertaking a highly novel study and wanted my thoughts as to how best to design it. If you have a recurrent depressive condition with a predictable time of onset, such as SAD, he reasoned, why not start treatment with an appropriate antidepressant *before* patients develop their symptoms? In the case of SAD, starting the antidepressant in the early fall could test this very theory. By doing so you might prevent the development of winter depression. The antidepressant could be discontinued in the spring after the season of risk was over, and people would not be required to take the medication during the spring and summer. The antidepressant of particular interest to him was Wellbutrin XL, a once-a-day formulation of a well-known antidepressant that might be particularly beneficial in people with SAD because it is not associated with the weight gain, sexual side effects, and lethargy more common with some other antidepressants.

Over the next three years Dr. Modell and his colleagues, myself included, went on to conduct three large-scale studies involving more than a thousand patients with SAD at dozens of sites across the northern United States and Canada. We compared the effects of Wellbutrin XL versus placebo in preventing winter depression. The results were positive, and the drug reduced the chance of developing a winter depression by approximately thirty-five to fifty percent. In general the drug was well tolerated, and the only side effects that were present to a meaningful degree were dry mouth, nausea, constipation, flatulence, and weight loss. To my knowledge, these are the first studies to show that depression can be prevented by starting an antidepressant before it begins.

Another interesting finding to emerge from the Wellbutrin XL prevention study was that patients did not relapse after the medication was discontinued at the beginning of spring. This finding shows how patients with SAD often need to be treated only during the fall and winter months, when they are particularly at risk. Their antidepressant medications can often be tapered toward the end of winter. Curiously, sometimes medications that are well tolerated in the winter begin to cause side effects when spring arrives, probably because the brain's chemistry is changing with the change of the seasons. This often is a signal that it is time to reduce medication dosage. On the other hand, some people with SAD may need continued medications throughout the year.

Arlene, a forty-five-year-old editor, was one of my patients who participated in the clinical trial. I had diagnosed her as suffering from SAD some three years earlier and had treated her with light therapy. It worked, but she hated it. The light box offended her aesthetic sensibilities and served as a constant unwelcome reminder to her that there was something "wrong" with her. The dawn simulator woke her husband, which he found unacceptable. She was thrilled at the prospect of an alternative. For Arlene, Wellbutrin XL turned out to work just as well as light therapy with no ill effects, and she has now used it happily for the past two winters, starting it in the fall and stopping it in the spring.

While some people may want to prevent the symptoms of SAD before they start, others may prefer to wait for symptoms to develop before initiating treatment. Arlene clearly fell into the first group and was unwilling to suffer even the beginning of her winter doldrums before starting treatment. But there is every reason to expect that antidepressant treatment will be effective even if initiated after symptoms begin. Even though no antidepressant has received FDA approval specifically for the treatment of SAD, available evidence and extensive clinical experience suggest the value of these drugs. Ideally they should be prescribed by a psychiatrist who has both skill with medications and knowledge of SAD. In practice, however, primary-care physicians might be able to manage as well for many people. Regardless of discipline, it is very important to find a knowledgeable and empathic physician to ensure that you get good care.

Common Concerns and Considerations About Taking Antidepressants

All sorts of reasonable concerns arise about taking antidepressant medications. Will the drugs harm you? Will you feel too good and get hooked on them? If you feel better, will it be the result of the pills or your own efforts? You may always have been told to examine the roots of your problems and solve them from the ground up. Now someone is telling you not to worry about roots and origins. Just take the pills and you'll feel better. Can it be so simple?

The thought of someone recommending a mood-altering drug may trigger associations with drug pushers, to whom you have been advised to "just say no." So why should you react differently to a doctor who urges antidepressant medications? For several reasons: Recreational drugs are taken in an uncontrolled way to change the mood of the moment, inducing an immediate high. They are addictive, and withdrawal is generally very difficult, often resulting in serious symptoms, including crashing depressions. Antidepressant drugs do not generally cause an immediate high, nor are they addictive, though they should not generally be stopped abruptly as this can result in unpleasant discontinuation symptoms (see p. 214). Recreational drugs often require increasing amounts to get the same mood-altering effect; not so with antidepressants. Once the desired dosage is reached, it is often possible to keep it constant for the duration of treatment.

Some people may feel that taking an antidepressant is the easy way out, an evasion of responsibility for uncovering the cause of a problem and rooting it out. This idea can actually be harmful as it readily triggers thoughts that you are somehow to blame for the depression and responsible for fixing it yourself. This way of thinking plays into the guilt that so often bedevils those afflicted by depression and runs counter to the modern understanding that clinical depression is an illness involving disturbed brain biochemistry.

Many people are afraid that an antidepressant will change them for the worse. This rarely happens. Rather, most people feel that the antidepressant allows them to be their best self. In the minority who experience unwelcome changes, for example a decrease in their range of emotions, the antidepressant can simply be changed or withdrawn.

One reason it may be difficult to accept the medical model of depression is that there is no good laboratory test for it. We have to depend on the patient's history for diagnosis, which in the case of SAD is much easier to make than in other depressions, both because of the seasonal history and because of the reactivity to changes in environmental light. Invest some time and energy in finding a good doctor who will take your SAD symptoms seriously and knows his or her medications. Consult with your doctor about which medication will be best for you, using the rest of this chapter as a guide in this discussion.

Many people are concerned about how long they will have to remain on medications. This is easier to predict for patients with SAD than for those with other forms of depression because SAD is usually a self-limiting condition. When summer comes, symptoms generally resolve. In some cases, however, medications may be helpful even in the summertime. Another concern that I have heard from time to time is a fear that antidepressant medications will cause some permanent change in, or damage to, the person who takes them. Fortunately, chronic side effects are rare, and there is no evidence whatsoever that any long-term damage to the brain occurs. In fact, some studies suggest that long-term antidepressant use may actually protect brain cells against the damage that can occur as a result of chronic untreated depression.

Side Effects of Medications

Concerns about side effects are common and valid. People vary greatly in their propensity to develop side effects. On one end of the spectrum is the individual who develops none at all; on the other end is the person who develops them toward a host of different antidepressants at dosages so low that no beneficial effects are possible. Because of this wide variability, many psychiatrists choose to start with low dosages of the medication of choice and to build up after seeing how well the patient tolerates it.

The side effects of antidepressant medications differ from drug to drug and are discussed at greater length under each specific heading. For many antidepressants, common side effects include sedation, weight gain, dizziness, sexual difficulties, and a cluster of symptoms known as *anticholinergic side effects*—such as constipation, dry mouth, urinary retention, and blurred vision.

Recently there has been a great deal of publicity about the development of suicidal ideas in children shortly after they begin taking antidepressants. In the early weeks after starting a new antidepressant, the neurotransmitters are in flux, which presumably accounts for the infrequently observed instances of disturbed thinking, such as suicidal ideas, that can get activated before the antidepressants start to work. This relatively rare effect of antidepressants has been observed for decades, long before the new generation of antidepressants entered the market. Yet it has recently caused sufficient concern that the FDA has issued a so-called "black box" warning concerning the use of antidepressants in children. The "black box" is a highlighted area on the package insert designed to prevent this potentially serious side effect from getting lost in the fine print. If suicidal thoughts, or any other disturbing thoughts for that matter, should develop off or on medications, be sure to communicate them to your doctor without delay. It usually takes a couple of weeks at the proper dosage before an antidepressant begins to show its effect.

Remember that sudden discontinuation of most antidepressants can have unpleasant effects, including abnormal dreams, "pins and needles," dizziness, mood changes, irritability, strange sensations, and recurrence of depression, to name just a few of many possible symptoms. For some antidepressants, those that leave the system quickly, this may be more of a problem than for others. I suggest that you discuss the question of discontinuation with your doctor ahead of time. Also, be sure not to stop your antidepressants abruptly without consulting your doctor first. When it is desirable to stop an antidepressant, it should be tapered, wherever possible.

The Pros and Cons
of Using Antidepressant Medications

A cost–benefit analysis should certainly be undertaken every time medications are used. What good is this medication likely to do? What
harm might result? In the case of antidepressant medications, this analysis should be a shared process between patient and doctor, perhaps to
an even greater degree than for other forms of medicine. The reason
for this is that many of the symptoms of depression, such as sadness,
guilt, and feelings of low self-worth, are hidden, known only to the patient. The same applies for side effects. The psychiatrist depends
largely on the patient's evaluation of how bad both symptoms and side
effects are. In addition, since the patient has to live with both the
symptoms of the illness and the side effects of the medicine, it seems
only fair that he or she should have the major say in whether to be on
the medications or not and which one to choose.

So where does the psychiatrist fit into the picture? He or she should
educate the patient about the nature of the illness, the available treatment
options, and their potential benefits and possible risks. The psychiatrist
should summarize his or her experience with both the drug and the illness and show how it pertains to the patient's particular situation. Although the psychiatrist cannot know for sure how a drug will work in
any particular case, an explanation should be provided as to why a certain
drug is being chosen over others at a particular time. The patient should
be given an idea as to what effects—both good and bad—the drug might
have and when these effects are likely to occur. In addition, the psychiatrist should explain where the medication fits into the overall game plan
for the treatment of the patient's problems and what other steps will be
taken if it does not work well enough. The patient, in turn, should feel
free to share his or her concerns about the medication, which may be influenced by earlier medication experiences. Ideally the doctor and patient should discuss the pros and cons of the medication together, and
through such a dialogue the best decision is likely to be made.

Although most medications *can* cause a wide array of side effects,
many of these are extremely unusual. In my own practice, I tend to
discuss the commonest side effects of a particular medication and note
that other side effects may occur. I also recommend that my patients
ask their pharmacist for the medication package insert, which they
may or may not choose to read, but which is useful to have if any

questions arise. If while on medications you develop any physical or psychological changes that have not been discussed fully, or about which you feel concerned, you should not hesitate to contact your psychiatrist by phone rather than wait for the next session.

In general, the cost–benefit analysis greatly favors the use of antidepressant medications, especially when depression is moderate to severe, the individual is relatively healthy, and nonmedical alternatives (such as light therapy) seem unlikely to do the job by themselves. In addition, people with seasonal depressions seem to respond well to medications, and I cannot think of one patient with SAD who was not able to be helped to some degree by a combination of light, antidepressant medication, and the other strategies outlined in this book. Despite the benefits of antidepressants, if symptoms can be treated successfully without medications, this course is often preferable.

Medications Commonly Used in SAD

As I have mentioned, antidepressants should be administered only by qualified professionals. The patient's efforts will be well spent in locating and consulting such a professional. Once the doctor has been chosen, it is generally wise to defer to his or her judgment on the best medication to use, but the patient is certainly entitled to an explanation of why that particular drug has been selected and to a discussion of its advantages and disadvantages compared with other possibilities. The discussion in this section is intended to inform you about some of the most useful medications available for the treatment of SAD in particular and depression in general so that you can participate in your doctor's recommended antidepressant treatment regimen in a more informed way. It should not, however, be construed as medical advice, which can be given only by a doctor.

Many different types of medications are available for treating depression. The choice of which drug to use first is an educated guess, based on the available literature, the clinical picture of the patient, and the therapeutic and side-effect profile of the medication. Because there is no scientific method at this time for reliably predicting the best antidepressants for particular patients, administering them often proceeds by trial and error. If the first choice doesn't work, the next should be tried. I have seen some patients who have tried several different drugs without success until we finally hit on the right one. It's a bit like having a large bunch of keys and trying each in turn until you find the one that turns a lock. But once the lock turns, the door opens, and new vistas appear. So it is for the depressed patient who finally feels better and is able to enjoy life once again. It may be helpful to bear this image in mind if the first or second antidepressant fails to deliver its promised effect; otherwise, it is easy to become discouraged and give up prematurely when the next key on the bunch may be the right one.

All antidepressants take time to work. At least three weeks should be allowed after the medication has been administered *in sufficient dosage* before making a judgment about its effectiveness. Because of the wide variation in susceptibility to side effects, psychiatrists often choose to start a medication at a low dose and increase gradually. This precaution obviously increases the time before the medicine can have its full effect. Therefore, in severely depressed people, it may be desirable to start at a higher dose and increase more rapidly. One minor problem with starting at a low dosage is that the final dosage may appear to be huge compared to the initial one, whereas in fact it was the initial one that was very small.

In patients with SAD, antidepressant medications may be used either instead of light therapy or to supplement it. Light therapy may be only partially effective in eradicating the symptoms of SAD, and this partial effect may be enhanced by medications. In addition, if light therapy is used in conjunction with antidepressants, it is often possible to get by with smaller doses and correspondingly fewer side effects. It is often necessary to adjust the dosage with the changing seasons—increasing it as the days become shorter and darker and decreasing it as the days become longer and brighter.

The ABCs of Neurotransmitters

The human brain consists of billions of neurons that communicate with each other at junctions known as *synapses*. At the synapse an electrical message passing along the transmitting neuron causes the release of chemical messengers known as *neurotransmitters* that drift across the space between two neurons and stimulate special receptors on the receiving neuron. That transmits the electrical signal that continues to pass along the neural circuit. So it is that these amazing molecules, *neurotransmitters*, drive the circuits that are responsible for every function mediated by the human brain, including the regulation of our moods. Once released, the neurotransmitters are taken back out into the transmitting neuron (a process called *reuptake*), where they are broken down. Most of our antidepressants work by inhibiting the reuptake of these neurotransmitters, three of which have come under the most prominent scrutiny—serotonin, norepinephrine, and dopamine. A major difference between available antidepressants is their signature pattern of influence on the various neurotransmitters.

Brain neurotransmitter systems govern too many functions to cover in this simple introduction, so I'll mention just a few. Serotonin is important for inducing a calm, good mood and helping to restrain impulses such as displays of bad temper. Dopamine is important for reward pathways, pleasure, attention, and motivation. Norepinephrine increases alertness and energizes. Now that you understand the symptoms of SAD, you can see why all these neurotransmitters might be important in its treatment. Table 7 shows how different available antidepressants affect different neurotransmitters. A few of these antidepressants are described below in greater detail.

Wellbutrin (Bupropion)

This drug is thought to work by influencing dopamine and norepinephrine. It comes in three different forms: immediate release (IR), sustained release (SR), and the new once-a-day extended release (XL). The first two versions, which require multiple daily dosing, are available in generic form, the last one only in brand name. The large SAD prevention study mentioned earlier in this chapter used the XL form of the drug.

Advantages of Wellbutrin are that it is energizing and not associated with weight gain, sexual side effects, lethargy, or sedation. It may be particularly helpful when lethargy and sluggishness are a prominent part of the picture. Side effects in the SAD studies included dry mouth, nausea, constipation, flatulence, and weight loss, which occurred in a small proportion of people taking the drug. An uncommon but disturbing side effect is the occurrence of seizures. Therefore, people with a history of seizures would be advised to avoid this drug.

Selective Serotonin Reuptake Inhibitors (SSRIs)

- Prozac (fluoxetine), Zoloft (sertraline), Paxil (paroxetine), Luvox (fluvoxamine), Celexa (citalopram), and Lexapro (escitalopram)

As their name implies, these antidepressants work by selectively inhibiting the reuptake of serotonin. They are extremely popular for treating depression in general. Evidence suggests that they are also effective

TABLE 7
Brief Overview of Antidepressants

Name: Brand (generic)	Neuro- transmitters affected	Potential advantages	Potential disadvantages
Wellbutrin (bupropion)	DA +++ NE ++	Less likely to cause sexual difficulties and weight gain. Can prevent depression if started early in season.	Not as good for anxiety; may increase risk of seizures in vulnerable individuals.

Selective serotonin reuptake inhibitors (SSRIs)

Prozac (fluoxetine)	SE +++		
Zoloft (sertraline)	SE +++	All are effective. Approved for some anxiety disorders as well as depression.	Side effects: Problems with sexual functioning, lethargy, weight gain.
Paxil (paroxetine)	SE +++		
Celexa (citalopram)	SE +++		
Luvox (fluvoxamine)	SE +++		

Serotonin and norepinephrine reuptake inhibitors (SNRIs)

Effexor (venlafaxine)	SE ++ NE ++	Approved for treatment of some anxiety disorders as well as depression.	Can cause increased blood pressure and some SSRI-type side effects.
Cymbalta (duloxetine)	SE ++ NE ++	May be helpful when there are physical symptoms of depression.	Can cause nausea, dry mouth, drowsiness, constipation, and insomnia.

Tricyclic antidepressants

Tofranil (imipramine)	SE ++ NE ++	All tricyclics are effective and may help anxiety as well as depression. Their sleep-inducing side effects can initially be an advantage for those with insomnia.	Tricyclics often have more side effects than modern antidepressants. These include dry mouth, constipation, blurred vision, fatigue, and weight gain. Dangerous in overdose.
Anafranil (chlorimipramine)	SE +++ NE +		
Elavil (amitriptyline)	SE ++ NE ++		
Norpramin (desipramine)	NE +++ SE +		
Pamelor/Aventyl (nortriptyline)	SE ++ NE ++		

Note. SE = serotonin; NE = norepinephrine; DA = dopamine; + = slight; ++ = moderate; +++ = marked.

for treating winter depressions in patients with SAD. There is no evidence that one of these is superior to any other in general, although in particular individuals one may prove to be better than others. Several of these are now available in generic form. They are particularly good when anxiety is a prominent part of the picture. Advantages include a low level of the type of side effects that bedeviled earlier antidepressants, such as constipation and dry mouth. Disadvantages include sexual side effects, fatigue, a sense of flattened emotions, and weight gain. These affect only some people taking these drugs, whereas others are lucky and experience no side effects at all. Sexual side effects may include decreased desire and greater difficulties with arousal and achieving orgasm.

Combined Serotonin and Norepinephrine Reuptake Inhibitors (SNRIs)

• Effexor (venlafaxine) and Cymbalta (duloxetine)

These drugs influence both serotonin and norepinephrine transmission. Effexor is available in both an immediate and extended release (XR) preparation. Effexor has been approved for some anxiety disorders as well as for depression. Cymbalta, the latest arrival on the antidepressant scene as of the time of writing, is given in a once- or twice-a-day dosage. Common side effects of Effexor include activation, sedation, increased blood pressure, sleep disruption, and sexual side effects. Common side effects of Cymbalta include nausea, dry mouth, drowsiness, constipation, and insomnia. In addition, Cymbalta might be harmful to the liver in those who drink excessively.

Tricyclic Antidepressants (TCAs)

• Norpramin (desipramine), Tofranil (imipramine), Pamelor (nortriptyline), and Elavil (amitriptyline)

These old workhorses date all the way back to the 1950s and for years were almost the only antidepressants available. They were superseded by the SSRIs and other modern drugs because they had many troublesome side effects such as dry mouth, constipation, blurred vision, seizures, and slowed-down conduction of electrical signals in the heart. If taken in overdose, they are far more dangerous than more modern drugs, and such overdoses can be fatal. Despite these problems, they remain useful drugs when newer ones are unable to do the job for one reason or another. In practice, though, I rarely use these medications for people with SAD.

Combining Antidepressants with Light Therapy

In clinical practice, I often find that using medications together with light therapy has its advantages. First, the combination is often more effective than either of the treatments administered alone. Second, it is often possible to get away with lower dosages of medications—and therefore fewer side effects—if light therapy is used as well. Finally, it may be possible to get away with less time in front of the lights if they are used together with medications.

A possible disadvantage of this combined strategy is that the treatments may accentuate each other's side effects. For example, a person may be more likely to experience hypomanic symptoms if on a combination of light therapy and medications than on either treatment alone. Although some experts have raised the possible concern that antidepressants may sensitize the eyes to light in a potentially harmful way, I have never heard of such an event occurring even though these treatments have been used together for more than twenty years.

Sara's Story: Throwing the Kitchen Sink at It

Every now and then I encounter a patient with SAD whose symptoms are either so severe or so resistant to simple remedies that every measure has to be taken to overcome them. You have to throw the kitchen sink at the problem. Sara was such a person.

Sara was a psychiatric nurse in her late thirties, married and without children, who lived and worked in rural Massachusetts. She had suffered from problems with the winter since she was seventeen years old and had received help for them in the form of psychotherapy and numerous medications, which helped to only a small degree.

Life became much more difficult for Sara in the two years before she consulted me, starting with a serious depression that occurred, quite uncharacteristically, during the summer shortly after she quit smoking. At first I wondered whether nicotine withdrawal might have triggered the depression, but on closer questioning it emerged that the nurses who smoked would get the chance to take those patients who were smokers out into the sunshine for frequent smoke breaks. Non-smokers like Sara, on the other hand, were required to remain indoors on a dark psychiatric ward for long hours and had little access to bright natural light. Sara remained depressed through the summer, into the next fall and winter, and was still depressed when I saw her at the end of the second summer.

What followed was an extensive series of interventions to help free Sara of her depressions. She kept a careful log of her moods so that we could accurately evaluate the effects of these interventions. Light therapy (10,000 lux for up to one and a half hours per day) plus regular aerobic exercise didn't help much. After a month I prescribed Prozac, and a few days later she went to Florida on a week's vacation. For the first time in months, her mood moved into the normal range. On her return, we increased her light treatment to two hours per day, one hour in the morning and one hour in the evening. She remained in reasonably good spirits until December, when her depression once again became a problem.

I raised her Prozac dosage and reminded her to keep exercising. Within a few weeks she was feeling somewhat better again, but that didn't last for long. In December she went down to Mexico on vacation and her depression lifted, only to return shortly after she returned home. She hooked a bright bedside lamp up to a timer, which she set to go on an hour before she was due to wake up in the morning. In addition, she worked at increasing the brightness of her indoor lighting both at work and at home. Although she managed to keep working, she suffered from fatigue and depressed mood, and winter felt like one long chore. Finally, in March of the next year, for the first time in over two years, she switched out of her depression in a solid way and we were able to discontinue all forms of treatment, including medications.

Given the serious difficulties that Sara had suffered despite multiple treatment interventions, she and I began to discuss strategies to minimize her SAD symptoms the next winter. I recommended that she purchase a dawn simulator and a portable light box, which would give her more flexibility and control over her environmental light the following winter. We brought her husband, an extremely supportive and understanding man, into our therapy sessions so that he would be involved in all discussions about plans that might affect him, as well as provide suggestions of his own. Sara decided to plan several brief trips to Florida as a "safety net" for the forthcoming winter when the depression became too bad. Not only did this strategy prove extremely valuable, but just knowing that the plan was in place was a great comfort. We also used the summer to work in psychotherapy on some traumatic experiences that Sara had suffered in early adulthood. Free of depression, she was able to obtain some relief from the burden of these painful experiences.

Sara began to feel depressed again in early August, and I started to treat her with a combination of light therapy (one to two hours per day) and Prozac, in escalating dosage. She exercised regularly and began to use a dawn simulator in an attempt to hold the time of dawn constant as the days became shorter. By mid-December her depression deepened once again and was severe enough to warrant the addition of Wellbutrin to the Prozac. On a combination of light therapy (two hours per day), daily aerobic exercise, Prozac, and Wellbutrin at maximum dosages, she felt reasonably well and was able to continue to work and to deal with issues in her psychotherapy. One of these issues was her need to learn to take good care of herself, especially given the stress of her serious SAD symptoms.

She did use her planned time away to good effect, and the three one-week vacations, scheduled for December, January, and February, all significantly lifted her spirits. She was able to tell her husband just how bad she felt at times during the winter, and he began to appreciate their need to make major lifestyle changes to accommodate her problem. Together they chose a community in Florida to which they relocated. Since Sara has lived in Florida, her moods have been considerably better, and she has never expressed a word of regret about her choice to leave her home, family, and friends for sunnier climes.

I have deliberately included a story of someone who has found neither a quick nor an easy path to recovery. I can think of several other people who, like Sara, have needed to combine multiple types of treatments, including relocation, to conquer their winter depressions. Despite these efforts and sacrifices, or rather because of them, almost everybody can resolve the problem of winter depression one way or another. The message of Sara's story for those of you out there whose path to recovery has also been difficult is "don't despair." There are all kinds of things that can help, either individually or in combination, and I recommend that you try different approaches at the advice and under the supervision of a qualified professional. Keep well informed and up to date on the latest research developments. Even if you don't completely overcome your SAD symptoms this winter, who knows what new discoveries next winter will bring?

To summarize, find a psychiatrist or other doctor with experience in the medical treatment of SAD. Discuss all your concerns about medications with him or her and decide together on the best medication for you. The choice of the right medicine is an educated guess, and if one does not work, the next one may or combinations of different treatments should be considered. If you have a regular history of troublesome winter depressions, consider asking your doctor to start you on Wellbutrin XL before you develop your fall symptoms. The outlines provided in this chapter are just descriptions of the effects these drugs may have and of my own experience with them; they are not intended as recommendations. It's important to remember that antidepressants frequently work well in patients with SAD in conjunction with light therapy and other treatments, allowing smaller doses of medications to be used.

ELEVEN

A Step-by-Step Guide
Through the Revolving Year

So far, we have considered the effects of the seasons in a number of ways, but there is one critical aspect that is worth bearing in mind if you are to understand the seasons and their effects on you. With some variation from year to year, the seasons revolve in a certain predictable rhythm, and we reflect these changes in our responses, which are also predictable to some extent. In this chapter, I examine these predictable changes and encourage you to do the same, examining your year as a whole and planning accordingly. Forewarned is forearmed, as they say, and nowhere is this more true than in understanding the predictable cycle of your seasonal changes.

When we think of the changing seasons, many different images come to mind. One image that has stayed with me since my colleagues and I published the first description of the syndrome of SAD is that of a staircase. We asked the first nineteen patients with SAD studied at the NIMH to think back over the course of their seasonal problems and note the months when they typically experienced their winter symptoms. Figure 9, reproduced from the initial publication that resulted from that study, illustrates when that first group of patients experienced their symptoms in relation to the daylength in Rockville, Maryland, which is at the latitude where the study occurred.

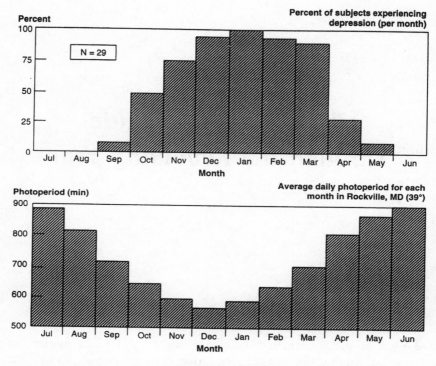

FIGURE 9. Relationship between symptoms of SAD and length of day (photoperiod). From Rosenthal et al. (1984). This figure is in the public domain.

As you can see, some difficulties began in September, and the frequency of symptoms rose progressively over the next four months, reaching a peak in January, remaining high in February and March, and then declining sharply in April and May. There is a correspondence between the frequency of symptoms and daylength, with symptoms increasing as daylength decreases toward the winter solstice and the reverse occurring as the days lengthen once again. I have often thought of the lower part of the graph as a staircase leading downward, with my mood—and that of my patients—declining with the waning light and then leading upward again as mood improves with the return of the sun. If you look at the graph carefully, you will note that there is not an exact correspondence between daylength and symptom frequency. Symptoms remain at high levels through January and February even though the days are getting longer through those months. We believe this happens because January and February are very dark and cloudy months, at least in Maryland, and even though the days are getting longer, the actual amount of sunlight to which people are exposed is often at its lowest after the winter solstice.

It is helpful to consider the typical progression of the symptoms of SAD using this image of a staircase. Although people differ as to when they get their symptoms over the course of the year—and indeed what symptoms they get—a very typical progression is shown in Figure 10.

As you can see, problems with mood do not usually occur early in the progression. Instead, the earliest problems usually involve sleep and energy difficulties, followed by appetite and weight changes, problems with concentrating, and reduced sex drive and socializing. It is often only after these changes are under way that people begin to feel depressed, anxious, and irritable.

Whenever I see a patient with SAD in consultation, one of the first things that I do is establish the pattern of his or her annual cycle. When do the first symptoms occur? What are these symptoms, and how do they progress through the revolving seasons? When does he or she begin to emerge from the depression, and what are the other seasons like? Establishing such a pattern helps me and my patient plan for the coming year and try to ensure that it is less troublesome and more enjoyable than the previous one.

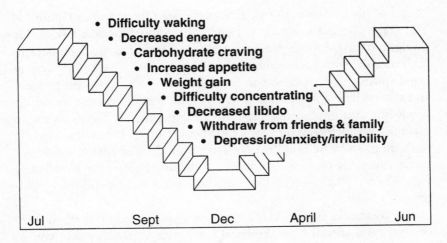

FIGURE 10. Symptoms of SAD.

One such patient is a man named Keith, a social scientist in his late thirties, who came to me about a year ago with a history of SAD going back at least twenty-two years. Trained in economics and law at the finest Ivy League universities, it is curious that he went so long without recognizing the nature of his problem and seeking help for it. He attributes this delay to two factors. First, he had a friend, a woman with debilitating SAD, who would routinely gain ten to twelve pounds each winter, sleep ten to twelve hours a day, and suffer tremendously from debilitating symptoms of SAD. He contrasted the relative mildness of his own symptoms with hers and failed to recognize that they were suffering from the same condition, but with different manifestations. Second, he had been strongly influenced by psychological and sociological schools of thought, which seek to explain behavior as a result of human interactions rather than a biological effect of the physical world.

Once Keith was able to make the paradigm shift from a psychological to a biological model, however, he applied his intellect to understanding his problem and communicated this to me in a way that was so illuminating and compelling that I have chosen his story to illustrate the predictable effects of the changing seasons on our minds and our bodies.

The History of Your Annual Cycle

In one of his first visits to me, Keith produced the graph in Figure 11. The graph shows the typical pattern of his annual mood changes. He thought back over the previous ten years and assigned numbers to each month, with higher numbers corresponding to when he was in good spirits, lower numbers to when he was in his depressed periods, and the midline corresponding to when he was in an even mood. In producing this graph, he created a valuable template for us to use in planning his forthcoming year's treatment. In fact, I first saw Keith in the spring, and based on the graph, we both decided that it would not be necessary for us to meet until the following September after Labor Day, when we would plan his course of action for the following winter.

If you suffer from SAD, I encourage you to map out the history of your own annual cycle. Figure 12 provides a grid that asks you to rate your mood for each month over the last five years. If you can't re-

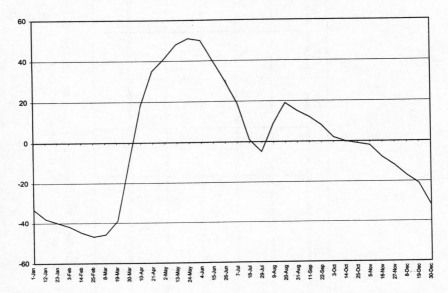

FIGURE 11. A typical profile of Keith's moods over the course of the year.

member that far back, three years will probably do just fine. If you have moved to a different latitude or climatic region in the last few years, the exercise may be less reliable since your seasonal pattern of mood and behavior will tend to change with latitude and climate. Once you have put numbers in all the squares of the grid, you should average the numbers for each month and enter them in the graph provided in Figure 13. That will give you a picture of your own annual cycle, which will help you plan out the coming year.

I recommend that you purchase a special journal or calendar for the year and mark in it some of the key points in your own annual cycle: when your mood begins to slide, when it crosses the midline, when it reaches its low point, when it begins to recover, and so on. As we look further into the predictable changes that the year brings, there will be other days and dates that you might want to mark on this calendar and that may help you with your planning. Be sure that there is room in the journal for you to make notes as well.

Once you understand your own seasonal pattern, you can consider how to incorporate the treatments described in earlier chapters into an overall treatment plan. The general principles of treatment are as follows:

Scale: +50 = The best I've ever felt
         0 = Even mood
       -50 = The worst I've ever felt

	Year	July	Aug.	Sept.	Oct.	Nov.	Dec.	Jan.	Feb.	Mar.	April	May	June
Last year													
2 years ago													
3 years ago													
4 years ago													
5 years ago													
Average													

FIGURE 12. A grid to help you develop numbers to graph your seasonal profile. From *Winter Blues*. Copyright 2006 by Norman E. Rosenthal. Permission to photocopy this figure is granted to purchasers of this book for personal use only (see copyright page for details).

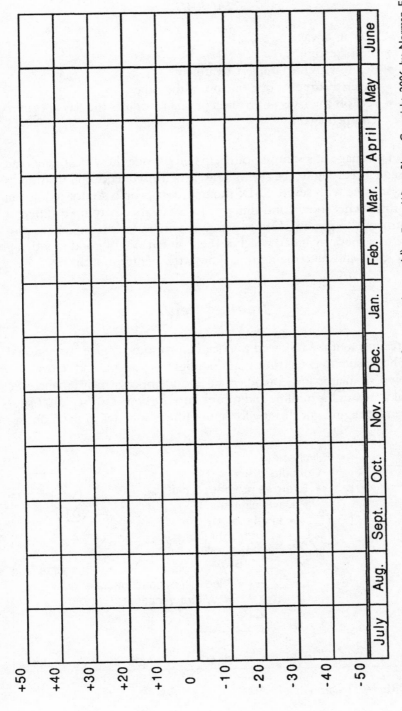

FIGURE 13. A picture of your seasonal profile (use average from previous grid). From *Winter Blues*. Copyright 2006 by Norman E. Rosenthal. Permission to photocopy this figure is granted to purchasers of this book for personal use only (see copyright page for details).

- Plan in advance.
- Start treating early.
- Begin with the simplest treatment.
- Layer treatments one on top of the other.
- Peel off the layers of treatment one by one as the days begin to lengthen again.

The image of a staircase can help you consider how treatments can be sequenced. Figure 14 shows how I might sequence the treatments for someone with severe SAD, though most people do not require all the treatments shown and differ as to when they may need different treatments. In general, I try to get away with as little treatment as possible to achieve my goal, which is the maintenance of good mood, energy level, and functioning throughout the winter months.

Treating Keith

In treating Keith, I followed the diagram to some degree. I suggested that he be sure to get as much outdoor light as possible and start to use a dawn simulator in September. In mid-October, which is where he usually crosses his midline and moves into the depressed region, I suggested he begin light therapy for about fifteen minutes in the morning

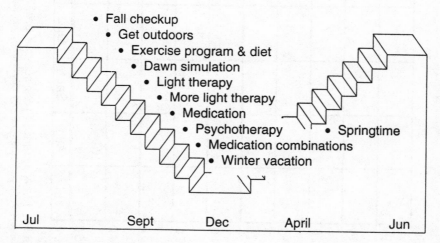

FIGURE 14. Treatment of SAD.

and fifteen minutes in the evening. It had an immediate effect of buoy-
ing him up, making him feel safe and warm. It also made him "very
jumpy." Within a few minutes of starting therapy, his pulse went up to
ninety beats per minute, his nasal passages dried up, and he developed
headaches, but after two weeks these side effects stabilized and he fell
into a more comfortable pattern of using the light. It is quite unusual
to experience such marked side effects so quickly after starting light
therapy.

This is how Keith describes the first winter of using lights.

On the one hand, mentally and emotionally I deployed all my
emotional reserve to prepare for the onslaught of winter—all
the signs were there—my memories of these winters were so
profound that I spent a good deal of the fall on guard. On the
whole, I had the sense that I still dipped and declined, still
slipped behind and coasted for a while—though it was not a
depression but a recession, as an economist would say. But all
the while I felt that there was a lifeline, that I was wearing a
harness, a climber's rope—that if I fell, there would be a stop
to the fall that would catch me a long time before I hit bottom—that there was a safety net.

Many of the symptoms returned in kind but to a lesser
degree. Tastes definitely changed—both musical and food
tastes—but I never became monotonic. I don't believe I ever
had trouble getting out of bed during the winter. I used a
dawn simulator; more important, I think, I opened the shutters at night for the first time in twenty years. But the dawn
simulator has been a balm. Many times I would wake up before the alarm, which would have been inconceivable in years
past.

This winter I had to be in charge of the most high-profile
and stressful piece of work in my life, the preparation of
which coincided with what have been the traditionally worst
weeks of my life—from the first weeks of November to the
middle of February—and I never faltered. Without treatment
I would still have managed but would have had no energy for
anything else; that was not the case this year. I managed to
get to the movies, go to parties, and even host a dinner party.

There were a couple of bad spells, but I could almost always link those to not having done the lights for several days

or critically depleting my energy through inadequate sleep or excessive stress.

The one thing that was very much absent this year was the feeling of being trapped in a tunnel and the sense that time has significantly prolonged itself. It felt as though May was a world away in the past; this year that long stretching out of time—to the point of feeling that every day did not get you closer to the spring—did not happen. The year kept its shape.

I remember waking up on a Saturday in early January, looking at the calendar, seeing that February ended on a Saturday, and thinking to myself, "Eight weeks; all right, here we go," and being surprised at how fast the time went.

Predictable Markers of the Revolving Year and What You Can Do About Them

Although the year has a certain rhythm to it, the exact nature of that rhythm will differ from person to person and, to some extent, from year to year. Take some time to think about your year as a whole and note the important markers: points when you can expect seasonal effects as well as predictable events such as when you plan to take your vacation; when the children get out of school, go off to summer camp, or come home from college; deadlines; and major life events or stresses. You might want to record these in your journal or calendar so that you can be sure to take them into account when you plan your year.

Summertime

In the words of the haunting Gershwin tune, the living is often easy during the summertime. To be sure, some people have predictable summer difficulties, and this may not be as exhilarating a time as spring or fall. If you look over Keith's annual profile, you will see a small downward notch in midsummer. Writers and artists also report that summer is a less creative time for them than spring or autumn, according to Dr. Kay Redfield Jamison, who has studied the subject of creativity and its relationship to mood disorders. Some people suffer from summer depressions, others from summer hypomania, and yet others do not emerge completely from their winter depression when summer arrives. But for most of us, summer is a carefree time, when we want to get away, to play and forget that winter was ever here and will ever come back again. But for those of us who, like the fabled grasshopper, would like to play all summer long, here are some pointers that could come in handy when the dark days of winter arrive.

- Don't spend all your vacation time during the summer. Save at least some of it for the winter, when you will need it more.
- If you have a major task to undertake, such as changing your job, moving house or moving to another city, do so in the summer, when you have more energy.
- If you do move in summer, check to make sure that your new house, apartment, or office is well illuminated all year round. It might be bright during the summer but dark as a dungeon during the winter.
- This might be a good time to plan for the winter, though in reality most people wait until the end of summer to do so.

September—The Beginning of Fall

Labor Day is often a reliable marker of the beginning of fall, in the culture and the natural world, even though the formal beginning of the season is the autumnal equinox some two to three weeks later. In September, some people are beginning to feel the onset of their winter symptoms—changes in appetite, sleep patterns, or energy level—while others are still fine at this time.

No matter how mild or severe your winter difficulties may be, I almost always recommend that people undergo a fall checkup. It is a good opportunity to do the following:

- Purchase necessary lighting equipment. If the light tubes in a light box are old, consider replacing them.
- Put your exercise and dietary program in place.
- Do what you can to keep predictable stresses to a manageable level over the winter.
- Plan one or more winter breaks in a southern place—if feasible and affordable.
- Inform family members, friends, and, when appropriate, colleagues or associates that you are soon going to enter your less

sociable season and become less dynamic than you have been during the summer. Engage their support ahead of time where appropriate. Obviously judgment needs to be exercised in deciding when it would be helpful for others at work to be informed about your seasonal difficulties and when you are better off keeping this to yourself.

- Consider consulting appropriate professionals—such as a therapist, physician, or dietitian—so that they are on board at the beginning of the winter season.
- Get outdoors and enjoy the beauty that nature has to offer at this time of year.
- Be sure to keep your bedroom shades up and your shutters open so that you can benefit from the first rays of morning sunlight.
- It is often a good time to start using your dawn simulator to offset the effects of the shortening days. The autumnal equinox is that time of year when days are shortening most rapidly.
- A special note for parents and homemakers: Look ahead to the section on December that follows and also see the suggestions about stress management on page 181. Make a list of things that need to be done for the holidays and do as much as possible ahead of time. This can include purchasing, writing, and addressing cards; assembling decorations for the Christmas tree or buying Hanukkah candles; buying gifts early; or informing people that this holiday season is going to be a bit different from others (that is, it will involve less work for you).

October and the Daylight Savings Time Change

In the North, October is a variable month. There are still some fine days, but winter is beginning to assert itself. Like Keith, many patients with SAD need to start using their light box during this month. I usually recommend that people start with short durations of light exposure—for example, fifteen minutes once or twice a day. As the month progresses, this duration may need to be increased, but it is always wise to use your own internal state as a guide to determine how much light is right for you.

The last week in October is when the clocks are usually set back an hour, a transition that often causes difficulties for people with SAD. For them, the extra hour of darkness in the evening is a heavy price to pay for the extra hour of light in the morning, which they are often unable to benefit from fully since they are generally asleep or indoors at that hour. At this time it may be useful to:

- Increase the amount of evening light therapy to deal with the extra hour of darkness at that time while continuing to use light therapy in the morning.
- Consider writing your holiday cards and doing some of your holiday shopping and planning, before you feel overwhelmed by the effects of the short, dark days.
- Consider doing bulk shopping for nonperishable goods to save yourself the effort later on.

November

> Whenever I find myself growing grim about the mouth;
> whenever it is a damp, drizzly November in my soul;
> whenever I find myself involuntarily pausing before coffin
> warehouses, and bringing up the rear of every funeral I meet;
> and especially whenever my hypos get such an upper hand of
> me, that it requires a strong moral principle to prevent me
> from knocking people's hats off—then, I account it high time
> to get to sea as soon as I can.
>
> —HERMAN MELVILLE, *Moby Dick*

In the northern United States and northern Europe, November seems to be the month when people with SAD really begin to feel bad. Their general sentiments toward this month were well expressed by Henry Adams, the famous chronicler of American life, who wrote to Charles Milnes Gaskell from Washington, DC, in November 1869:

Dear Boy:

I sit down to begin you a letter, not because I have received one since my last, but because it is one of the dankest, foggiest, and dismalest of November nights, and, as usual when the sun does not shine, I am as out of sorts as a man may haply be, and yet live through it. . . . This season of the year grinds the very soul out of me. My nerves lose their tone, my teeth ache, and my courage falls to the bottomless bottom of infinitude. Death stalks about me, and the whole of Gray's grisly train, and I am afraid of them, not because life is an object, but because my nerves are upset. I would give up all my pleasures willingly if I could only be a mouse, and sleep three months at a time. Well! one can't have life as one would, but if I ever take too much laudanum, the coroner's jury may bring in a verdict of willful murder against the month of November.

Recently a coroner in England did in fact bring in a verdict of murder against the month of November, or rather, the cause of death was given as SAD. The victim was an Englishwoman who had just returned to England in November from a vacation in some sunny place, when she became overwhelmed by symptoms of severe SAD, which drove her to suicide. It is always hard to think about someone taking his or her own life, but this is especially so when the condition driving the person to such extremes is completely treatable. No one should have to feel so cornered by SAD that suicide appears to be the only way out.

The following guidelines may help steer you through this difficult month.

• By now, most people need light therapy regularly. While the daily duration of therapy needed is variable, it is not at all unusual for people to need thirty to forty-five minutes in the morning and the evening.

• Be sure to maintain your exercise program. If you let it slip now, it may be hard to retrieve it through the rest of the winter. Light therapy will help you stick to your exercise routine.

• You may require medications at this time, but check with your doctor before starting them. I do not recommend, for example, that you simply pick up last year's medicine bottle and start taking the leftovers, calling your doctor only when you have run out of medications.

• Watch out for holiday foods and eating patterns. Once the weight tends to creep on this early in the season, it can career out of control in the months to come. See Chapter 8 for more information about this.

December and the Holiday Season

A person with SAD will often experience mixed feelings about December and the holiday season. It is no coincidence, of course, that major holidays, such as Christmas and Hanukkah, occur around the winter solstice and involve the kindling of light—the Yule log, the Hanukkah menorah, the Christmas tree. Rituals of renewal at the approach of the New Year, prayers for the return of the sun, and the need for holiday cheer, which is enhanced by illumination, feasting, and drinking, come together in the modern celebration of the winter festivals as they have for centuries. Even as people with SAD may struggle to keep up with the chores and expectations that attend the holidays, so their spirits may be buoyed up by the great carnival that overtakes our society at this time of year.

From the vantage point of the declining light, all the same principles that operated in November continue and all the same advice applies. Fortunately, less is often expected of people at work during the holidays, which can be a great relief to someone suffering from SAD. On the other hand, it can be a difficult season for homemakers, who not only have many additional chores and duties associated with the holidays but also feel an extra sense of responsibility for creating a convivial and joyous atmosphere. When one is feeling fatigued, withdrawn, and sad, that is a particularly tall order.

Advice to Homemakers Who Struggle with the Winter Holidays

• Now is the time to benefit from some of the plans put in place earlier in the season (see September, p. 235).

• Explain to your family why this season is difficult for someone with SAD; that you will be able to do only a limited number of things toward making the holidays special. Enlist their help and support. Remind yourself and them that what is really special about the holidays is being together and enjoying one another's company. Sometimes this is easiest to do and works best if the holiday season is kept relatively simple.

• Consider not making the winter festival the one when you do most of the work; for example, you might make less fuss over Christmas or Hanukkah and put on an extra-good Easter egg hunt or have Passover at your place next spring.

• Get as much help as possible. For example, maybe there is a service that delivers a Christmas tree to you. Paying someone to help clean the house at this time may be the best holiday gift you can give yourself. Divide up the work and organize the family to do different chores.

- Consider going to a restaurant for at least one of the Christmas meals.
- Actively work on not feeling guilty; remember, you never asked to get SAD.
- Consider increasing the amount of light therapy or other treatments you are receiving to help you get over the holiday season.

Travel Over the Holidays

If you need to leave home for more than a day or two from December through February, it is usually very important to take your light therapy apparatus (dawn simulator, light box, or light visor) with you. You will probably bridle at the inconvenience, but believe me, in most cases it is well worth it.

Despite his reservations, one young man with SAD decided to take his light box with him to his fiancée's home over the Christmas break. He found his fiancée's family to be interested and accepting of his predicament, and more important, he was able to enjoy his time with her and with them.

One problem with successful treatment of SAD is that you can easily forget that you have the condition at all. I have made this error myself, most recently and egregiously on a trip to Tromsö, a city north of the Arctic Circle, where I was to chair a conference on SAD during the depths of winter. I thought that I could manage without the lights for the three or four days of the trip and arrived in the city during its legendary dark days when the sun does not rise above the horizon. The very day I arrived there, I felt the energy drain out of my system, like blood running out of my veins, and all I wanted to do was to lie on my bed and stare at the ceiling.

The conference organizers informed me that it would be a day or more before they could have a light box sent in, and I was fortunate to be bailed out by Jennifer Eastwood, head of the SAD Association of Great Britain (SADA), a presenter at the conference who had made all the necessary arrangements to have a light box installed in her room from day one. This she was gracious enough to share with me. As I sat in front of the box, I felt energy returning to me within the hour and all of a sudden was buzzing with excitement at being in this famous northern city at a conference devoted exclusively to SAD and its treatments.

The moral of the story is: If I can forget my light box in a place and at a time when I desperately needed it, so can you. Don't deny the extent of your SAD symptoms and forget the degree to which you are being buoyed up by your light therapy (as I did), and be sure to see that you have adequate light exposure when you travel (advice I have every intention of taking myself in future).

The Holiday Blues and SAD

For therapists in clinical practice it is not unusual to see some feelings of sadness around the time of the holidays. Although this is a time when people are supposed to be happy, and many are, for some, the expected happiness does not arrive. Lonely people, people without family or friends, and people who grew up in dysfunctional families and have unpleasant associations with the holidays simply can't achieve the ideal that many commercial images of the holidays portray. Obviously, having SAD can only increase the suffering of people who also feel the holiday blues.

How can you tell which problem is plaguing you? The holiday blues are really quite distinct from SAD in that people with SAD are suffering from a clinical depression that arises largely from their special biology, whereas the holiday blues involve sadness that arises out of psychological conflicts. SAD typically lasts for several months, whereas the holiday blues are usually confined to the holiday season. Finally, patients with SAD typically experience a variety of physical changes— for example, in eating, sleeping, energy level, and daily functioning. There is no evidence that most people reacting to Christmas or the holidays show these changes.

Although a number of studies have tried to document the holiday blues by examining, for example, the frequency of visits to the emergency room for psychiatric help, or admissions to psychiatric units during the holiday season, it has proven to be an elusive entity to nail down. In fact, one study showed that presentations to psychiatric emergency rooms decreased in the few days before major holidays and increased in the few days after them. It is as though people did not want to spoil their holiday by going to the emergency room, so they waited until the holiday was over before doing so.

Despite the absence of studies demonstrating the existence of the holiday blues, they certainly do exist. I have never been more aware of this than during one holiday season when I was asked to participate in a radio program about the holiday blues along with a few other professionals. The radio station typically played music that appealed to a teenage audience, which might have accounted for why those who called in were predominantly teenagers. Many of them had heartbreaking stories, of being alone over the holidays, of not having the kind of holidays they imagined other families to have, of broken relationships, and other sources of grief, experienced with the intensity that is perhaps unique to adolescence. Hearing these stories one after the other was quite moving. I was impressed in particular by one young caller who described the great pain and hardship in her life around the holidays. During a commercial break, one of my colleagues on the show acknowledged that the young lady in distress was in fact her daughter. She said sadly that she had tried to do whatever she could to help her through the holidays, apparently to no avail. I was left with a feeling of how complex and difficult the holiday blues can be—sometimes for the whole family.

There is no reason, of course, why people might not suffer from both SAD and the holiday blues. As I have noted, the many chores and activities that surround the holidays pose a burden to those suffering from SAD. In addition, since SAD often runs in families, the holiday season may trigger memories of a parent who was unable to cope at that time of year and might have done so by withdrawing, being mean-spirited, or getting drunk.

If the holidays are a recurrent source of pain and difficulty for you, I strongly recommend that you seek out a therapist to help anticipate and deal with them, by helping you to understand the basis of your pain and learn how to heal it. Only when that is accomplished can the holidays become a time of genuine celebration. The advice I would give to those who suffer from both the holiday blues and SAD is to look beyond the commercial elements and the duties, chores, and conventional activities that attend the season and attempt to seize the essence of what is great about it—kindness, community, relaxation, and generosity of spirit. Since charity begins at home, you should start by being kind to yourself and not overloading yourself with social and other holiday responsibilities. That is a sure key to being more available to others at this time of year.

Anniversary Reactions

One factor that can affect the way a person feels at any time of year is the anniversary of some sad event that occurred at that time in a person's past. When such an anniversary comes at a season that is already difficult for a particular person, the hardship of the season is compounded.

Freud recognized the existence of so-called anniversary reactions and, in his description of Fraulein Elisabeth von R. (1895), he wrote: "This lady celebrated annual festivals of remembrance at the period of her various catastrophes, and on these occasions her vivid visual reproduction and expressions of feeling kept to the date precisely." Longfellow also recognized the "secret anniversaries of the heart, when the full river of feeling overflows."

In contrast to the symptoms of SAD, these anniversary reactions usually occur around the date of the anniversary and do not typically last for weeks or months. They do make life more difficult, though. One of my patients, a professional woman, would recall the anniversary of her mother's suicide in October many years before. She anticipated her memory of the shocking details for weeks in advance and it quite shook her for much of the month of October. It was very important for this woman to acknowledge and understand the power that this memory continued to have over her as a source of pain that was distinct from her SAD. On the other hand, I have seen people with SAD try to explain their recurrent winter symptoms purely as a reaction to the anniversary of some sad event in the past and this is, of course, an unsatisfactory approach both in terms of accounting for the extent of the symptoms of SAD and in planning a proper treatment plan for them.

- If you know that a certain time of year brings up painful memories, make a note of this date in your journal and planner.
- Let friends, family, and other supportive people know that the date is approaching and seek extra support from them at this time. They probably won't know how difficult the memories are for you unless you tell them.
- Plan activities that help you come to terms with the pain of the memory. For example, you may want to visit a special place that reminds you of a lost loved one in the company of a supportive and loving person.
- Recognize that you might not function as well over the days around the anniversary and cut yourself some slack.
- You will deal best with the anniversary if you acknowledge its power over you, the impact it has on you, and recognize that as the anniversary passes, the pain associated with the memory will diminish in its intensity.

January and February—The Dark Days

> These
>
> are the desolate, dark weeks
> when nature in its barrenness
> equals the stupidity of man
>
> The year plunges into night
> and the heart plunges
> lower than night
>
> to an empty windswept place
> without sun, stars or moon
> but a peculiar light . . .
> —WILLIAM CARLOS WILLIAMS, "These"

Now the time you have been planning for has arrived—the two worst months of the year. But if your plans are in place and if you handle them—and yourself—correctly, you should avoid the sentiments expressed in the preceding verse. I hope that you have the opportunity to travel toward the sun, even if it is for a short time. If you do not, you will need to soldier on through these weeks, but there are many things you can do to help yourself through the dark days. Some of these things I have already outlined in the previous chapters, though I will summarize them here again. Other strategies can be learned by examining the lives of those who have overcome their condition to some extent and have managed to find joy in this darkest of seasons. Meanwhile, though, the dark days are upon you. Look through the following checklist and see which of the guidelines you have already incorporated into your life and which may yet be worth trying:

- Get more light in any safe way you can:
  —Use your dawn simulator.
  —Keep your shutters open in the bedroom.
  —Go outdoors whenever you can when the sun is shining.
  —Drive around in your car when the sun is out.
  —Enjoy the sunlight reflected off snow.
  —Use your light box regularly.
  —Brighten up your home.
  —Spend time in the brightest room.

- Minimize your stress:
  —Don't undertake unnecessary chores.
  —Delay that which can be delayed.
  —Don't allow guilt to prevent you from saying no to new burdens and commitments.
- Explain to others what is going on and tell them how they can help make life easier for you.
- Exercise as much as you can.
- If you are not on medications and are still laboring under the burden of winter, discuss with your doctor the possibility of starting them.
- If you are on medications and they do not seem to be doing the job, discuss with your doctor the possibility of modifying your medication regimen.
- Keep a journal.
- Find out what brings you pleasure and do more of it.
- Find out what brings you displeasure and do less of it.
- Buy some forced bulbs and watch them grow and bloom in these dark months—reminders that spring is not so far away—what one of my patients called "tulip therapy." I find amaryllis plants especially encouraging because their rapid growth dramatizes the passing of time, while their brilliant flowers foreshadow the return of the sun.
- Accept that winter may never feel as good as the other seasons, no matter how hard you try to cope with it.
- Accept the downtime, the quiet of this dormant season.
- Wait for spring; it will arrive; it always does.

March and April—Spring

> At the end of winter there is a season
> in which we are daily expecting spring
> and finally a day when it arrives.
> A flock of geese
> now in the dark flying low over the pond ...
> I stood at my door and could hear their wings.
> —HENRY DAVID THOREAU

Spring comes in different ways in different places, and we each have our own way of feeling this crucial transition from the season of dark-

ness to the season of light. For most people with SAD, the arrival of
spring is met with exhilaration. It is like water to a dried-out desert
wanderer, or food to a starving man. It is an overwhelming relief. But
there are some who experience pain in this transition and feel left out
of the general carnival spirit that everyone around them appears to be
celebrating. My advice at this point is to:

- Pay attention to how you are feeling at this transition time, recognizing that not everyone experiences spring in the same way.
- It is a good time to pick up tasks left undone through the winter. It is no coincidence that spring cleaning occurs in spring.
- But be sure to enjoy the season; you have waited for it and la-
  bored long through the winter to get here.
- And don't pack away your lights, your winter ways, and winter
  paraphernalia too quickly. Spring is a volatile month, an observation eloquently made by the New England poet Robert Frost
  in "Two Tramps in Mud Time."

> The sun was warm, but the wind was chill,
> you know how it is with an April day
> when the sun is out and the wind is still,
> you're one month on in the middle of May.
> But if you so much as dare to speak,
> a cloud comes out over the sunlit arch,
> a wind comes off a frozen peak,
> and you're two months back in the middle of March.

TWELVE

"How Can I Help?"

Advice for Family and Friends

Other people can be a terrific source of comfort and support to someone with SAD. If you are a relative or friend of a seasonal patient, the following information should help you fill that role.

Things to Do

1. *Understand the problem.* Recognize that the seasonal mood problem is a real affliction. This may be hard to appreciate, especially for people who have never themselves been depressed. More mildly afflicted friends and relatives also have a hard time understanding how bad people with SAD can actually feel. It is important to realize that severity makes a big difference. I would encourage friends and relatives of the seasonal person to read some of the stories in the earlier part of the book to gain insight into how disabling the problem can be.

It can be helpful to think of SAD as similar, in certain critical ways, to a physical illness. We do not know what the underlying abnormality is in SAD, but it presumably resides somewhere in the brain, where some chemical process does not function normally, resulting in all the symptoms of the condition. Somehow, light that impinges on the eyes plays an important role in this key chemical process. During the short, dark days of winter, when there is not enough light in the environment, the brain-chemical abnormality becomes manifest in the form of SAD symptoms. Bright light reverses the symptoms, presumably by correcting the underlying abnormality. As a diabetic needs insulin shots and may need encouragement to go along with the program, your friend or relative with SAD needs extra light and can benefit tremendously from your support. You can help, for example, by keeping your friend or relative company while he or she is sitting in front of the lights.

Once you understand the mood and energy problems of SAD, you will be able to handle them better. If your spouse falls behind in paying the bills or carrying out various chores when winter arrives, it will be much easier for you to put up with the resulting inconvenience if you recognize that you are probably dealing with SAD symptoms rather than laziness. If you want to find out more about the condition and its treatments, you may find parts of this book helpful.

2. *Just be there*. Don't feel you have to do anything specific. Your undemanding presence and company will be experienced as soothing and helpful. Even though the seasonal person may appear withdrawn and unfriendly, he or she will often appreciate having company. As one patient I know puts it, "I want my friends to tolerate me sitting solemnly in a corner reading a magazine. I like people to be around but not asking very much of me, because I don't have very much to give." Another patient echoes this need for understanding, noting that when you are depressed, "you get into a place where it's hard for a person to relate to you unless he really cares about you, has known you for a while, and understands your seasonality." She recognizes that "people don't like their friends to change. It's hard for the people you live with," but she requests of her friends that they do not expect her to be "bubbly and full of myself like I am in the summer. . . . Just accept me the way I am."

3. *Encourage the seasonal person*. Remind him that this is a passing phase, that he has not always felt this way, and can and will feel better again. A person who is lethargic and uninspired during the depths of the winter may be kind, friendly, charming, or witty at other times of the year. Remind him about the good times. When you're depressed, it's easy to forget that they ever happened, as well as forgetting everything you have ever learned about depression. At such a time a friend or relative who understands what is happening can help tremendously

simply by saying "Hey, you're forgetting, this is your winter problem. It will pass."

4. *Help with simple things.* Sometimes even shopping or laundry can feel like a huge chore to the depressed person. Offers by friends and family to help out with these will generally be greatly appreciated. One family had a system of rotating household chores weekly, some of which were easier and others more difficult. During the winter, the children understood that their mother was not able to tackle the more difficult chores, and all agreed that she should be exempt from bathroom duty during those months.

The best way to find out what help is needed is to ask. Examples are going to the grocery store for a friend, fixing breakfast for your wife or helping her get the kids off to school while she sits in front of her lights, sitting and talking to a friend or loved one while he does the laundry or pays the bills, or helping him or her wake up in the morning (which is so difficult for a person with SAD). All these things will be remembered and rewarded by a deepening and strengthening of your relationship.

5. *Try to understand the seasonal person when he or she is in the hypomanic phase.* Sometimes it's difficult to understand the high side of SAD as well. Someone who has been hibernating all winter and suddenly springs into action with more energy than anyone else may be hard to take. As one patient puts it, "I think it's easier to love someone who's down and depressed and hurting in some way. But please remember to love her when she's happy and successful as well." It may also be helpful to point out *tactfully* that the seasonal person is going a bit fast for you and most other people and that it may be useful to get some help to slow down a bit. Encourage your friend or relative to avoid being exposed to too much bright light. Sleeping with the bedroom shades down or wearing dark glasses during daylight hours may help people slow down at such times if they are too wired.

When people are a bit high, they can become argumentative. The friend or relative exposed to such querulousness would do well to choose carefully what issues to bring up. The husband of one of my seasonal patients, who has learned the value of this strategy over the years, avoids confronting his wife on minor issues. He observes, "If we have a conflict, it's going to be over something worthwhile."

A seasonal person who is showing poor judgment, impulsiveness, or sleeplessness should be encouraged (or taken) to see his or her psychiatrist.

Things to Avoid

1. *Don't judge and criticize.* The seasonal person is already feeling bad about not functioning up to his normal standards and letting friends and family down. Very often he is his own harshest critic, measuring his own actions and finding them wanting. To have these criticisms confirmed by someone he loves and respects can be extremely painful, may further undermine his self-esteem, and could enhance feelings of depression and worthlessness. A tendency to judge and criticize the seasonal person is very understandable, but it stems from a fundamental misconception that the seasonal person is willfully declining to do certain things or is being self-indulgent and weak-willed and is giving in to things.

It may be helpful for you to think back to some time when you were feeling weak, tired, or out of sorts, perhaps due to a physical condition such as an infection or operation. Imagine how you would have felt to be criticized at such a time for not meeting your obligations with sufficient energy or enthusiasm. One young man who has been in and out of seasonal depressions for the past several years still finds it difficult to convince his friends that he has been suffering from an illness. They continue to regard his months of withdrawal and impaired functioning as a character disturbance or failure of will. As a result, he is beginning to reevaluate these friendships.

2. *Don't take the seasonal person's withdrawal personally.* You should not assume that he or she is mad at you or uninterested in being friends with you. One patient thinks back on friends who have called her during her down times and said, "Well, I've called you the last three times. Do you really want to be friends anymore?" She observes, "That kind of situation seems to pop up all the time in the winter. I understand that other people need certain things from a friendship, but it comes at a time when even getting up to answer the phone is a major effort: Who is it going to be? What do I have to talk about now? The best kind of friend is someone who is willing to keep calling you and to keep saying 'Do you feel like doing anything?' I'm not saying that friends should baby you, nor do they have to sit there and hold your hand. It's very simple: Just accept someone who is in a different place." The same person recalls hurtful conversations with friends who have not understood her difficulty. "They say, 'Oh, yeah, here you go again,' and it's sort of mocking. They just don't understand."

3. *Don't assume that it is your responsibility to make the seasonal person feel fine.* It's not likely to work, and you will probably end up feeling frustrated and irritated at your failure. When you feel responsible for bringing a person out of a depression and you have failed to do so, you are likely to feel angry. You have sunk so much energy into trying to reverse the situation that you may be inclined to see the depressed person as having caused you to fail. You will then be more likely to blame him for making you feel that way. You might attribute your "failure" to a willful attempt on his part to resist all help and, in your anger, feel inclined to say that if he is not willing to accept your helping hand, he deserves to remain in a slump. As I have noted already, anger tends to get turned on the depressed person just when he feels least capable of coping with even the most ordinary things in life, let alone problems with a dear friend or relative. The key to not getting angry is understanding the problem and not feeling responsible for fixing it. But do remember that simple things, such as being there for your friend or family member, can make an enormous difference.

Part III
Celebrating the Seasons

THIRTEEN

A Brief History of Seasonal Time

So far, I have discussed the discomfort and disability the seasons can cause and have considered light largely as a medication. These factors, however, account for only a small part of the effect that light and the seasons have on the mind. The seasons provided an impetus for the development of our solar calendar and helped us come to terms, both intellectually and emotionally, with the passing of time. The fluxes in mood, energy, and vitality that may be experienced with the changing seasons have infused many people with a creative energy that has been the source of many of their finest achievements. These internal changes, coinciding as they do with those in the natural world, have inspired artists and writers to express, in paint or in words, the shifting beauty of their landscape. It is these other aspects of light and the seasons that are the subject of this chapter.

Although the solar calendar may seem commonplace to us, since we use it on a daily basis, our earliest measure of time was based on the more obvious monthly cycle of the moon. The calendar helped ancient civilizations predict the changing seasons and decide when to plant their crops. A major problem with the lunar year, which consisted of twelve months, was that it fell short of the 365-day solar year

255

by several days. As a result, the lunar year shifted gradually out of phase with the seasons. In an attempt to correct these shifts, certain societies inserted extra months at intervals into their lunar calendar.

The Egyptians have been given credit for developing the solar calendar. They used their ability to predict where the sun would fall on a given day to illuminate their obelisks and add drama to their religious festivals. Many societies have since used the similar principle of knowing where a slab of light or shadow would fall on a particular day—for example, the winter or summer solstice—to enhance their sense of awe over a mysterious, yet predictable, universe. The solar calendar, as measured, for example, by the sundial, worked well, and still does, in predicting the changing seasons.

The problem of anticipating seasonal changes in the world around us has not been an exclusively human one. For many animals, especially those that live at some distance from the equator, it is crucial to be able to anticipate when it will be cold or hot, when food will be scarce or plentiful, and when to mate, migrate, or hibernate. As we have seen, from the lowly *Gonyaulax* to domestic animals such as sheep and horses, the organism must be able to anticipate the seasons so as to make the appropriate adaptive changes. To time such events correctly, all these animals have evolved complex physiological programs that depend for their accurate timing on information from the physical world. The environmental time cue of greatest importance across a multitude of species, including perhaps humans, is the length of the day, which is a function of the solar year. Thus our solar calendar and the calendar of our biological responses both follow the annual course of the sun across the sky. The discovery of the solar calendar by the Egyptians, the product of human intellect, and the seasonal patterns of biology, shaped over hundreds of thousands of years by the forces of evolution, have both used the sun and the seasons as the most dependable and meaningful markers for charting time over long periods.

Quite apart from the practical need to measure time, humans have also had to deal with the emotional impact of its passing. Over the course of time, we receive the gifts of life, health, youth, and children, and the rewards of our labors; yet in time we lose them all. We are subject to aging, disease, the destructive forces of our fellow human beings, and finally, death. How do we come to terms with all these losses, as well as with the burden of the errors we have made?

These are age-old problems, and ancient humans found a novel solution to them: Simply abolish time. Wipe it out and start all over again. Thus, in ancient times, at the end of each year, people engaged in cleansing rituals, purifying themselves of the dirt and sin they had accumulated over the previous year. They could then enter the new year fresh and clean. All manner of complex rituals were developed. For example, sins would be transferred to a goat, and the animal would be driven out of the area—the proverbial scapegoat. Not only were one's sins abolished, but the slate of time was itself wiped clean. Ancient humans lacked a sense that one year led to the next—a concept of time that has been termed *linear* or *historical*. Instead, they believed in cyclical time, "the myth of the eternal return," which happens to be the title of a fascinating book on the subject by Mircea Eliade.

Around the time of the winter solstice, it was traditional to extinguish and rekindle fire. Even in modern times, the festivals that take place around the time of the winter solstice are celebrated with lights: the colored ones on Christmas trees and the candles on a Hanukkah menorah. In some cultures, the winter solstice coincides with the new year, and the extinguishing and rekindling of fire could also be regarded as symbolizing the obliteration of time past and the start of new time. Alternatively, such activities might be viewed as a celebration of (or prayer for) the return of the sun's light following the winter solstice. The use of light in these rituals may also serve to lift our spirits during the darkest days of the year.

Cyclical time was common in many ancient societies. The Greeks conceived of history as cyclical and developed the idea of a "Great Year" many thousands of solar years in length. The Great Year, which they believed corresponded to the rotation of the heavens, had a Great Summer, when planetary forces would combine to destroy the earth by fire, and a Great Winter, when the world would be overwhelmed by water. The Indians had a similar concept of a cosmic cycle, called a *Mahayuga,* which was thought to last four million years.

It seems likely that the obvious seasonal changes in the world around us, and our internal changes in mood and behavior, together perhaps with the wish to abolish the past, all contributed to the development of a cyclical sense of time. In the last few centuries, however, a linear or historical one has prevailed. This sense of time is familiar to every schoolchild who has had to construct a dateline showing how certain events occurred over the years. An integral part of this concept is that these events took place in a certain sequence and that, in certain critical ways, the clock or calendar cannot be turned back. Thus, World

War II took place in part because of unresolved issues from World War I. Dropping the atom bombs on Japan put an end to World War II, an event that could not have happened four years earlier, since the atom bomb had not yet been invented. The dropping of the bomb ushered in an age in which nuclear warfare is an ever-present possibility. That has changed the nature of war and the whole way in which we view our world. Thus, nowadays, even schoolchildren become thoroughly familiar with the concept of linear or historical time that moves in one direction only.

The Jews have been credited with the development of the sense of linear time. Calamities that beset the children of Israel were interpreted by the prophets as the result of the wrath of God, proof that the people needed to reform their ways. The prophets thus forced the people to turn away from a purely cyclical and ever-renewing sense of time and face the consequences of their actions. This concept was continued in Christianity, which sees time as a straight line that traces the course of humanity from its creation through Redemption to the present. The Chinese, in their descriptions of successive dynasties, have been credited with independently coming up with a linear sense of time, and such a sense was surely present in the mind of the thirteenth-century Japanese sage Dogen, who observed, "Time flies more swiftly than an arrow and life is more transient than the dew. We cannot call back a single day that has passed."

According to Eliade, the conflict between the two different perceptions of time—cyclical and linear—continued into the seventeenth century, after which the latter view gained ascendance. This was in keeping with the development of science, the theory of evolution, and the idea of human progress, all of which were believed to proceed in a linear way. Despite this linear trend, both Jews and Christians have continued to celebrate cyclical time in the form of seasonal rituals and festivals. There was a renewal of interest in cyclical time in the twentieth century. Historians such as Oswald Spengler and Arnold Toynbee considered the problems of periodicity in history. The works of two important modern writers, T. S. Eliot and James Joyce, are, in Eliade's view, "saturated with nostalgia for the myth of eternal repetition and . . . the abolition of time."

One of the reasons it took modern scientists so long to recognize SAD might have been the ascendance of linear over cyclical time. According to a linear way of thinking, a psychiatrist might consider, for example, a patient with three episodes of winter depression as follows:

Three years ago, in October, she broke up with her boyfriend and became depressed for several months. By April, she recovered, moved, and found a new job. She was not able to function for long in this position, however, became depressed, and lost the job in December. The next March, she entered into a new relationship, which seemed to lift her spirits. She was well until about a month ago (October), when her relationship difficulties resurfaced, and she has since become markedly lethargic, withdrawn, and depressed.

In the last few decades, however, we have once again become interested in cyclicity in the form of biological rhythms. It was this developing interest that served as a major precursor to the recognition and description of SAD.

FOURTEEN

Polar Tales

The days are growing rapidly shorter and the nights, only too
noticeably longer.... It is this discouraging veil of blackness,
falling over the sparkling whiteness of earlier nights, which
sends a vein of despair running through our souls.
—DR. FREDERICK COOK, *Through the First Antarctic Night*

I have frequently been asked, "Have they studied SAD in Scandina-
via? Don't they get a lot of it over there?" In recent years, since our
work from the NIMH first appeared, Scandinavian research groups
have done considerable work on the subject. Before then, however,
there was little or nothing about it in Scandinavian medical literature.
Given the degree of light deprivation so far north, this gap was surprising. Were Scandinavians particularly resistant to the problems of
SAD? Had their researchers simply overlooked its importance? One
Swedish psychiatrist provided a witty answer: "Either everyone there
has it," he replied, "or no one does."

Since then, thanks to research by several Scandinavian researchers,
it has become apparent that approximately one in three adults in the
far north is affected adversely by the winter season. Icelanders might
be an exception, possibly protected biologically against the dark days,
as I mentioned earlier. Nevertheless, Dr. Andrés Magnusson, a psychi-

atrist from Iceland, notes that "everyone seems to have some relative who takes to bed for the whole winter." Cases that sound like SAD can also be found, according to Magnusson, in Icelandic myths. Seasonal changes in behavior are reportedly rife in the population as a whole; they are so widespread in the far North, according to some observers, that most people just take them for granted. This may be why they did not attract the attention of the medical community until reports started appearing from other parts of the world.

In fact, some of the best descriptions of the behavioral effects of circumpolar winters come from outsiders. Dr. Frederick Cook, for example, who went on a nineteenth-century expedition to Antarctica as ship's doctor to the *Belgica,* described how the crew suffered from isolation and harsh weather while trapped in the ice during the Antarctic winter. The sixty-eight consecutive days of darkness appeared to affect the men badly, and, according to Cook, they "gradually . . . became affected, body and soul, with languor." He described other psychiatric problems among the crew, concluding, "The root cause of these disasters was the lack of the sun." He found that treating his men with direct exposure to an open fire seemed to help them, perhaps more because of the light than the heat.

Dr. Cook also provided us with a description of seasonal rhythms of sexual drive among the Eskimos: "The passions of these people are periodical, and their courtship is usually carried on soon after the return of the sun; in fact, at this time, they almost tremble from the intensity of their passions and for several weeks most of their time is taken up in gratifying them."

Such shifts in sex drive, with a surge of interest in the spring, continuing into the summer, almost certainly affect people living at lower latitudes, though to a lesser degree. Many societies have created spring rituals that incorporate elements of sexuality or fertility, which coincide with the burgeoning of nature outside and rising sexual passions within.

An excellent description of the psychological effects of the dark days on the people of Tromsö in northern Norway was provided by Joseph Wechsberg, who wrote an article in *The New Yorker* called "Mørketiden," which means, "murky times." Tromsö, which lies 215 miles north of the Arctic Circle, has forty-nine sunless days during the winter. Wechsberg observed that "the people talked a lot about mørketiden, and at the same time protested that they were not affected by it." He reported that people felt tired, had difficulty getting up in the morning and accomplishing their work, and suffered from disturbed sleep, low energy level, and actual depression. In other words, many of these people complained of the symptoms of SAD. One man he interviewed even observed that the depression seemed to be a problem particularly among women.

Wechsberg described an opposite pattern of behavior in the summer. People rarely seemed to feel tired and often did not feel like going to bed. They were active at all hours of the night. There was widespread celebration as people headed for the country to "fish, hunt, have fun." As a result, it was difficult to get any work done.

Wechsberg observed that in winter the people of Tromsö kept their indoor lights on constantly during the day. One woman reported missing the sun so much that she gravitated toward the window. The return of the sun after forty-nine dark days was celebrated as *Soldag,* or Sun Day. Children were sent home early from school that day, and all work stopped by noon. The first rays were greeted with tears, prayers, and special wishes. Some people, unwilling to wait for this day, flew to southern Norway to see the sun.

Since Wechsberg's article, research into the effects of the seasons has been undertaken in earnest under the direction of Dr. Arne Holte. I have since visited Tromsö twice myself, once in the summer and once in the winter. In the summer, looking out of the window of my hotel across the bay, I could not tell whether it was day or night. Traffic crossed the bridge at all hours of the day, people walked about in the streets, and human behavior provided no clue as to the time of day. I felt euphoric at first and later unpleasantly revved up and exhausted, and sleep would not have been possible had I not pulled down the blackout shades installed specifically for that purpose. In the town there was merriment well into the early hours of the morning.

How different the town looked in winter. The streets were covered in snow under the dark purple-black cover of the sky. There was a silver rim on the horizon, a reflection off the clouds of the sun shining somewhere far away, south of the Arctic Circle. Tramping through the snow at night, there was a peaceful stillness in the crisp air, while overhead, the northern lights were faintly visible, like a diaphanous curtain waving gently in an impalpable breeze. Small wonder that the natives of the North believed that these mysterious lights were torches to guide the spirits of the dead to the world beyond.

Dr. Holte's findings that seasonal difficulties are common in Tromsö have not been universally appreciated. Many have commented that the story is greatly overblown and that a fuss is being made of nothing. Perhaps the stoicism of the North prevents many of these people from acknowledging their difficulties. The dramatic seasons have always been part of their lives, and they may accept them as a law of nature, immutable and therefore to be accepted without complaint. In contrast, perhaps my own upbringing, in a climate where the seasons were mild, enabled me to recognize the dramatic nature of the seasonal changes in North America. As in Edgar Allan Poe's story of the purloined letter, sometimes that which is right under one's nose is most difficult to observe.

FIFTEEN

SAD Through the Ages

*T*he relationship between depression and the seasons was first observed over two thousand years ago by Hippocrates, who noted, "It is chiefly the changes of the seasons which produce diseases." Aretaeus, in the second century A.D., recommended that "lethargics are to be laid in the light and exposed to the rays of the sun, for the disease is gloom." Yet it is only since the late twentieth century that seasonal depression has entered the diagnostic manual of psychiatric diseases and light therapy has been seriously considered as a treatment for winter depression. Why did it take medical science so long to rediscover the wisdom of the ancients? The elements needed to make this discovery—our powers of observation, the charting of mood changes over time, and bright light—have been available for ages. What brought about the rediscovery was not some technological breakthrough, as in so many other areas of medicine, but advances in our understanding of psychiatric diseases and our changing concepts of time.

The following are three historical cases of SAD, described over a span of some three centuries. Clinically, they have certain distinct resemblances to one another and to modern-day descriptions of SAD. One thing that I find fascinating about these cases is how they illustrate the different ways in which the physicians of various eras conceptualized SAD and what that can teach us about the changing concepts of the mind and mental illness over the centuries. During the era when the first case was described—the seventeenth century—medical science was still under the powerful influence of the humoral theories of disease that had held sway since the times of ancient Greece. The second case was described in the nineteenth century, when the impact of the physical environment on mental illness was considered of great importance to those suffering from mood disorders. The final case was described in the middle of our own century, when psychoanalytic theories had the greatest influence on our approach to the mind and its disorders.

Anne Grenville

She was the daughter of the bishop of Durham and the wife of a minister, but Anne Grenville, who lived in England in the late 1600s, is remembered instead for her extraordinarily well-documented psychiatric problems and the prominence of the physicians she consulted. We owe this thorough documentation to an ongoing battle between her father and her husband. Her father claimed that she had always been healthy, and according to her sister, she had been driven to madness by her husband. Her husband disclaimed responsibility, and his annoyance at Mrs. Grenville's psychiatric problems was compounded by financial difficulties, which were further aggravated by his father-in-law's reluctance to pay the expected dowry.

Mrs. Grenville appears to have suffered from a cyclical mood disorder. According to one physician she consulted, "There are twin symptoms, which are her constant companions, Mania and Melancholy, and they succeed each other in a double and alternate act; or take each other's place like the smoke and flame of a fire." Her problem would probably not have received so much medical attention—at least nine prominent physicians saw her—had it not been for the troublesome nature of her manic episodes. According to one physician,

> The first oncoming of this recurrent disease shows itself by mild insomnia, unusual talkativeness, propensity to laughter, practically continuously. . . . But as the illness increases, her periods of wakefulness become more extended, or if she does fall asleep, her condition is worsened as a result of the sleep; silence succeeds talkativeness, morosity, laughter . . . and finally, she sometimes rages against her attendants and attacks any-

one she meets in a petulant manner. [Dr. Peter Hunauld, Rector of the University of Angers, 1673]

It is not uncommon for mania to begin as a euphoric condition and progress to a state of irritability and anger. As the following description of the alternate phase of Mrs. Grenville's condition indicates, she also suffered from recurrent depressions:

> From time to time the symptoms of melancholia proper also put in an appearance; she carries on her ordinary tasks and duties in a gentler manner, sometimes taciturn, timid, and sorrowful, without a trace of savageness. . . . [physicians Stephen Taylor and Robert Wittie, York, 1670]

The seasonality of her symptoms—particularly her tendency to become manic in the summer—was well documented. For this reason, one of her doctors suggested special treatments "at the approach of the dog days." The dog days are the six hottest weeks of the year, named after the dog star, Sirius, the brightest star in the firmament. Once a year, the dog star rises in direct alignment with the sun, and the ancients believed that around this time its effects combined with those of the sun to produce the intense heat of July and August.

Mrs. Grenville's case is not exactly typical of most SAD patients I have seen, whose manic symptoms are generally less prominent. In addition, although her manias clearly occurred in the summer, and we are told that these alternated with her depressive episodes, we are not told specifically that the depressions occurred in the winter, though it seems likely that they did. Her depressions were probably less well documented than her manias, because depression is often regarded as less of a problem by a patient's relatives. The patient frequently takes the opposite point of view, seeking help when depressed but not when manic.

Many theories were advanced to explain Mrs. Grenville's condition, and on the basis of these, several treatments were suggested, all, unfortunately, to little avail. The diagnoses of her illness showed the continuing influence of the humoral theories of the ancient Greeks, according to which human beings were composed of four humors: blood, yellow bile (*choler*), black bile (*melanchos*), and phlegm. These humors were thought to be associated with the four seasons— spring, summer, autumn, and winter, respectively. Different types of climates—cold or hot, moist or dry—were thought to act on the different humors, altering their relative influence on a person. So were different constellations and planets. These influences on an individual's innate disposition were thought to result in one of four temperaments: sanguine, choleric, melancholic, or phlegmatic.

Melancholia, as its name implies, was considered to be due to an excess of black bile. The planet Saturn was thought to exert an influence on this condition. In one artistic portrayal of the four humors, the melancholic describes his nature as follows:

> God has given me unduly
> In my nature melancholy.
> Like the earth both cold and dry,
> Black of skin with gait awry,
> Hostile, mean, ambitious, sly,
> Sullen, crafty, false, and shy.
> No love for fame or woman have I;
> In Saturn and autumn the fault doth lie.

The idea of black bile being responsible for melancholia was extended by Aristotle to account for mania as well. According to him, black bile, which he regarded as being naturally cold, "produces apoplexy or torpor or despondency or fear." However, if the black bile became overheated, "it produces cheerfulness, accompanied by song and frenzy." In keeping with this thinking, several of Mrs. Grenville's doctors attributed her condition to "atrabilious ferment," in other words, black bile. According to one of the doctors,

> The whole aim of our treatment must be at least to blunt that ferment, if we cannot entirely destroy it, This was the purpose behind the treatments proposed by the learned Doctor Bellay of Cleves: namely, cooling medicines, aperients, gentle evacuants, and occasionally hypnotics. The hope is, by these remedies to be able to suppress the force and energy of that atrabilious humour; for which purpose, especially as a preventive measure, you must see that every year at the beginning of spring you use the well-established remedies to provoke a flow of the haemorrhoids by the application of leeches.

The twin legacies of the ancient Greeks to the treatment of Anne Grenville were the humoral theory of disease, which tied melancholia to the seasons, and a cyclical view of time, whereby the rotation of the stars in the heavens resembled the rotation of the seasons, but on a much larger scale. With these theoretical views of the world, it was quite natural for them to emphasize the influence of the seasons on human lives.

The Case of M

Approximately 150 years after Anne Grenville was treated for her problems, a patient we know only as "M" consulted the famous French psychiatrist Jean Etienne Esquirol, who described his case as follows:

> M, a native of Belgium, forty-two years of age, of a strong constitution and transacting a very large business, consults me at the close of the winter of 1825. Observe the account which is given me by him. "I have always enjoyed good health, am happy in my family, having an affectionate wife and charming children. My affairs are also in excellent condition. Three years since, I experienced a trifling vexation. It was at the beginning of autumn, and I became sad, gloomy, and susceptible. By degrees I neglected my business, and deserted my house to avoid my uneasiness. I felt feeble, and drank beer and liquors. Soon I became irritable. Everything opposed my wishes, disturbed me, and rendered me insupportable, and even dangerous to my family. My affairs suffered from this state. I suffered also from insomnia and inappetence. Neither the advice nor tender counsels of my wife, nor that of my family, had any more influence over me. At length, I fell into a profound apathy, incapable of everything except drinking and grieving. At the approach of spring I felt my affections revive. I recovered all my intellectual activity, and all my ardor for business. I was very well all the ensuing summer, but from the commencement of the damp and cold weather of autumn, there was a return of sadness, uneasiness, and a desire to drink, to dissipate my sadness. There was also a return of irascibility and transports of passion. During the last autumn and the present winter, I have experienced for the third time the same phenomena, which have been more grievous than formerly. My fortune has suffered, and my wife has not been free from danger. I have now come to submit myself to you, sir, and to obey your directions in every thing."
>
> After many questions, I offered the following advice. A hospital will not benefit, but on the contrary, injure you. . . . In the month of September, you should go to Languedoc [in the South of France] and must be in Italy before the close of October, from whence you must not return until the month of May. This counsel was closely followed. At the close of De-

cember, he was at Rome. He felt the impression of the cold, and the beginnings of a desire to drink were manifest, but shortly disappeared. He escaped a fourth attack by withdrawing himself from the coldness and moisture of autumn. He returns to Paris in the month of May, in the enjoyment of excellent health.

This beautiful early description of SAD and the inspired treatment, so successful in the case of M, is impressive. It appears that Esquirol's treatment of patient M with climate modification was not an isolated event, for he observed that it was the practice of English physicians to send their melancholic patients into the southern provinces of France and Italy, "thus protecting them against the moist and oppressive air of England."

Esquirol acquired his enlightened approach from his mentor, Phillipe Pinel, the French psychiatrist renowned for removing the chains from patients in a Paris mental hospital. Pinel had strong reservations about "the usual routine of baths, bloodletting, and coercion," the standard treatment for mood disorders at the time, but suggested instead a "moral treatment" that relied more on empathy, understanding, and encouragement.

Pinel also drew attention to the importance of the physical environment in modulating mood. For melancholics, he pointed out "the urgent necessity of forcibly agitating the system, of interrupting the chain of their gloomy ideas, and of engaging their interest by powerful and continuous impressions on their external senses."

With such a renowned mentor behind him, Esquirol went on to make his own original contributions to psychiatry. He noted that depression could result from many different causes and ought to be treated in different ways, "not . . . limited to the administration of certain medicines." In his view, "Moral medicine, which seeks in the heart for the cause of the evil, which sympathizes and weeps, which consoles, and divides with the unfortunate their sufferings, and which revives hope in their breast, is often preferable to all other." However, he also stressed the importance of the physical environment, recommending "a clear sky, a pleasant temperature, an agreeable situation with varied scenery."

The late nineteenth and early twentieth centuries saw the development of bright artificial light as a therapeutic modality. In fact, Niels Finsen of Sweden was awarded one of the first Nobel prizes for medicine for his work on the effects of artificial light on the tubercle bacillus. Bright light was used for many conditions, including depression. A leading British psychiatrist observed:

> Since the energising influence of sunlight on all living matter is so well known, it is surprising that therapists have not made greater use of this natural curative agent.
>
> In the province of psychological medicine it is generally accepted that no institution, from a structural point of view, is complete without its solarium. . . . In addition . . . several mental institutions have already installed apparatus for the production of artificial sunlight.
>
> Even to the lay mind, it is obvious what a stimulating and beneficial influence artificial sunlight can exert on those whose fund of energy is seriously depleted by nervous or mental disorder, especially during the dull, sunless, and depressing months of our British winter. [Dr. J. G. Porter Phillips, Bethlem Hospital, London, 1923]

The Unmarried Clerk

The next published case of SAD was reported one century after Esquirol's description of patient M, and on the other side of the Atlantic. In the United States, in 1946, a certain Colonel George Frumkes published in the *Psychoanalytic Quarterly* the case of a thirty-year-old clerk. Dr. Frumkes describes the patient's history as follows:

> [He] was recovering from a depression of a type he had had each year for the past ten years. Although he knew he would be better in the spring and summer, he wanted to be treated so that the depressions would not recur. They began in August or September and continued about six months. During the spring and summer he was overactive and too confident, without excitement or unseemly behavior. After the recurrence of the first few cycles, he was never free from the fear of the autumnal depression. This constant threat interfered with his freedom of action in his business and in his relationship with women.
>
> The depressions were heralded by the observation that he was sweating excessively; then he felt vague anxiety, followed by the fear that he would not be able to do his work. Later came feelings of unworthiness and inefficiency. He was convinced his work suffered because he was slow, because he had to check his work four times, and he dreaded anything new and avoided making decisions. He tried to evade as much work as possible without attracting attention, and he avoided contact

with superiors and fellow workers. Despite the great effort it cost him, he never missed a day's work. He felt he had no right to indulge himself. He was certain that his deficiencies were apparent to everyone. If he could have afforded to do so he would have remained in hiding in the South for six months. If criticized, he would suffer keenly and be incapable of defending himself. Praise or affection caused him suffering because he felt he was an impostor not deserving such consideration.

He was especially uncomfortable in cold weather, but there was not a constant relationship between the depth of the depression and the drop in temperature. Certain signs foretold his recovery: he would take out his camera, make strokes as if he were playing tennis, and become interested in girls. In his overactive phase he was with as many as four girls a week; he was restless, prided himself on doing the work of three men, and devised new office systems.

Dr. Frumkes follows up this excellent description, which will sound familiar to all SAD sufferers, with an extensive history of the patient's background: His parentage, family relationships, childhood, and employment background are all reviewed. His sex life is a particular focus of attention. His sexual development, the sleeping arrangements in the family, masturbatory practices, dating patterns, and dreams and fantasies about sex take up well over half the article.

In attempting to explain the patient's depressions, Dr. Frumkes departs from the simple and straightforward prose used to describe the patient's symptoms and launches into a convoluted psychoanalytic interpretation. According to his formulation, the patient's depressions

> began about the time he learned that masturbation was not a unique sin of his; when there was a decrease in the intense, conscious feeling of guilt. The depressions represented a redistribution of the punishment in the psychic economy. . . . Masturbation for him was an unconscious infantile sexual striving for his mother, and the associated hostile impulses connected with this drive.

Dr. Frumkes also suggests that the depressions might have represented "memorial observances of the births of his brothers and sisters." Such explanations for the development of manic and depressive episodes were frequently offered by U.S. psychiatrists in the 1950s and 1960s. I have read through many medical records of manic–depressives treated at the New York Psychiatric Institute during these years, and was impressed by some of the ingenious formulations, which purported to explain both depressions and manias in terms of childhood experiences.

Dr. Frumkes treated his patient with psychoanalysis. Although he did not specify the frequency of sessions and length of treatment in his paper, I would assume he met with the patient four or five times a week over several years, as is customary in traditional psychoanalysis. Dr. Frumkes reports that "as the treatment progressed, the depressions diminished in regularity and intensity. The patient undertook work of a nature he had formerly dreaded. A year following treatment, he wrote that he had had no disturbances of mood, that he was married and felt well."

It is difficult to know quite what to make of this reported outcome. It seems as though the patient did indeed have sexual conflicts, and it is quite conceivable that the analytic therapy was helpful for them. However, my experience with SAD makes me question the likelihood that the treatment made a significant impact on his annual depressions, though he might have worried less about them.

It is interesting to consider that in the same year in which Dr. Frumkes published his case, a German physician, Dr. Helmut Marx, reported using bright artificial light to treat four men who had become depressed in the dark days of an arctic winter. Marx's work was impressive in that he recognized the recurrent nature of winter depressions and even described the overeating that often accompanies the condition. Not only did he identify light deficiency as a trigger for this condition—and bright light as an effective treatment—but he also correctly suggested that light acted via the eyes to influence the hypothalamus. All these insights are in agreement with our views of SAD and light therapy some forty years later. Marx's report, however, was unknown to modern psychiatrists until very recently and had little influence on patterns of psychiatric treatment or research.

How, in the course of the century between the cases of Esquirol and Frumkes, did the importance of the physical environment get lost? In my view, the main reason for this was the powerful influence of Sigmund Freud. Although the discovery of psychoanalysis contributed enormously to our understanding of the human mind, it also obscured our consideration of alternative hypotheses—for example, the simple possibility that depressions could be related to regular changes in climatic variables.

Freud also made his mark on our view of time. He had two opinions on the subject. First, he asserted that the information that was repressed into the unconscious mind remained unaltered by the passage of time. This was a linear, historical view—of time as an arrow. Like the Dead Sea Scrolls, resting in their earthen jars in a cave until they were discovered, unaltered by time, so the repressed memories of childhood were buried in the unconscious, to be discovered later by the analyst. Freud's second opinion on time perception in the mind was that "in the id there is nothing corresponding to the idea of time." He summarized these two views as follows: "The processes of the system *Ucs* (the unconscious) are timeless; i.e., they are not ordered temporally, are not altered by the passage of time, in fact bear no relationship to time at all." Although his colleague Fliess believed in the importance of cyclical processes in the mind, there is little evidence that Freud regarded such a cyclical sense of time as being of any major importance.

So it was in the United States, as the second half of the twentieth century unfolded, that psychiatry lost its grip on time as an important consideration in evaluating psychiatric conditions, and this applied to both cyclical time and the longitudinal evaluation of individuals over time. Rather, the psychological associations of the moment were what mattered. Like a hologram in which a fragment contains an image of the whole picture, everything was contained in the present, in the cross-section of the mind that appeared there and then to the analyst.

As for the biological developments in psychiatry in the second half of the twentieth century, the biggest news was the development of psychotropic drugs, which could reverse psychosis, depression, and mania. These were the single most important factor in emptying out our state mental hospitals and "deinstitutionalizing" their patients. The consequences of such deinstitutionalization—for example, homelessness and street people—have caused new problems, but there is little question that the discovery of effective psychotropic drugs was a major breakthrough for psychiatry.

However, these drugs were regarded as suitable only for more disturbed patients, whereas those who were able to function in the outside world, like Dr. Frumkes's patient, were more likely to receive only psychotherapy. To some degree, a two-class system of psychiatric patients resulted. Since most patients with SAD do not require hospitalization, most would have been grouped in the healthier class and given insight-oriented psychotherapy.

Two trends in modern psychiatry were responsible for paving the way for the rediscovery of SAD and light therapy. First, standard ways of identifying discrete psychiatric conditions were developed; and second, cyclical time was rediscovered. The development of criteria for identifying psychiatric syndromes came from a group of psychiatric diagnosticians at Washington University in St. Louis. This group emphasized the importance of examining the longitudinal course of an illness, rather than relying primarily on the mental state of the patient as presented to the psychiatrist at any given moment. As to cyclicity and behavior, the great strides made in the last few decades in understanding biological rhythms in animals were applied to people. Pioneering human studies in Germany and the United States showed that humans had an endogenous circadian system resembling that of other animals—the medical importance of cyclical time had been rediscovered.

The NIMH group, led by Dr. Thomas A. Wehr, expanded on earlier observations by other circadian rhythm experts to develop the idea that disturbances of biological rhythms may underlie cyclical mood disorders. The cycle of day and night, light and dark, is crucially important in modulating daily rhythms in animals. It was logical, therefore, that light should recapture the interest of psychiatric clinicians and researchers, who had abandoned it some fifty years before. Into this environment came Herb Kern, scientist and patient, with fifteen years of documented seasonal cycles of depression and hypomania, to usher in the modern era of SAD and light therapy.

SIXTEEN

Creating with the Seasons

Great Wits are sure to Madness near ally'd,
And thin Partitions do their Bounds divide.
—JOHN DRYDEN

*T*he association between genius and insanity is ingrained in our culture. We are told about the "thin line" that exists between the brilliant artist and the madman. Is there any truth to this assertion? Have great artists of the past indeed suffered from psychiatric disturbances and, if so, what forms have these disturbances taken? Where do seasonal responses fit into this picture, if at all? Does sensitivity to light—a cardinal feature of patients with SAD—seem to go along with sensitivity to our exterior and interior worlds?

The Link Among Mood Disorders, Creativity, and the Seasons

The concept that genius and madness are somehow connected goes back at least to the time of Aristotle, who observed that "no great genius was without a mixture of insanity." He added, "Those who have become eminent in philosophy, politics, poetry, and the arts have all had tendencies toward melancholia." The Roman playwright Seneca echoed this view, noting that "the mind cannot attain anything lofty so long as it is sane." For centuries this belief persisted, and melancholia was somehow endowed with cultural value. Genius was regarded as a "hereditary taint," transmitted in families, along with mental illness.

It is only in our century, however, that the subject has been a matter of serious study. Dr. Nancy Andreasen was the first researcher to study the relationship between creativity and mental illness, using modern psychiatric diagnoses. She interviewed thirty creative writers at the prestigious Iowa Writers' Workshop about their own backgrounds and those of their close relatives and compared their responses with those of thirty control subjects. She found a substantially higher rate of mental illness among the writers and their family members. She had approached the study with the belief that there would be an association between schizophrenia and creativity. To her surprise, it was not schizophrenia but disorders of mood regulation—especially those involving a tendency to mania or hypomania, in addition to depression—that distinguished the writers from the control group. She concluded that the traits of creativity and mood disturbance appeared to run together in families and could be genetically mediated.

More recently, Dr. Kay Redfield Jamison studied a group of eminent British writers and artists for evidence of psychiatric illness, seasonal variations in mood and productivity, and the perceived role of intense moods in their creative processes. She selected these artists and writers on the basis of objective acclaim, in the form of prestigious prizes and other types of acknowledgment. She interviewed them extensively and found very high rates of mood disorders in the group. Over one-third had been treated for mood problems, the great majority with medications or hospitalization. Poets were most likely to require medication for depression and were the only group to require treatment for mania. Playwrights had the highest total rate of treatment for mood disorders, but a high percentage of this group had been treated with psychotherapy alone. Exceptional among the writers in regard to their mood stability were biographers, who reported no history of mood swings or elated states. Although these writers were as outstanding as the others, in terms of their objective achievements, they were perhaps a less creative group.

Almost all subjects—with the exception of the biographers— reported having had intense, highly productive, and creative periods. Most of these lasted between one and four weeks. These episodes were marked by "increased enthusiasm, energy, self-confidence, speed of mental association, fluency of thoughts, elevated mood, and a strong sense of well-being." They sound very much like "hypomanic" episodes, without the behavioral disturbance that term implies. Ninety percent of Dr. Jamison's group reported that very intense moods and feelings were either integral to or necessary for the development and execution of their work.

Investigating the association among seasons, mood, and productivity, Dr. Jamison found a strong seasonal pattern of mood changes among artists and writers, with highest mood scores in the summer and lowest in the winter. Peak periods of productivity, while also seasonal, occurred in the spring and the fall. It seemed that as mood increased from spring to summer, so productivity declined to some extent, picking up again in the fall. Those who had been treated for mood disorders had a sharper decline of productivity in the summer than the other subjects.

A few possible explanations for this drop-off in creativity in the summer, as mood continues to improve, come to mind. When people are too euphoric, they are often not best able to produce. Their thoughts may race too quickly, and their focus may be scattered. There is a tendency to start many tasks but not to follow through— distractibility is a problem. Those subjects in Dr. Jamison's study who had been treated for mood disorders might have experienced more marked highs during the summer, with greater associated difficulties in focusing and carrying out tasks. Another possibility is that the artist might not wish to be creative during the summer. One writer with SAD, whom I know, said that she has so much fun in the summer that she doesn't want to spend her golden, sunny days bashing away at a word processor.

A novel way of measuring creativity has been developed by Drs. Ruth Richards and Dennis Kinney, researchers at Harvard University. The advantage of their Lifetime Creativity Scale is that it can be used to measure creativity in anyone, not just in those of exceptional talent. By means of this scale, these researchers were able to show a higher rate of creativity among manic–depressives (bipolar patients) than expected. But even greater creativity scores were found among the relatives of bipolar patients—those with milder mood swings or no clear-cut mood swings at all. This heightened level of creativity found in relatives of bipolar patients may explain why the illness has been transmitted so successfully from generation to generation. People who carry bipolar genes may be at an advantage to survive and reproduce by virtue of their creative abilities. People with bipolar tendencies and their relatives seem more likely to take risks, such as emigrating, which may be highly adaptive in crisis situations.

All these studies suggest that Aristotle was correct in linking mood disturbance and creativity. It seems as though the most creative people are those with milder forms of mood disturbance, which is in keeping with my clinical experience. Severe depressions or wild manias are not conducive to productivity. The opposite is true for mild depressions alternating with hypomania. During hypomanic periods, thoughts and associations flow rapidly, energy and confidence levels are high, the need for sleep is reduced, and ideas are more readily generated and pursued. During mild depressions, these ideas can be evaluated critically. Ideas that are too grandiose or unlikely to succeed can be discarded, and those that look most promising in the more sober light of depression can be retained and developed. Mild depressions may be conducive to the drudgery that is required for any creative venture—the daily plodding necessary for the execution of any grand scheme.

The seasonal person will easily recognize this pattern of mood swings and its relationship to creativity, for the depressions of SAD are often relatively mild in severity, the hypomania restrained and productive. As we now know, the mood changes in SAD patients are often driven by the amount of daylight present. Many creative artists have recognized the connection between changes in environmental light and their mood and productivity. The following section deals with famous creative people who suffered from mood disorders—especially those for whom there is evidence of strong seasonality or light sensitivity.

Moody and Famous:
Sensitive to Seasons and Light

The list of famous people with mood disturbances is impressive. Although there was no psychiatrist with a modern diagnostic handbook around to record the mental status of most of the people in this section, abundant evidence for mood disorders exists in most cases. It is not my purpose here to be comprehensive, only to select some illustrative examples of famous creative people with mood disorders. Among artists we have Michelangelo, Albrecht Dürer, and Vincent van Gogh; composers include George Frideric Handel, Gustav Mahler, and Robert Schumann; writers include John Milton, Edgar Allan Poe, Ernest Hemingway, and Virginia Woolf; politicians include Abraham Lincoln and Winston Churchill, who referred to his depressions as his "black dog." Sir Isaac Newton was perhaps the most eminent scientist to have suffered from manic–depression.

How many of these people were strongly seasonal in their mood swings or sensitive to changes in environmental light is hard to say with any clinical certainty, especially since SAD as a distinct entity was first described long after most of these artists were deceased. Statistically, it is highly likely that many of these people were seasonal. Figures for the rate of SAD among clinics of recurrent depressives range from one in six to one in three. Highly creative people with mood disorders are more likely to have SAD than other forms of mood disorder, most of which are more disruptive to productivity. Beyond such general statistical information, however, we do have specific clues about seasonality and light sensitivity in several cases.

Among writers, Emily Dickinson is a likely candidate for a diagnosis of SAD (see Chapter 17). T. S. Eliot might be another patient for this distinguished clinic. His poetry sparkles with references to light. We learn that Eliot was instructed by his doctors to go south each winter. Could that have been to treat his SAD? We can only speculate. Milton is reputed to have suffered from summer SAD and, according to his biographer, was able to work on *Paradise Lost* during only half the year, between autumn and spring.

Another writer with a mood disorder was Guy de Maupassant. Toward the end of his life he attempted suicide and went on to die in an asylum. The following extract is from a story called "Who Knows?" in which the narrator, who ends up in an asylum, recalls how he went to Italy, where the sunlight made him feel good. After that, he recounts,

I returned to France via Marseilles, and in spite of the gaiety of Provence, the diminished intensity of sunlight depressed me. On my return to the Continent, I had the odd feeling of a patient who thinks he is cured but who is warned by a dull pain that the source of illness has not been eradicated.

Was de Maupassant seasonal? It seems like a fair bet.

Among musicians, Handel and Mahler were most clearly seasonal. Both, we are told, did most of their creative work during the summer months. One of the most prodigiously rapid feats of composition was Handel's *Messiah,* which he completed in twenty-three days, between late August and mid-September. Mahler, who called himself the "summer composer," was fortunately an avid letter writer. His seasonal mood changes are clearly reflected in his letters. Contrast the following two letters, one written in summer and one in winter.

To Joseph Steiner, Puzsta-Batta, June 19, 1879

Dear Steiner,

Now for the third day I return to you, and today I do so in order to take leave of you in merry mood. It is the story of my life that is recorded in these pages. What a strange destiny, sweeping me along on the waves of my yearning, now hurling me this way and that in the gale, now wafting me along merrily in smiling sunshine. What I fear is that in such a gale I shall someday be shattered against a reef—such Mae stem grazed!

It is six o'clock in the morning! I have been out on the heath, sitting with Fárkas the shepherd, listening to the sound of his Shawn. Ah, how mournful it sounded, and yet how full of rapturous delight—that folktune he played! Ah, Steiner! You are still asleep in your bed, and I have already seen the dew on the grasses. I am now so serenely gay and the tranquil happiness all around me is tiptoeing into my heart, too, as the sun of early spring lights up the wintry fields. Is spring awakening now in my own breast?! And while this mood prevails, let me take leave of you, my faithful friend!

Contrast that with a winter postcard, sent to Friedrich Löhr, January 20, 1883.

Dear Fritz,

Simply cannot find time to write to you properly. Sending the stuff soon. My address is:. . . . Am extremely depressed.

Very best wishes to you and your family,

Yours,

Gustav

But two years later, in spring, Mahler wrote to the same friend:

My dear Fritz,

My windows are open and the sunny, fragrant spring is gazing in upon me, everywhere endless peace and repose. In this fair hour that is granted me I will be together with you. . . .

   With the coming of spring all has grown mild in me again. From my window I have a view across the city to the mountains and woods, and the kindly Fulda wends its amiable way between; whenever the sun casts its colored lights within, as now, well, you know how everything in one relaxes. That is the mood I am in today, sitting at my desk by the window, from time to time casting a peaceful glance out upon this scene of carefree calm.

There are many other letters that suggest that Mahler suffered from SAD.

Painters and sculptors are more difficult to diagnose in retrospect than writers, but Jamison's work would suggest that they are as susceptible to mood disturbances. Artists, perhaps more than any other group, have struggled to portray light. In fact, the works of some can be instantly recognized by the distinctive quality of the light they portray: Turner's swirls of light; Rembrandt's splashes of *chiaroscuro,* illuminating the pensive faces of his models; and, of course, the dazzling colors of Vincent van Gogh.

Of these three painters, the only one with a clear history of a mood disorder is van Gogh. It seems very likely that he suffered from manic–depression, although his clinical picture was complicated by intoxication with absinthe, the French liquor that at that time had a toxic ingredient in it. Van Gogh's intimate understanding of depression is apparent in his famous sketches, *Sorrow* and *The Old Man in Sorrow.* In contrast to these sad figures is *The Reaper,* a young man striding boldly across a field with a huge, luminous sun shining in the background. Van Gogh's wonderful use of light and color might make one suspect that he was extremely sensitive to light, and indeed, his letters to his beloved brother Theo appear to bear this out. They are filled with descriptions of his feelings of sadness and joy, and of his sensitivity to the weather, and to light and darkness in particular. Here are a few selections (reprinted from Irving Stone's *Dear Theo*):

[Autumn in Drenthe, 1883]

When I look around me, everything seems too miserable, too insufficient, too dilapidated. We are having gloomy days of rain now, and when

I come to the corner of the garret where I have settled down, it is curiously melancholy there; through one single glass pane the light falls on an empty co lour box, on a bundle of brushes the hair of which is quite worn down. It is so strangely melancholy that it has, luckily, almost a comical aspect—enough not to make one cry over it.

As long as the weather was fine I did not mind my troubles, because I saw so many beautiful things; but with this rainy weather, which we must expect to continue for months, I see more clearly how I have got stuck here, and how handicapped I am. . . .

[Winter in Nuenen, 1883]

Hardly ever have I begun a year of gloomier aspect, or in a gloomier mood. It is dreary outside; the fields are a mass of lumps of black earth and some snow, with days mostly of mist and mire. . . . This is what I see in passing, and it is quite in harmony with the interiors, very gloomy these dark winter days.

[Spring in The Hague, 1892]

Spring is coming fast here. We have had a few real spring days; last Monday, for instance, which I enjoyed very much. I think the poor people and the painters have in common this feeling for the weather and the change of the seasons.

In February 1888, Vincent van Gogh left Paris for Arles, in the south of France, at least in part to escape the darkness of the North and seek out the brilliant and dazzling light of Provence. In van Gogh's own words,

I came to the south for a thousand reasons. I wanted to see a different light, I believed that by looking at nature under a bright sky one might gain a truer idea of the Japanese way of feeling and drawing. Finally, I wanted to see this stronger sun . . . because I felt that the colors of the spectrum are misted over in the north.

Here is a description to his brother Theo, written from Arles in the summer of 1888:

The loneliness has not worried me, because I have found the brighter sun and its effect on nature so absorbing. . . .

Yesterday at sunset I was in a stony heath where some very small and twisted oaks grow, in the background a ruin on the hill and corn in the valley. It was romantic, like a Monticelli; the sun was pouring bright yellow rays upon the bushes and the ground, a perfect shower of gold, and all the lines were lovely. . . .

Here is another description of the sun by van Gogh:

> Now there is a glorious fierce heat, a sun, a light which for want of a better word I can only call yellow, pale sculpture yellow, pale lemon gold. How beautiful yellow is.
>
> Life is almost an enchantment. Those who do not believe in the sun here are without faith!

To sum up, creativity appears to be more common among patients with mood disorders, especially those whose condition is relatively mild, as well as among the relatives of such patients. It is quite conceivable that genes for creativity and mood disorders are transmitted together. It is important for treating psychiatrists to understand this. Eradicating all mood swings may diminish creativity in some people, though it is likely to improve matters greatly for those whose mood swings are severe. Nowadays, when an understanding of the human genetic makeup is close at hand, and the possibility of preventing certain undesirable genes in the new generation is scientifically conceivable, we would do well to consider the beneficial aspects of certain types of emotional disturbance, while never forgetting the pain they can cause. Had the birth of all depressives in history been prevented successfully, the world we live in would be a far different place today, though not necessarily a better one.

Prominent seasonal changes in mood and behavior seem particularly conducive to creativity, and there is evidence that many creative artists, both past and present, have experienced them.

SEVENTEEN

Words for All Seasons

*F*or centuries, the seasons have inspired poets and songwriters, who have left us a glorious legacy describing the changes that occur, both in the world around us and in ourselves as, year after year, the tilted earth rotates around the sun. What is it that has so inspired writers over the ages? I believe it is, first, the intense feelings with which the changing seasons imbue us; second, the capacity of seasonal images to evoke memories in us; and third, the appeal of the cycle of the seasons as a metaphor for a person's life.

The seasonal changes in energy, feelings, and drives that we now recognize to be a common part of the human experience are accompanied by prominent changes in the world around us: varied colors, fragrances, temperatures, and sounds. By reminding us of these specific sensations, the poet can evoke in us the feelings that often accompany them. Beyond the re-creation of these feelings, and the nostalgia that comes with them, the seasons remind us of cyclical time, loss and recovery, birth, death, and renewal.

In poetry, spring has usually been portrayed as representing reawakening, rebirth, sexuality, and joy, and for some this is true. Yet others find spring to be a difficult and painful season. Summer is seen as a time of happiness and generativity. Autumn engenders mixed feelings: Nature is intensely beautiful and summer's harvest abounds, but there are also hints of the approach of winter, and melancholy often accompanies them. Then winter comes, and with it the death of vegetation; cold, inhospitable temperatures; food shortages; the disappearance of birds and animals; and, of course, the waning of the sun's light.

The cycle of the seasons has often been compared by writers and artists to a person's life. This is a strange metaphor. One might think that a person's life would be better conceptualized as linear—a straight line from birth to death. But perhaps it is more difficult for us to think of our lives in such a linear way—as a segment snipped out of a long string, with a finite beginning and end. Instead, we once again embrace the concept of cyclical time—ashes to ashes, dust to dust—to create the more comforting image of life as a ring, round and complete.

In connecting the seasons with the cycles of a person's life, poets have linked spring with youth, summer with the prime of life, autumn with declining powers, and winter with old age.

Seasons and Passion

In spring, as the saying goes, a young man's fancy lightly turns to thoughts of love, and this applies to women, too. So it has been since biblical times, when Solomon, poet and lover, sang out to his beloved:

> For lo, the winter is past,
> the rain is over and gone.
> The flowers appear on the earth,
> the time of singing has come
> and the voice of the turtledove
> is heard in our land.

The passions of spring continued unabated for thousands of years. As Shakespeare observed:

> Between the acres of the rye
> With a hey, and a ho, and a hey nonino,
> These pretty country folks would lie,
> In the spring time, the only pretty ring time,
> When birds do sing, hey ding a ding, ding:
> Sweet lovers love the spring.

Yet the spring has not always been associated with unmixed joy. With spring comes the revival of desire, which has lain dormant through the winter. There may be an inertia to overcome before the energy of spring can be fully enjoyed. Emily Dickinson, one of our most seasonal poets, described this sensation:

> I cannot meet the Spring unmoved—
> I feel the old desire—
> A Hurry with a lingering, mixed,
> A Warrant to be fair—

T. S. Eliot, in his famous lines, expressed a more painful form of spring fever:

> April is the cruelest month, breeding
> Lilacs out of the dead land, mixing
> Memory and desire, stirring
> Dull roots with spring rain.

Summer has been regarded by some as a season of heady delight. Emily Dickinson writes:

> Inebriate of air am I,
> And debauchee of dew,
> Reeling, through endless summer days,
> From inns of Molten Blue.

She compares herself to a bee, drunk on the light of the sun, an influence more intoxicating than any liquor brewed.

Although autumn has been regarded by some, like Keats, as a "season of mists and mellow fruitfulness," a time of beauty and fulfillment, others have seen it as a sad time—a time of waning light and a harbinger of the coming winter. Matthew Arnold, for example, wrote:

> Coldly, sadly descends
> The autumn evening.
> The field Strewn with its dank yellow drifts
> Of wither'd leaves, and the elms,
> Fade into dimness apace,
> Silent.

While poets have had their differences in their views of autumn, winter has been almost universally treated as a season of despondency and unremitting gloom. According to Shakespeare, "a sad tale's best for winter." James Thomson, in his poem "Winter," in 1726, encapsulated the common view of this season:

> See! Winter comes, to rule the varied Year,
> Sullen, and sad.

Seasons and Memories

The poet can depend on the reader to have powerful memories and emotions associated with the seasons. The distinctive colors, smells, and characteristics that each brings serve as cues to memories of poignant events that have occurred in that season. Conversely, the memory of a significant event is often colored and modified by the season in which it happened. We can perhaps recall the quality of the sky, the weather, and the specific smells of the season. Associations such as these were emphasized by Freud in his models of how the mind works. The importance of such associations continues to be recognized by both writers and mental health professionals. They are in no way incompatible with our more recent understanding of the biological changes in mood and behavior associated with the seasons.

Such memories, reawakened by a particular time of year, are described, for example, by Edgar Allan Poe in his poem "Ulalume":

> The skies they were ashen and sober;
> The leaves they were crisped and sere—
> The leaves they were withering and sere;
> It was night in the lonesome October
> Of my most immemorial year,

As the poem continues, it emerges that the poet, driven by some compulsion that he does not understand, seeks out a path to the tomb of his beloved, whom he buried on that same October day the year before. He has repressed this memory until he comes across the tomb with the name of his beloved, Ulalume, upon it. At this sight, the sad memory of her loss penetrates him and he recalls now why the autumn, with its crisped and sere leaves, sent such a chill through his heart. Poe thus provides us with a powerful example of how we associate important events in our lives with the seasons in which they happen.

So does Shelley in his poem "Adonais," where he laments the death of Keats, which occurred in late winter. He writes:

> Ah, woe is me! Winter is come and gone,
> But grief returns with the revolving year.

The Seasons of a Person's Life

The seasons as metaphor for the stages of a person's life was succinctly expressed by Keats:

> He has his lusty Spring, when fancy clear
> Takes in all beauty with an easy span:
> He has his Summer, when luxuriously
> Spring's honey'd cud of youthful thought he loves
> To ruminate, and by such dreaming high
> Is nearest unto heaven; quiet coves
> His soul has in its Autumn, when his wings
> He furleth close; . . .
> He has his Winter too of pale misfeature,
> Or else he would forgo his mortal nature.

Shakespeare also compares the final stages of a person's life to winter and finds both barren and dreary:

> That time of year thou may'st in me behold
> When yellow leaves, or none, or few, do hang
> Upon those boughs which shake against the cold,
> Bare ruin'd choirs, where late the sweet birds sang.

Seasonal imagery has also been used to evoke feelings about an era, as Dickens did when he labeled the period of the French Revolution as "the spring of hope . . . the winter of despair." Likewise, Thomas Hardy, looking out over the landscape at the end of the nineteenth century, saw in its dreary, wintry features a metaphor for the dead century and a confirmation of his sense of hopelessness for the future:

I leaned upon a coppice gate
When Frost was spectre-grey
And Winter's dregs made desolate
The weakening eye of day. . . .

The land's sharp features seemed to be
The Century's corpse outleant;
His crypt the cloudy canopy,
The wind his death lament.

The ancient pulse of germ and birth
Was shrunken hard and dry,
And every spirit upon earth
Seemed fervourless as I.

The Loveliness of the Light

Just think of the illimitable abundance and the marvelous
loveliness of light, or of the beauty of the sun and moon and
stars.

—St. Augustine, *City of God*

Light has many meanings for us, and poets and authors have used images of it to illustrate them. Besides revealing our world to us, light can, in itself, influence the way we feel. In addition to the effects of light shining from the world outside, much has been written about the "inner light."

The capacity of light to induce in us a sense of wonder and joy may be new to scientists, but writers have recognized it for centuries. In the second verse of Genesis, we are told:

And God said, "Let there be light"; and there was light. And God saw that the light was good.

Later on in the Bible, in Ecclesiastes, we are advised:

Truly the light is sweet, and a pleasant thing it is for the eyes to behold the sun.

Just as light has been associated with joy, so has darkness been associated with sorrow. Perhaps no poet could understand darkness so well as the blind Milton, who wrote:

Seasons return, but not to me returns Day, or the sweet approach
    of ev'n or morn,
Or sight of vernal bloom, or summer's rose,
Or flocks, or herds, or human face divine;
But cloud instead, and ever-during dark
Surrounds me, from the cheerful ways of men.

But even to the sighted, the dim light of winter could prove de-
pressing. If the reader is not by now convinced that Emily Dickinson
suffered from SAD, the following verse should settle the question:

> There's a certain Slant of light,
> Winter Afternoons
> That oppresses, like the weight
> Of cathedral tunes.
>
> Heavenly hurt, it gives us;
> We can find no scar,
> But internal difference
> Where the meanings are.

Dickinson's intuitiveness is astonishing. She not only connects her
mood with the quality of the light—specifically, its low angle—but recognizes that one can be hurt without external manifestations; that inside the mind are places where the meanings of things are recorded,
where joy and suffering are experienced. Although Dickinson points
out that weak and fading light can be oppressive, she also observes that

> We grow accustomed to the Dark—
> When Light is put away—
> As when the Neighbor holds the Lamp
> To witness her Goodbye—
>
> Either the Darkness alters—
> Or something in the sight
> Adjusts itself to Midnight—
> And Life steps almost straight.

Again, this brilliant poet is observing something within herself
that corresponds to the physiological changes that occur in the eye—
and perhaps the brain—when we are surrounded by darkness. The eye
adapts to the dark—the pupil enlarges and the rods, the most light-

sensitive receptors in the retina, take over from the cones, which are responsible for ordinary vision. It is quite conceivable that a corresponding adaptation to the dark occurs in the brain.

Flooding the dark-adapted eye (and perhaps brain) with light may have a powerful effect on mood. Such an effect, as is produced by bright snow on a dark winter's day, was described by T. S. Eliot in "Little Gidding":

> Midwinter spring is its own season . . .
> When the short day is brightest, with frost and fire,
> The brief sun flames the ice, on pond and ditches. . . .
> A glare that is blindness in the early afternoon—
> And glow more intense than blaze of branch, or brazier,
>
> Stirs the dumb spirit: . . .
> In the dark time of the year . . .
> The soul's sap quivers.

The capacity of light to affect mood was recognized by William James in his book *The Varieties of Religious Experience*. He cites an example from the autobiography of J. Trevor, in which the author describes how, one Sunday morning, he felt unable to accompany his wife and sons to church, "as though to leave the sunshine on the hills, and go down there to the chapel, would be for the time an act of spiritual suicide. And I felt such need for new inspiration and expansion in my life." So reluctantly he bid his wife and sons farewell and headed for the hills with his stick and his dog.

> In the loveliness of the morning, and the beauty of the hills and valleys, I soon lost my sense of sadness and regret. . . . On the way back, suddenly, without warning, I felt that I was in Heaven—an inward state of peace and joy and assurance indescribably intense, accompanied with a sense of being bathed in a warm glow of light, as though the external condition had brought about the internal effect—a feeling of having passed beyond the body . . . by reason of the illumination in the midst of which I seemed to be placed. This deep emotion lasted, though with decreasing strength, until I reached home, and for some time after, only gradually passing away.

Architects have recognized the important influence of interior lighting of a building on the way its inhabitants feel. For example, in a recent restoration of a small London church designed by Christopher Wren, the architects went to great lengths to create the effect of daylight in the church's dome. One lighting consultant noted that he was seeking "that magical moment when you feel light becomes a material rather than something only to be in." Had similar pains been taken with the lighting in the church of Mr. J. Trevor, who was just quoted, he might not have chosen to spend his morning in the sunlight of the hills.

Mr. J. Trevor's response to the sunlit hills is reminiscent of the reactions of the people of Tromsö on *Soldag* or, for that matter, of the reports by many patients with SAD following treatment with bright light therapy. Just as the darkness oppressed Emily Dickinson by acting on the place "where the meanings are," so perhaps the light exerts its uplifting effects by acting on the same part of the brain to reverse the oppressive effects of darkness. It seems reasonable to postulate, as Emily Dickinson did, the existence of a part of the brain capable of being stimulated by light entering the eyes and thereby registering feelings of wonder and joy. The same part of the brain, if deprived of light, might lead to sadness and despair. I would speculate that this part of the brain, so sensitive to the presence or absence of light, is located in—or influenced by—the hypothalamus at the base of the brain.

Besides the many descriptions of the way in which light from the world outside affects our mood, there are also many reports of internally perceived light, often associated with powerful emotions and, at times, with religious conversions or other major life changes. Eliade, who called this experience "the mystic light," described many reports of such experiences by holy men of all religions, as well as by apparently ordinary people. Famous examples of mystic light experiences appear in the New Testament, where Saul of Tarsus, on the road to Damascus, experienced blinding light, which resulted in his conversion to Christianity; and in the Bhagavad Gita, where Krishna appeared to Arjuna "with the effulgence of a thousand suns." The poet Henry Vaughan (1622–1695) described such an experience as follows:

> I saw Eternity the other night
> Like a great *Ring* of pure and endless light,
> All calm as it was bright.

How can we understand mystical visions of light if we do not ascribe these experiences to divine intervention? I believe that the clue may lie in their resemblance to the euphoriant effects of bright light therapy in patients with SAD or to the effects on those in the far North or South when the sun returns after many weeks of darkness.

During light therapy, light enters via the eyes and acts on a part of the brain "where the meanings are," inducing feelings of energy, re-awakening, tranquillity, harmony, and joy. Under certain circumstances, the same part of the brain might perhaps be activated either spontaneously or by some stimulus other than light.

Whatever the mechanism of such mystical light experiences, and whatever their influence on the individual might be, there seems to be little question that they occur. Their profound emotional effects are compatible with the idea that light can powerfully modify mood and behavior—a lesson I have learned from my experiences with the treatment of patients with SAD.

EIGHTEEN

Winter Light
Life Beyond SAD

One must have a mind for winter
To regard the frost and the boughs
Of the pine-trees crusted with snow;

And have been cold a long time
To behold the junipers shagged with ice,
The spruces rough in the distant glitter

Of the January sun; and not to think
Of any misery in the sound of the wind,
In the sound of a few leaves,

Which is the sound of the land
Full of the same wind
That is blowing in the same bare place

For the listener, who listens in the snow,
And, nothing himself, beholds
nothing that is not there and the nothing that is.
—WALLACE STEVENS, "The Snow Man"

As this beautiful poem suggests, one must have a mind for winter.
The joys of the season are not easily acquired, especially for those
whose biology makes them want to flee from winter. They are joys

that must be earned. And so, gentle reader, having reached the end of this book, you have earned the right not only to endure winter, but to enjoy it; not only to treat the maladies that it brings, but to seek out its hidden pleasures. By now, we have a generation of people who have grown up since SAD was described and light therapy has been available. There are SAD veterans of many winters, those who have been unable or unwilling to flee to the sunny South, who have nevertheless made good lives for themselves in the North. I count myself among these fortunate individuals. This chapter deals with what we have learned about life beyond SAD and how we have found light in this dark season.

Winning My Own Battle with Winter

Winter no longer fills me with foreboding. All the evidence of its impending presence is still there in the world around me: the encroachment of dark at either end of the day, like a rat nibbling away at a piece of cheese; the leaves turning color; the odd angle of the sun. But the feeling is different. There is a stirring inside me, a sense that this is what I have been waiting for, the winter, a wild frontier, alien and familiar as the wilderness, provoking me to react, create, survive, and triumph. Perhaps that is what it feels like to raft down the white waters of an untamed river or scale a sheer cliff. I have no idea. I have never done either of these things and probably never will. No matter. Winter is adventure enough for me.

I have been told by rock climbers of the surge of adrenaline they feel when they gaze down hundreds of feet, especially those who hang from the cliff by their bare hands without the help of tools. I know of some who have even felt the need for such death-defying exploits to feel alive, a vital part of their world. Perhaps winter has offered that sort of adrenaline rush to humans ever since they wandered from the sundrenched savannahs and ventured into the glacial regions of the North.

I was amazed to read of the ice man, excavated recently from a glacier in which he had been buried for over five thousand years. He was well equipped for life in that unfriendly climate. Dressed in bearskin clothes and a grass cape, he carried a copper axe, and a bow and arrows, housed in a deerskin quiver. Among the many things found with the frozen man were two birchbark canisters, which might have held the embers from a fire, a sloeberry—no doubt his food—and two mushrooms strung on a leather cord, perhaps a type of primitive anti-biotic. Of course, no one is fully protected against bad luck, and all his tools and preparations were of no help to him on the fateful day of his death. I like to think that it was swift, a sudden blast of ice or snow and quick oblivion while he was asleep, dreaming of how best to snare some animal or find his favorite berries higher up the slopes. In any event, we are the beneficiaries of his untimely fate as nature, acting as museum curator, embalmed him for our scrutiny.

Harsh environments foster creativity, and winter in the North is about as harsh an environment as you can find on our planet. Animals that live at some distance from the equator must generate energy for all their body functions, against the gradient of the freezing cold, when all the usual sources of energy in our physical world—plant and animal life—are at their lowest ebb. This challenge of survival is dramatized in the book *Two Old Women*, a moving story by Velma Wallis, in which she describes how two elders are abandoned by their tribe at the ap-proach of winter. For these two frail people, being forced to confront the Alaskan winter without food, shelter, or electricity is virtually a death sentence. After absorbing the shock of this betrayal, one woman says, "If we are going to die, let us die trying, not sitting." And slowly, painfully, they try, compensating for their lack of strength and agility with a lifetime of accumulated wisdom and experience. Ultimately they succeed not only in surviving the winter but also in accumulating enough food to help feed the entire tribe.

Many people with SAD will surely be able to relate to the old women in Wallis's book. Even though you may not be old or live above the Arctic Circle, and though you may have adequate heat and food all year round, winter remains a difficult season. But as with the old women, the urge to fight against winter can triumph over the longing to give up and succumb to it. Nowadays, when asked how se-vere my SAD is, I am always at a loss for an answer, simply because for many years I have not allowed the condition its full expression. I have used every means at my disposal to overcome it, and as a consequence, each winter has become a little easier for me. Age and experience have been my allies, as have the testimonies of those who claim winter is the best time of year for them. I have tried to learn what they enjoy about winter so that I can experience it too. So far have my skills at manag-ing the winter developed that I have even come to the point of looking forward to the winter, a state of mind I never thought possible.

One aspect of the winter that has been a source of joy for me is my research. Winter has been a critical part of my business. In this regard, I have found myself sharing an unexpected kinship with purveyors of space heaters, sweaters, and furs, with ice fishermen and ski instructors. I have researched the effects of darkness, and the success of such research depends on bad weather, which brings patients into a research program. Unseasonably clement winter weather, on the other hand, may keep potential research subjects away and may threaten studies by altering the biology of those involved in experiments. During one recent winter, my group did exceptionally well in recruiting patients for our program as the northeastern United States was hit by one ice storm after another. I would wake up each day, check the weather conditions, and respond with glee at the news of the latest storm. My wife was not amused.

Don't get me wrong, though. Such euphoria is not to be depended on, and winter still has the power to buffalo me. Every winter brings with it at least a few dark days when I feel a sort of stasis of the blood, a sludging of all my biological processes, especially my thinking. I am in slow motion in relation to the rest of the world and compared to how I feel at all other times of the year. I have come to accept these days, but I still dislike them. I wake up on such dark days stirring like a hedgehog disturbed from his hibernating state. I am in conservation mode and do and say only what is essential. Fortunately, with good self-care these days become fewer with each passing winter.

But when the winter stasis is upon me, I lose the capacity to process multiple things at the same time. I become linear. One idea has to be completed before there is room in my brain for the next one: one action at a time. Finish this before starting that. What a pain in the neck! So I proceed through my daily activities. Exercise is essential, coupled with light; yet motivation is hard to muster. On days of ice and snow, I ride my stationary bicycle in front of a light box and the morning news.

By now, I have been through this cycle almost thirty times since my arrival in North America. I understand its biological basis and, more important, that it will pass in time, provided I use light and exercise and limit the stresses that can be controlled. Above all, I need to accept my need to hibernate (albeit to a much reduced extent). I must let go of some of my driving demands. If I lower my expectations of myself, I have to acknowledge that my functioning is quite acceptable, and for now, that has to be good enough.

The holiday season brings its round of social activities. When I am not in my dark days, I am a very sociable person, but when the stasis of the blood sets in, I want to sit at home, to brood and ruminate. Now it is time for some dinner engagement, and I am paralyzed before my clothes closet, fixated over what shirt to pick out, over the ordinary things that have to be done to get out of the house and on my way. "I have no energy," I mutter under my breath. "I don't think I can possibly have any fun tonight."

But I usually do. People energize me. And so I am off again, carried forward by the remedies I both prescribe and use. And I do enjoy the parties, the friends, the fact that even though the sun has abandoned us yet again, there is still life to be had in winter. Or else, of an evening, I curl up with some good book, poetry perhaps that can be read in snatches. On one occasion, my wife and I chose to spend New Year's Eve in the bedroom in front of the television. We had the bright lights on and dozed and watched television intermittently. And then, all of a sudden, "Auld Lang Syne" was playing and the ball was falling in Times Square. We gave each other a hug, and at that moment I had the distinct impression that somewhere in the heavens, the sun had passed its nadir and begun to climb.

Recapturing the Winters of Childhood

For most people who develop SAD, its symptoms begin after adolescence. Many of them have happy memories of the winters of their childhood, but these are buried under years of suffering. After they overcome their SAD symptoms, one of the unexpected gifts of this healing is to be able to access these memories once again and feel a sense of reintegration with their childhood selves. I have interviewed several such people with SAD, who grew up in different parts of the United States, and here are three of their stories.

Skating in New England

The winters of New England, made famous in writings such as those of Robert Frost, are known for their snowy landscapes, icy ways, frigid temperatures, and the tough-mindedness of those who have made it their home. Kathleen, now in her thirties, remembers growing up in a Catholic neighborhood of Boston. For her, the joyful memories of winter are inextricably entangled with skating. She recalls:

> When I was eleven or so, I got my first pair of skates. There was a field nearby—technically more of a swamp—and in the fall, the boys would go down and burn up the field, and the fire department would come and put out the fire. All the reeds would have been burned down below the water level, and it would freeze over in the winter. We'd all go shovel it off and skate. The boys would play hockey, and the girls would try to do figure skating.
>
> We would occasionally get ice storms and ice would freeze on the trees, and it would be very dangerous. But one of the most fun memories I have of winter was of one such ice storm. Of course we didn't have school that day and the streets froze over to such an extent that we all grabbed our skates and went skating up and down the streets of the neighborhood and had a grand time.

As an adult, Kathleen controls her SAD well by a combination of light therapy and outdoor exercise. She continues to run, ski, and, of course, to skate. She notes:

> With skating, there comes a moment, after your body has warmed up and you're not rusty anymore, particularly if you are skating outdoors and there are not a lot of people around, when everything comes together. I'm just skating, and there's the sky and the sun and the trees, and it's not even like praying anymore. I become the prayer. You become graceful, moving, but part of all the scene around you, the frozen pond, the soul of the trees and the sun.

Making a Wood Fire in Winter

> Wood warms you twice—once when you cut it and once when it burns.
>
> —Henry David Thoreau

James, a man in his thirties, formerly a mathematician, now owns and runs a flower and herb farm with his wife in the mid-Atlantic region of the United States. He recalls a lifelong love of wood fires in the winter.

> We'd always have a fire when we got back home: that's always been a big thing for me. I love the fire in the fireplace. I like gathering and cutting the wood. It's almost as much fun as the fire itself. I've always liked the wood—the smell, the feel, cutting, organizing and stacking it, making use out of something that's already there, the resourcefulness of it. Not just turning on some kind of appliance. I like starting the fire in the fireplace, the challenge, knowing how to do it. You learn about bark, which wood not to burn, how to watch out for poison ivy, which you can get even worse in the winter than in the summer. I like cooking over fires and the direct heat of the fire, better than devices like heat pumps. I like its different phases or stages—as the thing dies down a little, it just sort of glows. A lot of times you'll get sleepy after a while; the fire kind of corresponds to your level of activity.

As an adult, James has handled his own seasonality by choosing a career that allows for varying levels of work at different times of year. He works with the sun—long hours in the summer and short hours in the winter. He has resisted growing too much in a greenhouse because that would defeat his wish to slow down during the winter. And there is no preserving, because everything fresh is purchased rapidly. He feels the changing seasons almost as he imagines a plant might feel them, waiting for the wild blackberries to come back each year and the appearance of every fruit and flower at its predicted time. By fitting his lifestyle to his biological rhythms, James has found peace and contentment.

Drinking Tea in the Snow in Alaska

Beth, an Athapaskan Indian, was born in Alaska in a small village at the junction of the Yukon and Tanana Rivers. She recalls the special respect her people had for the land and all its animals, even those they hunted for sustenance. For example, when her brothers set out to kill a moose, they would never say out loud what they were planning to do. If they did, they believed, the moose would hear that boastful statement and evade them. Instead, they would say, "We're going to look around," and everyone knew what they meant. In the same way, telling a story about how they shot the moose would be frowned on.

Dealing with winter is a dominant theme in the lives of the Athapaskan Indians. The people would make intense preparations for the onset of winter. Her family would boat up to Fish Lake to pick the high- and lowbush cranberries to make jellies and jams for the winter. In late summer, they would catch salmon in fishnets and fishwheels. The fish would be taken to the smokehouse and smoked to last through the long winter months. Each family would shoot one moose at the start of the season. You shot only as much as you needed—no more.

Winters were tough in many ways. The family had only a woodstove for warmth and cooking. Her father and brothers would go out to cut birchwood, often in the waist-deep snow, wearing caribou-skin boots, tied with leather thongs below the knees. For additional food, they would hunt ptarmigan and rabbit in the snow.

Beth and her friends enjoyed outdoor things, even though at midwinter in Alaska there were only four hours of light a day. The lake would freeze over, smooth as a mirror, and they would skate on it or go sledding. They would hitch up the dogs and sled into the woods to build a campfire, make tea, and drink it with crackers and dry fish. Those were peaceful times.

Night was a time for visiting, telling funny stories, and playing wild card games in which the cards flew about in all directions. Then there were special occasions, when family-oriented activities and square dances would take place. She remembers winters as a time enjoyed by all.

Nothing in her childhood would have prepared Beth for the onset, later in life, of seasonal depression, inherited perhaps from her Caucasian father, who had married an Athapaskan woman. For this she was successfully treated with light therapy. She moved to Colorado, which she thought would be better for her because of the greater abundance of light at that lower latitude. Feeling culturally isolated from her people, however, she elected to return to Alaska, where she currently works and functions well throughout the year. Back in Anchorage, she is close to her family, her traditions, and her personal history, which she can now enjoy all winter long thanks to brief post-Christmas vacations in Mexico and the successful treatment of her SAD symptoms.

The Joys of Winter

As the preceding stories indicate, many joys can be found in winter, if only one has the inclination and energy to seek them. Here are some that I have encountered in my own experience of winters in the North. I encourage you to pursue whatever it is that gives you pleasure in the dark season.

Festivals, Stories, and Gifts

Winter is a fine time for festivals, storytelling, and gifts. Given the natural dreariness of the season, it is not surprising that different cultures have chosen to celebrate this time of year with festivals, many of which have ancient origins. Christmas, for example, is said to have its roots in pagan times, Hanukkah to hark back to the time of the Maccabees. Aside from these winter solstice festivals, there are a host of other ritualized celebrations to cheer up the dark days: Halloween, Thanksgiving, Oktoberfest, Valentine's Day, Groundhog Day, and the Ice Festival are all ways of marking the passing of winter in a spirited manner. According to one Minnesotan I spoke with, "The Ice Festival is a time when we go out and shake our fists at winter."

Giving and receiving gifts is a great way of remembering that we love and are loved even during winter. They are a natural addition to the winter festivals. Sometimes the best gifts are those that cost very little but mean a great deal. For example, one winter holiday when an ice storm caused our pipes to burst, I called a friend who is a building contractor, lamenting this sorry turn of events. He came right over, and we set out together to the hardware store to purchase the parts needed to fix the pipes. My friend, who would much rather be a counselor than a contractor, decided it was a good opportunity to improve my low self-esteem as a repairman and insisted on doing no hands-on work himself, but rather on guiding me through all the steps involved in fixing the pipe. To my amazement, I did it—and watched his delight as I bragged to him about my newfound technical prowess over dinner at a Chinese restaurant afterward.

Another time, over a Christmas lunch with my friend Kay Redfield Jamison, who had just completed her remarkable memoir *An Unquiet Mind*, we traded our usual gifts. The gift I remember most, though, from that day was the story she told me of the characters Rat and Mole from Kenneth Grahame's *The Wind in the Willows*, a story of friendship between two small creatures caught in a snowstorm. After lunch, she insisted on taking me to the nearest bookstore to buy a copy of the book that told this story of empathy and understanding between friends on a winter's day.

So stories can be gifts and gifts can generate stories, and both are excellent ways of bringing joy to the dark season. One of the great Christmas stories that connects giving with the season is O. Henry's "The Gift of the Magi," in which a husband and wife each sacrifice a prized possession to purchase a gift for the other. The husband sells his watch to buy combs for his wife's hair; she sells her hair to buy a chain for his watch. The wisdom of these two is that they understood that love itself is a great gift, surpassing material possessions. This theme is repeated again and again in the most popular stories and movies of the Christmas season, and it deserves to be. It helps us look beyond the material and into the spiritual, which is the special gift of winter.

It is not only in Western culture that storytelling thrives particularly in winter. Among the Lenape Indians, for example, the time for storytelling began with the first frost and ended with the last frost. The Indians were superstitious about telling stories during the summer for fear that the creatures of the forest might hear the storyteller talking about them and take revenge on him. Or the crops might stop and listen to the storyteller and forget to grow. They believed that stories carry great power, and so do we. Think, for example, how far people are willing to go out of their way for a well-told story, be it at the theater, at the opera or the movies, or in a book. The most powerful stories are those that stay with us and continue to affect us long after the last word is spoken or the last sentence read.

In some cultures and climates, for example in the Far North, gifts in winter can make the difference between life and death. Beth, the Athapaskan woman mentioned earlier, told me how in her village they always saw to it that no one went through the winter without enough food to eat. Psychiatrist Andrés Magnusson remembers how in the town in Iceland where he grew up they would round up the homeless on Christmas Eve and take them to the jail, where they would be sure to be warm and have a decent meal. Even farther south, we are enjoined around Christmastime to remember the neediest. There is something about this season of scarcity that has the capacity to bring out the best in us: witness the transformation of Ebenezer Scrooge in the perennial classic, *A Christmas Carol*.

Other Pleasures

Once the symptoms of SAD have been treated, even if only partially, all kinds of winter pleasures become possible, such as sports, socializing, reading, travel, solitude, and walking.

For the sports fan, winter presents many opportunities for both observing and participating. It is basketball and Super Bowl season for those whose preferred position is on the couch in front of the television. For the more active, snow and ice offer many opportunities for physical exercise, and the glittering light reflected off snowy surfaces is sure to elevate the spirits further.

When the symptoms of SAD are treated, thinking becomes sharper and it is easier to read again, to concentrate on another person's thoughts. Curling up in front of the fireplace with a good book can be a special treat on a winter day. Much has been written about winter. To the untreated SAD sufferer, such books may provide cold comfort, but once symptoms are treated, they may spark your interest. I have listed some of my favorite winter books in the bibliography. Edwin Way Teale, in his prize-winning *Traveling Through Winter*, describes winter as "a hundred seasons in one." In his charming book *Winter*, Rick Bass chronicles how he traveled to Montana to experience winter in the North. We read how he rides out his SAD-like symptoms, which he regards as part of the authentic winter experience. Donald Hall, in an essay on winter, describes himself as a lover of winter, one of those who is "partly tuber, partly bear."

An extraordinary amount of poetry has been written about winter, perhaps more than about any other season. One good thing about poetry is that it's short and therefore doesn't unduly tax one's attention span, which may be a boon if one is suffering from the symptoms of SAD. The Japanese haiku may be particularly appealing at this time, because one of the rules of haiku is that each poem should have only seventeen syllables. Another rule is that each poem should allude to one of the seasons. Somehow, in the spareness of the wording and references to nature, winter haiku has the amazing capacity to evoke the beauty, peace, and solitude of the season. Although winter is a season of parties and socializing, it is also conducive to solitude, whether for the reader by the fire or the skier on the slopes. In this regard as well, it is a season of contrasts.

Although I have warned against stressful travel during winter if you have SAD, once the symptoms of SAD are relatively well controlled, travel in winter can also be a great diversion. I am not referring only to trips to the Caribbean or other points south, which are designed specifically to get away from winter, but rather to traveling through winter and sometimes actually into winter. One such trip that I took was a book tour to some of the darkest cities in the United States. With the help of the light visor, I was not only able to get through the trip successfully but actually managed to enjoy it as well.

Winter has the capacity to surprise one. For example, when I reached Seattle, one of the darkest cities in the country, this beautiful town was awash in dazzling sunshine. There were clear views of the Cascade and Olympic mountain ranges, and not a cloud was to be seen over the huge Mount St. Helens. As I think of that day, I can still see the turquoise color of the sky that to me typifies the mystical beauty of the Pacific Northwest.

In Portland, Oregon, on the other hand, where it rarely snows, I arrived in the midst of the first snowstorm in a very long time. The flakes were small and feathery at first but later turned into a blizzard that paralyzed a city ill equipped to deal with it. Luckily, my tour guide had a four-wheel drive, so I was able to enjoy the way the snow had transformed the landscape, frosting the gingerbread roofs of the Victorian houses and freighting down the blackberry canes with cotton-white mounds. The sculpted fir trees, tufted with snow, were still festooned with red tinsel streamers from the holiday season. Red, white, and green: the official colors of Christmas. From the city park, a bronze deer, icicles hanging from its nose, gazed out at me, unmoved by the wintry spectacle.

The day of interviews went off without a hitch despite the weather, thanks to both my intrepid guide and the tenacity of the journalists involved, all of whom had gamely made it to their stations. By the day's end, the snow had turned to slush, and as I stepped into the truck I could see the brilliant reds and golds of autumn leaves shining through the melting crystals. The words of Albert Camus came to mind: "Even in the midst of winter, there is within me an invincible summer." That is the challenge of winter—somehow to hold on to our reserves of hope, cheer, and energy even when the dark and the cold drain us of much of our good humor and vitality.

Thoreau has written about the special joy of walking in winter. It is a joy I share with him. Although life may seem to have largely deserted the cities, there is much to be seen in the wilderness and parklands all around. The architecture of the trees can be seen best without their summer greenery. Where flowers once bloomed, the winter weeds hold on to their intricately crafted seed cases. Many birds remain behind in the North. In Maryland, for example, there are chickadees, Canada geese (not all of which migrate to the far South), great herons, and bald eagles. Pairs of eagles will return to build their nest in the same location, year after year, in January and have their young in February. You can hear the sound of water running over stones, fed by underground streams or ice cracking at the edge of a pond. Deer and foxes walk between rocks covered with moss and lichen, as green as jade.

You may not need to stray far to enjoy walking in winter. As I walk through the familiar streets of my own neighborhood, I am reminded of how the different gardens looked last summer and compare that with their present dormancy. I enjoy the purple hearts of decorative cabbages or the red berries of holly at a time of year when any flash of color provides a welcome relief against the background of grays, browns, and conifer green. The air has a bracing quality.

Winter nights are especially good for walking and for stargazing when it is cloudless. One recent winter night, I stared through a friend's telescope and saw the moons of Jupiter and the rings of Saturn for the first time. As I wander through the streets, I am reminded of lines from George Meredith's poem "Winter Heavens":

> Sharp is the night, but stars with frost alive
> Leap off the rim of earth across the dome
> It is a night to make the heavens our home
> More than the nest whereto apace we strive.
> Lengths down our road each fir-tree seems a hive,
> In swarms outrushing from the golden comb.
> They waken waves of thoughts that burst to foam.

The darkness of the night is broken by the stars and the light of human habitation—streetlights, incandescent lights, flickering television screens, computer terminals, and, at the end of my walk, the intense blue-white fluorescent light shining through the curtains of my own home. And as I return to the beginning again, I think of winter and its many, many facets. It has been a difficult season, for me and so very many others, but in the difficulty there is the opportunity to bring out that which is best in each of us. Winter is a stimulus to creativity and to sharing the fruits of our creation with others. I write this book in that spirit, and if it brings you even a shaft of light on a winter's day, my mission has been accomplished.

Afterword

The End of an Era, 1979–1999

Between 1979 and 1999, research into SAD and light therapy flourished in the Seasonal Studies Program at the National Institute of Mental Health in Bethesda, Maryland. The work that was done during those years formed the basis of this book. It was a collaboration among many people: investigators (who are named below), nurses, social workers, research coordinators, assistants, and, of course, the research subjects themselves. All this required a considerable investment of funds, the result of which was the development of a field and the discovery of new treatments for an illness previously undescribed. At the same time the NIMH, through its extramural program, funded research grants throughout the northern United States, where critical work was done by many researchers whose contributions are described in this book.

The last decade has seen a radical change in funding priorities. The Seasonal Studies Program was closed down and SAD is no longer a subject of research at the intramural program of the NIMH. At the same time, the number of grants funded for research on this subject in other parts of this country shriveled so severely that, by the latest count, only three researchers were doing government-funded work on SAD or light therapy. It is understandable that funding priorities change over time. Yet it would be a great error to imagine that we have all the answers when it comes to understanding and treating SAD. It is interesting to speculate on the reasons for the dramatic change in funding. Perhaps it is the result of changing fashions or politics, but certainly not because the job has been done.

There are some encouraging signs of reawakening. A recent lead article in the *American Journal of Psychiatry* validated the benefits of light therapy for both SAD and nonseasonal depression. In addition, pharmaceutical companies have begun to take an interest in the area. But these efforts are only a new beginning. Much more is needed.

To all those for whom SAD is an important consideration, to all who would like to see it receive more attention and funding, I would once again offer a modest suggestion. Coordinate your efforts and develop a support organization to provide comfort and support to people with the condition and to promote research in the area. Such collective efforts could well stimulate a resurgence of interest in, and funding for, a disorder so near and dear to so many of us.

Fellow Investigators in the Seasonality Studies Program, 1979–1999

Fred Goodwin, Tom Wehr, Al Lewy, Dave Sack, Chris Gillin, Wally Duncan, Steve James, Fred Jacobsen, Barb Parry, Bob Skwerer, Siegfried Kasper, Jean Joseph-Vanderpool, Karen Kelly, Dan Oren, Doug Moul, Ellen Leibenluft, Norio Ozaki, Diego Garcia-Borreguero, Paul Schwartz, Erick Turner, Susana Feldman-Naim, Pam Madden, Alex Neumeister, Teo Postolache, Jeff Matthews, Ling Han, and Leo Sher.

Part IV
Resources

Where to Get Further Help
for Seasonal Problems

You can find further information about my work and my writings on my website, at *www.normanrosenthal.com*. I update the website from time to time.

Where to Purchase Light Fixtures

The following companies have excellent, long-term track records for delivering high-quality products, standing by their products with service, and keeping up to date with the latest developments in the field. All should offer a thirty-day, money-back guarantee on their products. There are, however, other light box companies that may work out equally well for you. Remember, my preference is for larger light boxes that deliver white light from fluorescent bulbs housed behind plastic diffusing screens with special UV light filters. These are the boxes with the longest track record for safety and effectiveness.

The Store at *www.cet.org*
   This Web-based supplier provides a variety of light fixtures, the type of negative ion generator used in SAD research studies, and other devices. The cet.org website contains a wealth of useful information and is worth checking out in its own right.

SunBox Company
19217 Orbit Drive
Gaithersburg, MD 20879
Phone: (301) 869-5980
Toll-free: (800) LITE-YOU (548-3968)
Website: *www.sunbox.com*
E-mail: sunbox@aol.com
Contact: Neal Owens
   Besides light boxes, dawn simulators, light visors, light pipes, and negative ion generators can also be obtained from SunBox.

Apollo Health, Inc.
352 West 1060
Orem, UT 84058
Phone: (801) 226-2370
Toll-free: (800) 545-9667
Website: *www.apollolight.com*
Contact: Henry Savage, Jr.
   Well known for their light boxes, some of which have a furniture-type finish.

Bio-Light by Enviro-Med
1600 SE 141st Avenue
Vancouver, WA 98683
Toll-free: (800) 222-3296
Website: *www.bio-light.com*
E-mail: info@bio-light.com
Contact: Sherrie Lindstrom

Bio-Brite, Inc.
7315 Wisconsin Avenue, #1300 W
Bethesda, MD 20814-3202
Phone: (301) 961-8557
Toll-free: (800) 621-LITE (621-5483)
Website: *members.aol.com/biobrite/bbhome.htm*
E-mail: biobrite@aol.com
Contact: Kirk Renaud
   Light visors are manufactured and distributed by Bio-Brite. This company also sells the SunRise clock.

Northern Light Technologies
8971 Henri Bourassa West
St. Laurent PQ, H4S 1P7
Canada
Phone: (514) 335-1763
Toll-free: (800) 263-0066
Fax: (514) 335-7764
Website: *www.northernlighttechnologies.com*
E-mail: info@northernlight-tech.com
Contact: Joe Ronn or Steve Nador

In the United Kingdom

Outside In (Cambridge) Ltd.
3 The Links, Trafalgar Way
Bar Hill, Cambridge CB3 8UD
England
Phone: +44 (0) 1954 780-500
Fax: +44 (0) 1954 780-510
Website: *www.outsidein.co.uk*
E-mail: info@outsidein.co.uk
Contact: Steve Hayes

More information about light therapy and SAD can be obtained from:

Society for Light Therapy and Biological Rhythms
P.O. Box 591687
174 Cook Street
San Francisco, CA 94159-1687
Fax: (415) 751-2758
E-mail: sltbrinfo@aol.com
Website: *www.sltbr.org*

How to Find a Doctor or Therapist Who Can Treat SAD

Now that SAD has been recognized for over two decades, I hope that many more practitioners are equipped to treat it well. If you have trouble finding a provider with expertise in this area, I recommend that you contact your nearest university department of psychiatry for a suitable referral.

Support Groups for SAD and Mood Disorders

As of the time of writing this book, the National Organization for SAD (NOSAD), which still has a website, *www.nosad.org*, is no longer a viable entity. I recommend that those who are interested in resuscitating this worthwhile group coordinate their efforts to do so.

Depression and Bipolar Support Alliance (DBSA; formerly known as
   National Depressive and Manic–Depressive Association [NMDA])
730 North Franklin Street, Suite 501
Chicago, IL 60610-7224
Phone: (312) 624-0049
Toll-free: (800) 826-3632
Website: *www.dbsalliance.org*

Depression and Related Affective Disorders Association (DRADA)
2330 West Joppa Road, Suite 100
Lutherville, MD 21093
Phone: (410) 583-2919
Phone: (312) 624-0049
Website: *www.drada.org*

Seasonal Affective Disorder Association (SADA)
P.O. Box 989
Steyning BN44 3HG
England
Website: *www.sada.org*

National Alliance for the Mentally Ill (NAMI)
Colonial Place Three
2107 Wilson Boulevard, Suite 300
Arlington, VA 22201-3042
Phone: (703) 524-7600 (main)
Toll-free: (800) 950-NAMI (member services)
Website: *www.nami.org*

Dietary Advice, Menus,
and Recipes

*I*n Chapter 8, I offered advice for preventing the typical winter weight gain experienced by people with SAD, centering on ways to thwart the carbohydrate craving that often accompanies the winter blues. Here are some more specifics, from shopping tips to a week's worth of menus and recipes. As you review the possibilities that follow, keep in mind these caveats:

• Some people need to restrict their carbohydrate intake to a far greater degree than others to lose weight or maintain their weight at an appropriate level. Others can handle higher proportions of complex carbohydrates without triggering cravings. I have included recipes for both types of people. *An asterisk (*) next to a recipe or menu item indicates that it has a higher proportion of carbohydrates than many of the others. A double asterisk (**) signifies a particularly high carbohydrate content*. In some recipes I offer two versions and star the higher-carbohydrate one or star a carbohydrate-rich ingredient that you may either include or omit. That way you can choose a diet that's best for you.

• At this time experience suggests that limiting carbohydrates helps many SAD sufferers, and menus and recipes like the ones that follow have worked for me and many of my patients. But, as mentioned in Chapter 8, extreme carbohydrate restriction may be unwise. And, in fact, it is best to view this type of dietary approach as a *reduced*-carbohydrate plan rather than a *low*-carbohydrate plan. Some low-carbohydrate diets have been criticized for being too high in protein and also too free with fat. You'll notice that this diet goes to neither of these extremes. For example, omelets and egg dishes call for egg whites or egg substitute rather than whole eggs.

   • I happen to be satisfied with a menu that does not vary much from day to day, but you may want to ensure that you don't get bored with your diet, which could tempt you to add carbohydrate-rich items that will perpetuate cravings. So pay close attention to the lists of ingredient options in the recipes and be creative. There is a wealth of vegetables and proteins to choose from, as well as infinite ways to combine them. Also, be adventurous with seasonings that contain no salt and feel free to substitute to taste for any of the seasonings listed in the recipes.

   • Dietary restrictions alone are never as effective as diet and exercise. *Be sure to get at least thirty minutes of total-body-movement exercise three times a week, as well as at least twenty minutes another two or three days a week.*

   • If trying a new approach to daily meals seems like an onerous task in the winter, keep in mind that you can prepare many individual foods (such as hard-boiled eggs) and many recipes in advance and have them ready to serve.

Shopping Tips

When you're planning your menus, it may be a good idea to make an initial shopping visit to the various grocery stores, health food stores, and natural or organic food markets in your area and check out the items you will need. Take a copy of the following guidelines with you for help in choosing items. You will not need to follow the recipes like a chemist in a laboratory; use your judgment in coming up with variations that are right for you. In other words, I don't expect you to count blueberries on a hectic morning; you know how large a portion is too large, and you are in charge.

How to Choose Groceries That Will Promote Your Winter Health

Health food is now readily available, even in large supermarkets, but especially in those grocery stores designed to attract educated and health-conscious shoppers in all seasons. Many of the menus listed in the chart call for ingredients that fit into general categories (cereal, yogurt, etc.) in which you can find wonderful, suitable products or, if you don't read the labels and choose carefully, you can accidentally buy products that are not good for you. Rather than dictate which brands you should buy, nutrition counselor Bette Flax recommends that you adopt a few rules of thumb to guide your shopping. That way you will find brands that fit the description and appeal to your individual taste.

Cereal

One serving should have:

- NOT MORE than 10 grams of sugar (the less, the better!).
- NOT LESS than 2 grams of fiber.
- NOT MORE than 4 grams of fat.
- NOT MORE than 250 milligrams of sodium.
- NOT LESS than 4–5 grams of protein.

Yogurt or Cottage Cheese

- The best yogurt will say "fat free" or "nonfat."
- Plain rice and soy yogurt is available for nondairy diets.
- Make sure it has NO ADDED SUGAR and no added salt.
- Total sugars should be less than half of the total carbohydrate content. (In other words, if there are 33 grams of carbohydrates, total sugars should equal 16 grams or less.)
- Labels for yogurt will say "lite" or "low-fat" or "nonfat" or "fat free." ("Lite" indicates sugar substitute, which is fine in many cases.)
- Labels for cottage cheese will say "low fat" or "1 percent fat"; WATCH SALT CONTENT!

Tortillas

- Sugar should be less than 4 grams per tortilla (the less, the better).
- Sodium should be 300 milligrams or less (the less, the better).

- Fat should be 3½ grams or less.
- Fiber should be 5 grams or more.

Protein Bars

One bar should have:

- NOT MORE than 6 grams of fat.
- NOT MORE than 6 grams of sugar.
- BETWEEN 15 and 26 grams of protein.
- NOT MORE than 250 milligrams of sodium.

Protein-Based Shakes

A single-serving shake should have:

- NOT MORE than 5 grams of fat.
- NOT MORE than 300 milligrams of sodium.
- NOT LESS than 150 milligrams of potassium.
- NOT MORE than 6 grams of sugar.
- BETWEEN 15 and 26 grams of protein.

Crackers

- Whole grain.
- Nonfat or low fat (the less, the better).
- Each serving should have less than 250 milligrams of sodium.
- Sugar should be 20 percent or less of total carbohydrate content.

Salad Dressing

- The clearer, the better.
- No added sugar (except for honey mustard, in which case look for low sugar content).
- Low fat, but in all cases less than 8 grams of fat per serving.
- Low sodium (the less, the better).

Canned Soup or Chili

It takes a lot of perusing and studying to find acceptable canned foods. Look for the lowest fat content you can find, no added sugar (add your own powdered seasonings for flavor), and definitely avoid high sodium content. If you shop carefully, you can find some canned foods that say "no salt added" and "no sugar added."

Frozen Vegetable Burgers or Breakfast Grillers

- Fat per serving should be less than 5 grams per burger.
- Sugar per serving should be under 6 grams.
- Sodium per serving should not exceed 380 milligrams.

Cheese

- Protein content should be at least 7 grams per serving.
- Fat content should be UNDER 5 grams per serving.
- Label may say "reduced fat" or "low fat" or "light" or "lite" or "part skim."
- LOOK FOR DETAILS: grams of fat per serving is what counts.
- It should also be low in sodium, less than 300 milligrams per serving.

You can also find lactose-free, soy-based cheese alternatives. They are tasty, but they do not contain much protein, and watch the sodium content! If you choose such an alternative, be sure to stay UNDER 300 milligrams of sodium per serving.

Acceptable Substitutes for Less Desirable Condiments

- Instead of ketchup, try hot sauce (diluted to taste).
- Instead of mayonnaise, you can get some very tasty soy dressings.
- Rather than using salt, you can find wonderful spices and even prepared seasoning mixes containing no salt.
- For sugary salad dressings, you can substitute a clear, low-sodium vinaigrette or a tasty balsamic vinegar.[1]

---

[1]People who are allergic to, or sensitive to, aspirin should not use balsamic vinegar.

Menus for a Week

	Sunday	Monday	Tuesday
Breakfast	*French toast with extras	"Crêpes" with sautéed spinach	Winterfest omelet with cheese
Midmorning snack (if necessary)	String cheese and nuts	*Fresh fruit (not banana)	*Yogurt
Lunch	Dark-green salad with fish, chicken, or turkey	*Stuffed sandwich with turkey	*Lunch tortilla wrap with salmon
Midafternoon snack	*Protein bar	2–3 hard-boiled egg whites	String cheese and nuts
Dinner	Baked chicken breast with vegetables	Salmon/tuna burgers with vegetables	Seafood salad deluxe and steamed vegetables
Evening snack	*Rice cake with almond butter	*Fudgsicle	Almonds or walnuts
Throughout every day, drink . . .	8–12 glasses of water	8–12 glasses of water	8–12 glasses of water

Menus for a Week (cont.)

Wednesday	Thursday	Friday	Saturday
*Yogurt/cereal bowl	Cheese scramble with mushrooms	*Cottage cheese/ cereal bowl	Winterfest parsley/ tomato omelet
2–3 egg whites	*Protein-based shake	1 slice "Lite" cheese/celery wrap or can of sardines	*Cottage cheese
Protein-filled lettuce wraps with tuna and onion	*Potato chili	Lunch omelet with spinach and cheese	*Stuffed sandwich with tuna
*Protein bar	1 slice turkey wrapped around string cheese	*Protein-based shake	"Crêpe" filled with asparagus
Overstuffed winterfest omelet with veggies and cheese, side salad	Grilled salmon with salad and vegetables	Turkey meatloaf with vegetables, side salad	Turkey or veggie burger with salad
1 egg white and blueberries	*Yogurt	String cheese and nuts	*Popsicle
8–12 glasses of water	8–12 glasses of water	8–12 glasses of water	8–12 glasses of water

Recipes

Breakfast

*French Toast

> 3 beaten egg whites or the 2-egg equivalent in egg substitute
> 1 tablespoon unprocessed bran
> 1 slice whole wheat bread

> *Extras*
> *Unsweetened all-natural applesauce (optional)
> Ground cinnamon[2]
> 2 small frozen veggie breakfast grillers or links

> —Beat the egg whites or pour the egg substitute into a small bowl. Stir in the bran and let sit for a minute or two. Heat a nonstick skillet and spray with vegetable spray.
> —Dip the bread into the egg–bran mixture. Transfer it to the pan and fry the French toast on both sides.
> —Meanwhile, microwave the veggie breakfast grillers or links according to the package instructions.
> —Serve with applesauce sprinkled with lots of cinnamon.

"Crêpes"

These can be made in advance and refrigerated for up to one week in a covered container. Make 2 or 3 for one breakfast serving. The following makes one crêpe.

> 1 egg white or the 1-egg equivalent in egg substitute

> —Heat a small skillet or crêpe pan and spray with vegetable spray. Beat the egg white or vigorously shake the egg substitute. Quickly pour it into the pan and tilt it to make sure the liquid spreads out. As soon as the edges of the egg pull away from the pan, lift the crêpe and quickly flip it to the other side for 5–10 seconds.
> —Slide the crêpe off the pan onto a warm plate and fill with any combination of chopped vegetables, bean sprouts, cooked tuna, salmon, shrimp, hard-boiled egg white or crabmeat salad, leftover shredded fish, chicken, or turkey, and/or "lite" cheese.

[2]Cinnamon helps lower your cholesterol!

Winterfest Omelet

*with Toast and Almond Butter

Any vegetables you like, cubed, diced, or sliced
2–3 egg whites or the equivalent in egg substitute
Onion powder, black pepper, oregano, and/or any no-salt spice, to taste[3]
1 ounce low-fat, reduced-fat, or "lite" cheese,[4] broken up
*1 slice whole wheat bread or 1 small tortilla or pita (optional)
*1 teaspoon all-natural almond butter[5] (optional)

—Steam the vegetables in the microwave; do not overcook.
—Spray a medium skillet with vegetable spray and heat over medium heat.
—Slide the beaten egg into the pan and sprinkle on the chosen seasonings. When the edges begin to solidify, carefully fold them into the center and tilt the pan so the uncooked egg runs out to the edges. Turn the heat down to low and repeat the edge-lift process several times. When the top is no longer liquid but not yet firm, gently turn the omelet over.
—Immediately scatter the cheese onto the omelet. Tuck the vegetables into the center and fold the omelet over to form a semicircle.
—Serve with whole wheat toast, pita, or tortilla, if desired, with the almond butter.

[3]Be adventurous with spices, but be cautious when stocking your shelves. Make sure the spices and seasonings you choose contain no salt, sugar, or MSG.

[4]Many fine reduced-fat, low-fat, or "lite" cheeses are available at most grocery stores, but especially at natural food, organic food, or health food markets. Investigate what is available in your local area and run some "taste tests" to see which ones satisfy your palate.

[5]For nut butter or preserves, check the list of ingredients carefully to make sure that they do not have added salt or sugar. Any ingredient that ends in the letters *ose* (for example, *sucrose, lactose, fructose, glucose, maltose*) or any form of syrup (such as corn syrup) is a form of sugar.

*Yogurt/Cereal Bowl

1 small individual fat-free or "lite" plain, lemon, or vanilla yogurt (you may also use acidophilus or organic low-fat yogurt)
1 tablespoon unprocessed bran
½ cup (for women) or 1 cup (for men) any acceptable breakfast cereal (you may also use raw amaranth, oat, or other flakes)
¼ cup unsweetened frozen or fresh blueberries
Ground cinnamon

—Place the yogurt in a bowl and sprinkle the bran onto it; mix well. Add the cereal of your choice, pour on the blueberries, and sprinkle on plenty of cinnamon.

Cheese Scramble

*in Wrap

Handful of chopped fresh spinach or other greens
½ cup sliced mushrooms
¼ cup diced green, red, and/or yellow bell pepper or other veggies of your choice
2–3 egg whites or the equivalent in egg substitute
1 slice low-fat, reduced-fat, or "lite" cheese, broken up (optional)
Seasonings and spices to taste
*1 whole wheat tortilla (optional)

—Microwave the vegetables; do not overcook.
—Spray a skillet with vegetable spray and heat it over medium heat.
—Slide the beaten egg into the pan. When the bottom surface and sides of the omelet have solidified somewhat, push the edges toward the middle of the pan with a spatula and gently repeat this process until the eggs are about half cooked.
—Before the center is firm, fold the vegetables in; sprinkle the seasonings on top.
—Continue pushing the edges toward the middle until the eggs are as dry as you like.
—To make a wrap, microwave the tortilla for 30 seconds, then fold the scrambled eggs into the tortilla, wrap, and enjoy.

*Cottage Cheese/Cereal Bowl

½ cup or 1 small individual container fat-free cottage cheese or lactose-free, fat-free cottage cheese
1 tablespoon unprocessed bran
½ cup (for women) or 1 cup (for men) any acceptable breakfast cereal (you may also use raw amaranth, oat, or other flakes)
Small handful of blueberries or 6 strawberries, sliced (or ⅓ cup diced fruit—but not bananas)
Ground cinnamon

—Place the cottage cheese in a bowl and sprinkle the bran onto it; mix well. Add the cereal. Toss the fruit or berries on top; sprinkle with plenty of cinnamon.

More Breakfast Choices

**Oatmeal Pudding

1 serving cooked 5-minute oatmeal, made with water
1 tablespoon unprocessed bran
3 heaping tablespoons vanilla or lemon yogurt or 1-percent cottage cheese
1 small container unsweetened all-natural applesauce
Lots of ground cinnamon

—Mix all ingredients together and enjoy.

*Breakfast Tortilla Wrap

1 whole-wheat tortilla
Filling of your choice

—Heat the tortilla in the microwave for 30 seconds. Fold it around a filling of any combination of chopped vegetables, "lite" cheese, bean sprouts, canned tuna, salmon, or crabmeat, cooked shrimp, hard-boiled egg white or crabmeat salad (use low-fat yogurt or fat-free soy dressing), and/or leftover shredded fish, chicken, or turkey.

Midmorning Snack

Take this snack about 2½ to 3 hours after breakfast, only if you really are hungry. *Do not repeat* what you had for breakfast.

1 or 2 sticks of "lite" string cheese plus small handful of unsalted almonds or walnuts

1 sliced cucumber sprinkled with onion powder and a stick of string cheese

*Celery (several stalks) with 1 tablespoon cottage cheese, fat-free yogurt, or all-natural almond butter used as dip

Celery with 3 or 4 sardines, mashed and used as dip

Celery stalk wrapped in 1 slice of "lite" cheese

*1 fresh fruit (other than banana)

2 or 3 hard-boiled egg whites

*1 small unsweetened applesauce with 1 or 2 sticks of "lite" string cheese

*Protein-based shake

1 thin slice turkey breast wrapped around 1 stick of string cheese

1 small can of sardines packed in water

1 piece of unsalted gefilte fish (no sugar added; not the "sweet" variety)

*1 individual container or ½ cup fat-free vanilla, plain, or lemon yogurt

*1 individual container or ½ cup 1-percent cottage cheese

*4 no-sodium crackers with 1 slice "lite" cheese, or 1 tablespoon all-natural peanut, almond, or cashew butter

Protein-Based Shake

This is not for children under 16 years old, since the high mineral content is not good for them.

1 envelope vegetable-based non-dairy (soy or rice) protein shake or whey (dairy) protein shake

1 cup water

½ cup lactose-free, fat-free milk

Several ice cubes

10–15 blueberries or 6–8 strawberries

—Put all the ingredients into a blender, in the order listed. Blend for 2 minutes.

Hard-Boiled Eggs

Up to a dozen eggs

—Take the eggs out of the refrigerator and let them warm on the counter to room temperature for about a half hour; then place them in a saucepan and add enough cold water to cover them completely. Bring to a gentle boil over medium heat, and then turn the heat down to low. Simmer the eggs for about 10 minutes. Turn off the heat, bring the pot to the sink, dump out the boiling water, and run cold water over the eggs for a minute. Let the eggs come to room temperature and then refrigerate immediately. They will keep for up to 4 days. Don't peel them until you are ready to eat them or use them in a recipe.

Lunch

Dark-Green Lunch Salad

The base of this salad should be a dark-green form of leafy vegetable.

Mass of romaine lettuce, arugula, red-leaf lettuce, spinach, or field greens
Any or all of the following:
   Artichoke, asparagus, bok choy, broccoli, Brussels sprouts, cabbage, cauliflower, celery, chives, cucumbers, garlic (all kinds), green beans, leeks, mushrooms (all kinds), onions (all kinds), parsley, peppers (all colors), radish (red or daikon), scallions, spinach, sprouts, tomatoes, zucchini (all kinds)
   *1 tablespoon well-rinsed canned or cooked black, pinto, kidney, or soy beans (optional)
   2–4 ounces grilled or roasted chicken or turkey breast, no skin; or sardines or other canned fish (no swordfish or tuna for pregnant women, though), or chopped hard-boiled egg whites; or any leftover fish, turkey burger, or veggie burger, broken up

For dressing:
1 tablespoon olive or canola oil
Any vinegar you choose
Lots of no-salt seasonings
OR make your own salad dressing by peeling a cucumber, dicing it, and blending it in a blender on high for 30 seconds with a bit of vinegar and some spices added for taste.

OR 1 tablespoon plus 1 teaspoon of the clearest vinaigrette dressing available (nothing white or orange; no Caesar dressing)

OR If you are using canned fish in this recipe, you can use the water from the can and add a touch of vinegar and a teaspoon of oil for taste.

—Toss the salad ingredients and serve with *4 low-sodium whole wheat crackers (you may want to crumble the crackers and throw them onto the salad as croutons).

Variations on the green theme:

Fresh baby spinach salad with chopped hard-boiled egg whites and salmon, with vinaigrette

Romaine and red-leaf lettuce salad with cucumber spun in blender and chopped shrimp

Mustard greens shredded finely with zucchini and tuna, with olive oil and white vinegar

Chopped chicken in halved head of Boston or bibb lettuce, with diced yellow and red bell peppers, with vinaigrette

*Stuffed Sandwich

3–4 ounces cooked turkey or chicken breast or 3–6 ounces any cooked fish

2 slices whole wheat bread, 1 tortilla, or 1 pita

Lettuce, spinach, shredded cabbage, any other vegetables you like

1 slice "lite" or low-fat cheese

—Assemble the meat or fish on the bottom slice of bread. Add the vegetables. Lay the slice of cheese on top and place the sandwich under the broiler or into toaster oven just long enough to melt the cheese. (If you use a tortilla, fold it over and grill it for a minute or less, or microwave it for about 35 seconds; if you use a pita, stuff it and heat for a minute or less.)

—Put the top slice of bread on top and serve with raw or steamed veggies.

*Lunch Tortilla Wrap

1 whole wheat or spelt or sprouted-grain tortilla[6]
A bit of mustard
1½ slices fat-free, reduced-fat, or "lite" cheese
One 3-ounce or 6-ounce can tuna (packed in water, drained) or chicken
   or turkey
Nonstarchy vegetables of your choice

—Spread the tortilla sparingly with mustard. Place the whole slice of
cheese on the tortilla. Crumble the tuna or dice/slice the turkey or
chicken on top of that. Add any vegetables you like—for example, tomato, onions, mushrooms, spinach, sprouts. Place the remaining ½
slice of cheese on top of that.
—Microwave the tortilla for 40 seconds, remove from the microwave,
and wrap up, folding in the sides and then rolling it up.
—Serve with a small green salad or cup of low-sodium, no-sugar-added
soup.[7]

Protein-Filled Lettuce Wraps

8–10 whole romaine or red-leaf lettuce leaves
½ cup chopped salad made of white-meat chicken, tuna, turkey, shrimp,
salmon, crabmeat, veggie burgers, sardines, any other fish, hard-
boiled egg whites, and/or any nonstarchy chopped vegetables
Up to 1 tablespoon fat-free plain yogurt, low-fat mayonnaise, low-sugar
honey mustard, soy dressing, or clear vinaigrette

—Wrap about a tablespoonful of chopped salad in a lettuce leaf and enjoy.

---

[6]You can purchase these, frozen, at a health food store or natural foods section of your super-
market.
[7]Beware of canned soups, beans, and vegetables. Read the ingredients carefully to make sure
the sodium content is very low and there is no added sugar or MSG.

**Potato Chili

Serve this with a small green salad.

> 1 sweet potato or white baking potato
> ½ can any spicy, low-sodium, fat-free vegetarian chili with black beans

> —Preheat a toaster oven or conventional oven to 425°F. Microwave or bake the potato until cooked.
> —Meanwhile, microwave or otherwise heat the canned chili. Remove the potato, slice it open, and mash the chili into it.

Lunch Omelet

Serve this with a small green salad or fruit on the side.

> 2–3 egg whites or the equivalent in egg substitute
> 1 slice low-fat, reduced-fat, or "lite" cheese, broken up
> Any or all of the following:
>> Handful of chopped spinach
>> ½ cup sliced mushrooms
>> ¼ cup diced green, red, or yellow bell pepper
>> Diced scallions, leeks, chives, or onions
>> Finely shredded red cabbage
>> Chopped parsley, cilantro, or other fresh herbs
>> Diced zucchini and/or tomatoes
>> Asparagus spears

> —Spray a skillet with vegetable spray and heat over medium heat. Toss in the vegetables, raise the heat to high, and cook, stirring, for 2 minutes. Remove and set aside in a bowl. (You can also microwave the vegetables while you make the omelet.)
> —Respray the pan if necessary, turn the heat to medium, and slide in the beaten eggs. Cook the eggs, gently lifting the edges of the omelet all around the pan to allow the uncooked eggs to slide under the solidified eggs, until the omelet is almost firm.
> —Carefully turn the omelet over in the pan and begin to cook the other side. Scatter the cheese on top of the omelet. Place the vegetables on top and flip half of the omelet over the other half so the filling is covered. Lower the heat and continue to cook the omelet until it is as solid/dry as you like.

Chopped Luncheon Salad

Frozen cooked tail-off shrimp
Dark-green lunch salad (see recipe above), without meat or fish
Any chopped nonstarchy vegetables
5 unsalted almonds, sliced
12 blueberries

—Assemble the salad as directed. Sprinkle the nuts and berries on the salad and toss.
—Soak a handful of the frozen shrimp in cold water for 6 minutes to thaw. Add to the salad and top with "lite" vinaigrette dressing.

Another Lunch Choice

Midwinter Green Soup

This makes 10–12 servings, but it keeps beautifully if you refrigerate it as soon as it cools to room temperature.

1 tablespoon vegetable oil
1 large red or white onion, diced
Up to 1 head of garlic, peeled and coarsely chopped
1 cup or more of any of the following vegetables, diced: asparagus, bok choy, broccoli, Brussels sprouts, cauliflower, green beans, leeks, mushrooms (all kinds), bell peppers (all colors), tomatoes, zucchini
½ head of cabbage (optional)
½ head of romaine or other dark-green lettuce and/or one 10-ounce bag of fresh spinach or one 10-ounce package frozen spinach
4 stalks celery, cut into large chunks
4 large carrots, cut into large chunks
A few black peppercorns
1 small turnip, diced
Your choice of herbs (fresh or dried) and seasonings (powdered) but no salt
2 tablespoons unprocessed bran
1 bunch fresh parsley, finely chopped

—Put the oil in a large soup pot. Add the onion and garlic and cook, stirring, over high heat for a minute or two. If you're using mushrooms, add them and cook for another minute or two. Add at least 3 quarts of water, making sure you cover the vegetables. You can always add more water later. At this point, add the cabbage if you're using it, and the lettuce, other greens, and/or spinach, and bring to a boil.

—Reduce heat and add the celery, carrots, peppercorns, turnip, herbs, and seasonings. If you need more water to cover all the vegetables, add it now and bring the soup back to a boil once more. Then simmer for an hour or more.

—Add all the other vegetables, the bran, and finally the parsley. Again, if you need to add water, bring the soup back to a boil after doing so, and then turn down the heat. Simmer for half an hour or more.

Variations

For tomato-based soup: Add unsalted tomato or V-8 juice with the water.

For bean soup: The night before you make your soup, soak ½ cup dried black-eyed peas or beans in water. When you are ready to start your soup, drain off the water you soaked the beans in. Add the beans when you add the first water.

For split pea or lentil soup: Drop in ½ cup split peas or lentils when you add the celery and carrots.

For a sour soup: Add ½ cup apple cider vinegar with the celery and carrots, and 1 teaspoon dry mustard with the seasonings.

For a "hot" soup: Add ¼ cup finely diced horseradish with the celery and carrots; use the red seasonings (cumin, cayenne) and toss in a finely diced jalapeño pepper with the parsley.

For a comforting chicken soup: Use twice as much onion, garlic, spinach, celery, carrots, and parsley. Add a whole bunch of chopped scallions with the onions. Remove all visible fat and skin from a whole chicken. As the onions are sautéing, add the chicken and stir it around rapidly with a wooden spoon. Bring at least 4 quarts of water to a boil in a separate pot or kettle. Pour it onto the chicken/onion mixture and boil for 10 minutes, then reduce the heat. Add spinach (and other greens if you like), celery, carrots, turnip, herbs, and seasonings. Simmer for 2 hours. If you need to add more water, add boiling water at this point. Then add any other vegetables you choose, parsley last. Simmer for half an hour more, then turn off the heat and let the soup cool until you can handle the chicken. Lift out the chicken and remove the meat from the bones. Discard all but firm, meaty portions. If you like, you can puree several cups of the soup (minus the meat) in a food processor or blender, and then pour it back into the pot for a final 20-minute simmer.

For egg-drop soup: After the soup is finished, strain the vegetables out and bring the liquid to a slow boil. Slowly pour in 2 well-beaten egg whites or the equivalent amount of egg substitute while stirring the soup with a fork. Simmer for 5 minutes and then add the vegetables back into the soup.

Midafternoon Snack

Take this snack about 3 hours after lunch. *Do not repeat* the morning food choices.

- *Protein bar with 15–25 grams of protein, no more than 6 grams of fat, 6 grams of sugar, and 200 milligrams of sodium. *CAUTION: NEVER MORE THAN ONE BAR PER DAY!*
- *1 small container low-fat, no-sugar-added plain, vanilla, or lemon yogurt
- *4 no-salt crackers with 1 or 2 "lite" string cheese sticks
- *½ cup lactose-free, low-sodium, or 1-percent cottage cheese with a bit of fruit (for example, 10 blueberries)
- *½ cup fat-free soy milk plus 1 small container unsweetened applesauce with plenty of cinnamon
- *Protein shake (never more than one shake per day)
- Lettuce wrap with 3 tablespoons protein salad (tuna, turkey, chicken, fish, egg white)
- 2 hard-boiled egg whites
- 2 skim-milk mozzarella string cheese sticks
- 1 "Crêpe" (see recipe above) with 2 tablespoons salmon salad or tuna salad filling

Note: If you're not having dinner until 7:00 or 8:00 P.M., have one afternoon snack at around 3:00 P.M. and a second one at about 5:30 P.M. or even somewhat later. For example, you could have a protein bar at 3:00 and a string cheese stick at 5:30, then eat the second stick of string cheese on the way home to keep yourself from getting ravenous. When you have two snacks, though, don't choose two with asterisks (**) or you will be having too much carbohydrate before dinner.

If you're starving, you can add a fruit (*) other than banana to the 3:00 P.M. snack.

Dinner

Baked Chicken Breast

Serve this with a small green salad or steamed vegetables.

> 1 boneless, skinless chicken breast
> Any seasonings, such as onion powder, garlic powder, minced onion, minced garlic, black pepper, paprika, oregano, and/or parsley
> *1½ tablespoons apricot fruit spread (sweetened with fruit juice only)

> —Preheat the oven to 350°F. Spray a small baking dish with vegetable spray.
> —Mix the seasonings in a small bowl. Dredge the chicken breast in the seasoning mix, then place in the baking dish.
> —Add water to the bottom of the baking dish to a depth of about 1½ inches.)
> —Place the apricot spread into a cup and microwave briefly to liquefy. Pour the apricot sauce over the chicken and bake for 20 minutes.

Seafood Burgers

Serve these burgers with steamed vegetables and a green salad. NO BUN!

> One 6-ounce can of tuna or crabmeat, or half a 15-ounce can of salmon
> 2 tablespoons egg substitute or egg whites
> 1 tablespoon low-sodium soy dressing or other fat-free mayonnaise-like dressing
> 1 tablespoon low-sodium, no-sugar-added mustard dressing
> ¼ cup oatmeal
> ½ teaspoon black pepper
> 1 teaspoon paprika
> ½ teaspoon dried oregano
> ¼ teaspoon onion powder
> ¼ teaspoon garlic powder
> ¼ teaspoon minced fresh or dried onion
> ¼ teaspoon minced fresh or dried garlic
> (You can use the seasonings you like best; this list is just one example; NO SALT!)

> —Combine the first 5 ingredients in a small bowl and mix well. Combine the seasonings in another small bowl.
> —Spray the skillet with vegetable spray and put half of the combined seasonings into the pan.

—Form the seafood mixture into 2 or 3 patties and fry them over medium heat on one side until they solidify enough to turn easily.

—Toss the remaining spices into the pan, turn the burgers, and cook on the other side until browned and heated through.

Seafood Salad Deluxe

Zucchini, yellow squash, green or red cabbage, green beans, celery, green or any other color bell peppers, leeks, and/or any other nonstarchy vegetables

Green leafy vegetables such as lettuce, kale, or spinach

Steamed shrimp, scallops, or any fish (leftover grilled or steamed fish is fine)

*1 heaping tablespoon rinsed canned or cooked black or kidney beans or 2 low-sodium whole wheat crackers, crumbled (optional)

1½ tablespoons "lite" or low-fat vinaigrette dressing

4–5 strawberries or 10–15 blueberries

—Steam the vegetables and then refrigerate them for an hour or more to chill.

—Assemble a tossed salad from the green leafy vegetables. Add the chilled vegetables and seafood. Sprinkle the beans or crumbled crackers over the salad.

—Add the dressing and then toss the berries onto the salad or serve them on the side.

Overstuffed Winterfest Omelet

1 winterfest omelet or lunch omelet (see recipes above)

*2 tablespoons rinsed canned or cooked black beans, kidney beans, or black-eyed peas

Unsalted spicy salsa

1–2 ounces additional salmon, tuna, sardines, shrimp, or crabmeat

Extra vegetables

—Follow the directions for preparing the winterfest or lunch omelet, adding the extra ingredients to make this a generously stuffed dinner omelet. (The extra vegetables can either be added to the omelet or served on the side.)

Grilled Salmon

Serve this with a green salad and/or raw or steamed vegetables.

* 1–2 tablespoons apricot fruit spread (sweetened with fruit juice only) (optional)

One 6-ounce piece fresh salmon fillet or salmon steak, preferably wild

Black pepper, onion powder, garlic powder, paprika, and/or other spices of your choice

1 tablespoon minced fresh or dried onion and/or 1 tablespoon minced fresh garlic

Frozen vegetables (optional) or fresh vegetables of your choice

Margarine spray

—Preheat the oven to 400°F.

—Microwave the apricot spread in a paper cup for about 20 seconds, until liquefied.

—Place the salmon in a baking dish or on a sheet of heavy-duty aluminum foil cut large enough to enclose the fish. Dust with the seasonings. Place the chosen vegetables on top. Spray with margarine spray and, if using aluminum foil, wrap and seal, poking a small hole in the foil tent. If you don't use foil, bake uncovered. Bake for 15–20 minutes, until the salmon is cooked to your liking.

*Turkey Meatloaf

If you want to prepare this dish with minimal carbohydrates, omit the potato and milk.

The recipe serves 4–6 people, or you can refrigerate (up to 4 days) or freeze (up to 1 month) individual portions for future use.

1 large white baking potato

2 pounds ground turkey or ground turkey breast

¼ cup balsamic vinegar or dry red wine

½ teaspoon black pepper, plus more to taste

1 teaspoon dried oregano

1 tablespoon minced fresh or dried onion

1 teaspoon onion powder, plus more to taste

1 tablespoon minced fresh or dried garlic

1 teaspoon garlic powder

⅓ cup (for ground turkey) or ½ cup (for ground turkey breast) no-salt tomato juice, no-salt V-8 juice, or no-salt tomato sauce

2 tablespoons egg substitute or egg white

⅓ cup oatmeal

Margarine spray

¼ cup skim milk

—Preheat oven to 350°F. Meanwhile, peel, dice, and boil the potato until tender.

—Place the ground meat in a large mixing bowl. Add the vinegar or wine and all the seasonings. Mix well with your hands. Add the oatmeal and mix again. Pour in the tomato or V-8 juice and the egg substitute or egg white. Mix the whole mixture very thoroughly with your hands and pack into an ungreased loaf pan.

—Drain the cooked potato, place in a bowl, and mash with pepper and onion powder to taste, 4 sprays of margarine, and the skim milk. Spread the mashed potato mixture on top of the meatloaf and bake for about 45 minutes, until it's cooked through and the top is browned.

Turkey Burgers

Serve this with steamed vegetables and/or a green salad.

2 pounds ground turkey or ground turkey breast

1 teaspoon minced fresh or dried onion

1 teaspoon minced fresh or dried garlic

2 tablespoons egg substitute or egg whites

¼ cup unprocessed bran or wheat germ

⅓ cup no-salt tomato juice or no-salt V-8 juice

½ teaspoon black pepper, or to taste

½ teaspoon dried oregano, or to taste

1 teaspoon onion powder, or to taste

1 teaspoon garlic powder, or to taste

Any spicy no-salt, no-sugar-added salsa, mustard, ketchup, or similar condiment (preferably low-sodium salsa)

—Thoroughly mix the ground meat, minced onion and garlic, egg, bran or wheat germ, and tomato or V-8 juice in a large bowl.

—Mix together the seasonings in a small bowl. (Season to taste, but use *no salt!*) Then add half of the mixture to the meat and blend very well with your hands.

—Spray a skillet with vegetable spray, then add the remaining spice mixture and heat the pan over medium heat.

—While the pan is heating, form the meat into patties. Add to the pan and cook, turning frequently until cooked through. Serve the salsa on the side.

Veggie Burgers

The freezer section of your local health food store will have many varieties of veggie burgers for you to choose from. This recipe makes a serving of 2 burgers; you can cut all the ingredients in half if one is enough for you for dinner.

½ cup sliced mushrooms
½ onion, quartered and sliced
2 frozen veggie burgers
2 slices low-fat, reduced-fat, or "lite" cheese
Diced bell peppers, 2 tomato slices (1 per burger), and/or sliced cucumber, zucchini, spinach, or other veggies of your choice

—Spray a skillet with vegetable spray, add the mushrooms and onion, and cook, stirring, over medium heat for 2 minutes. Push to the side of the pan if it's big enough or transfer to a plate.
—Add the burgers to the pan, cook until done on the bottom, then turn. Place the mushrooms and onions on top, melt the cheese over the vegetables and burger, and cook until heated through. Or microwave the burgers, top with the cheese, and microwave again to melt, then serve the burgers on top of the onions and mushrooms. Or make a double veggie cheeseburger by first cooking the veggie burgers in either pan or microwave, then stacking burger, veggies, cheese, burger, cheese, microwaving it again to melt the cheese, and then holding it all in place with a lettuce wrap. Whichever method you choose, serve the additional, raw vegetables on top of the burgers or on the side, but serve the burgers *without buns*.

More Dinner Choices

**Sweet Potato Meal

Serve this with a green salad and steamed vegetables. This is a very flexible meal. You can use ½ can of low-sodium, no-fat vegetarian chili instead of yogurt, or you can use the canned chili as a sort of salad dressing for the green salad, or you can mix the steamed vegetables into the chili for a veggie casserole.

1 large sweet potato
1 tablespoon nonfat vanilla or plain yogurt or 1-percent cottage cheese
Chopped onion and paprika or ground cinnamon, to taste

—Bake the potato in a conventional oven, toaster oven, or microwave until done. Cut it open, add the yogurt or cottage cheese, then sprinkle with lots of cinnamon or chopped onion and paprika, depending on your taste.

Pale-and-Lite Egg Salad

Up to 4 hard-boiled eggs, including only one of the yolks
1 tablespoon soy dressing, light clear vinaigrette, low-sodium, low-sugar
   mustard dressing, plain nonfat yogurt, or other condiment
1 cup chopped celery, chopped red cabbage, and/or other crunchy vegetable (such as onion, cucumber, daikon)
*¼ green apple, chopped

—Mix all the ingredients; be adventurous. Serve on a bed of lettuce.

Evening Snack

1 hard-boiled egg white with a small handful of blueberries
*2 tablespoons "lite" yogurt or nonfat (1-percent) cottage cheese, with a
   small handful of blueberries if you like
*1 no-sugar-added Fudgsicle or Popsicle or 2 low-sodium whole wheat
   crackers with fruit spread (sweetened only with fruit juice)
1 "lite" string cheese stick and a small handful of unsalted almonds or
   walnuts
*Baked apple or pear with 2 tablespoons nonfat yogurt heaped into mid-
   dle of fruit or ½ glass of skim milk or soy milk poured over the fruit
*1 level tablespoon all-natural almond butter on brown rice cake (op-
   tional)
10–15 unsalted almonds or walnuts
*½ cup skim milk or soy milk (no sugar added)

Baked Apples or Pears

*Keep up to a week in the refrigerator. You can make a single serving in the micro-
wave or toaster oven.*

2 to 4 apples or pears
Ground cinnamon

—Wash and core the apples or pears. If you are baking apples, make a slit in
   the peel of each apple in a horizontal circle. For pears, puncture a few
   holes in the skin of each. Put the fruits into a small glass baking dish (for
   conventional or toaster oven), or paper bowl (for microwave).
—Put a few tablespoons of water into the pan (about 1 tablespoon of
   water per fruit). Microwave on high for 2 minutes or bake in the oven
   for 40–45 minutes at 400°F.
—Serve warm or cold; use tons of cinnamon but no sugar or sweetener.

Further Reading

*T*his is not intended to be a comprehensive bibliography, but rather a list of some texts that the general reader might find useful and interesting.

Part I. Seasonal Syndromes

Chapter 2

Lam, R. W. (1998). *Seasonal affective disorder and beyond: Light treatment for SAD and non-SAD conditions*. Washington, DC: American Psychiatric Press.

Partonen, T., & Magnusson, A. (2001). *Seasonal affective disorder: Practice and research*. New York: Oxford University Press.

Rosenthal, N. E., Sack, D. A., Gillin, J. C., Lewy, A. J., Goodwin, F. K., Davenport, Y., Mueller, P. S., Newsome, D. A., & Wehr, T. A. (1984). Seasonal affective disorder: A description of the syndrome and preliminary findings with light therapy. *Archives of General Psychiatry, 41*(1), 72–80.

Chapter 3

Wehr, T. A., Duncan, W. C., Jr., Sher, L., Aeschbach, D., Schwartz, P. J., Turner, E. H., Postolache, T. T., & Rosenthal, N. E. (2001). A circadian signal of change of season in patients with seasonal affective disorder. *Archives of General Psychiatry, 58*(12), 1108–1114.

The original reference to the Seasonal Pattern Assessment Questionnaire (SPAQ) can be found in:

Rosenthal, N. E., Genhart, M., Jacobsen, F. M., Skwerer, R. G., & Wehr, T. A. (1987). Disturbances of appetite and weight regulation in seasonal affective disorder. *Annals of the New York Academy of Sciences, 499,* 216–230.

Papers that deal with how to score the SPAQ include:

Kasper, S., Wehr, T. A., Bartko, J. J., Gaist, P. A., & Rosenthal, N. E. (1989). Epidemiological findings of seasonal changes in mood and behavior: A telephone survey of Montgomery County, Maryland. *Archives of General Psychiatry, 46*(9), 823–833.

Rosen, L. N., Targum, S. D., Terman, M., Bryant, M. J., Hoffman, H., Kasper, S. F., Hamovit, J. R., Docherty, J. P., Welch, B., & Rosenthal, N. E. (1990). Prevalence of seasonal affective disorder at four latitudes. *Psychiatry Research, 31*(2), 131–144.

Chapter 5

Giedd, J. N., Swedo, S. E., Lowe, C. H., &Rosenthal, N. E. (1998). Case, series: Pediatric seasonal affective disorder. A follow-up report. *Journal of the American Academy of Child and Adolescent Psychiatry, 37*(2), 218–220.

Rosenthal, N. E., Carpenter, C. J., James, S. P., Parry, B. L., Rogers, S. L., & Wehr, T. A. (1986). Seasonal affective disorder in children and adolescents. *American Journal of Psychiatry, 143*(3), 356–358.

Swedo, S. E., Allen, A. J., Glod, C. A., Rosenthal, N. E., Teicher, M. H., Richter, D., Hoffman, C., Brown, C., & Clark, C. H. (1997). A controlled trial of light therapy for the treatment of pediatric seasonal affective disorder. *Journal of the American Academy of Child and Adolescent Psychiatry, 36*(6), 816–821.

Swedo, S. E., Pleeter, J. D., Richter, D. M., Hoffman, C. L., Allen, A. J., Hamburger, S. D., Turner, E. H., Yamada, E. M., & Rosenthal, N. E. (1995). The rates of seasonal affective disorder in children and adolescents. *American Journal of Psychiatry, 152*(7), 1016–1019.

Part II. Treatments

Chapter 7

Campbell, S. S., Dijk, D. J., Boulos, Z., Eastman, C. I., Lewy, A. J., & Terman, M. (1995). Light treatment for sleep disorders: Consensus report. III. Alerting and activating effects. *Journal of Biological Rhythms, 10*(2), 129–132.

Dijk, D. J., Boulos, Z., Eastman, C. I., Lewy, A. J., Campbell, S. S., & Terman, M. (1995). Light treatment for sleep disorders: Consensus report. II. Basic properties of circadian physiology and sleep regulation. *Journal of Biological Rhythms, 10*(2), 113–125.

Golden, R. N., Gaynes, B. N., Ekstrom, R. D., Hamer, R. M., Jacobsen, F. M., Suppes, T., Wisner, K. L., & Nemeroff, C. B. (2005). The efficacy of light therapy in the treatment of mood disorders: A review and meta-analysis of the evidence. *American Journal of Psychiatry, 162*(4), 656–662.

Lam, R. W., Carter, D., Misri, S., Kuan, A. J., Yatham, L. N., & Zis, A. P. (1999). A controlled study of light therapy in women with late luteal phase dysphoric disorder. *Psychiatry Research, 86*(3), 185–192.

Lam, R. W., Goldner, E. M., Solyom, L., & Remick, R. A. (1994). A controlled study of light therapy for bulimia nervosa. *American Journal of Psychiatry, 151*(5), 744–750.

Lewy, A. J., Bauer, V. K., Cutler, N. L., Sach, R. L., Ahmed, S., Thomas, K. H., Blood, M. L., & Jackson, J. M. (1998). Morning vs. evening light treatment of patients with winter depression. *Archives of General Psychiatry, 55*(10), 890–896.

Lewy, A. J., Sack, R. L., Miller, S., & Hoban, T. M. (1987). Antidepressant and circadian phase-shifting effects of light. *Science, 235,* 352–354.

Lewy, A. J., Sack, R. L., & Singer, C. M. (1985). Treating phase typed chronobiologic sleep and mood disorders using appropriately timed bright artificial light. *Psychopharmocology Bulletin, 21,* 368–372.

Oren, D., Reich, W., Rosenthal, N. E., & Wehr, T. A. (1993). *How to beat jet lag: A practical guide for air travelers.* New York: Holt.

Parry, B. L., Mahan, A. M., Mostofi, N., Klauber, M. R., Lew, G. S., & Gillin, J. C. (1993). Light therapy of late luteal phase dysphoric disorder: An extended study. *American Journal of Psychiatry, 150*(9), 1417–1419.

Rosenthal, N. E., Sack, D. A., Carpenter, C. J., Parry, B. L., Mendelson, W. B., & Wehr, T. A. (1985). Antidepressant effects of light in seasonal affective disorder. *American Journal of Psychiatry, 142*(2), 163–170.

Rosenthal, N. E., & Wehr, T. A. (1992). Towards understanding the mechanism of action of light in seasonal affective disorder. *Pharmacopsychiatry, 25*(1), 56–60.

Sack, R. L., Lewy, A. J., White, D. M., Singer, C. M., Fireman, M. J., & Vandiver, R. (1990). Morning vs. evening light treatment for winter depression. *Archives of General Psychiatry, 47,* 343–351.

Terman, M., Lewy, A. J., Dijk, D. J., Boulos, Z., Eastman, C. I., & Campbell, S. S. (1995). Light treatment for sleep disorders: Consensus report. IV. Sleep phase and duration disturbances. *Journal of Biological Rhythms, 10*(2), 135–147.

Terman, M., Terman, J. S., Lo, E. S., & Cooper, T. B. (2001). Circadian time of morning light administration and therapeutic response in winter depression. *Archives of General Psychiatry, 58*(1), 69–75.

Terman, M., Terman, J. S., Quitkin, F. M., McGrath, P. J., Stewart, J. W., & Rafferty, B. (1989). Light therapy for seasonal affective disorder: A review of efficacy. *Neuropsychopharmacology, 2*(1), 1–22.

Terman, J. S., Terman, M., Schlager, D., Rafferty, B., Rosofsky, M., Link, M. J., Gallin, P. F., & Quitkin, F. M. (1990). Efficacy of brief, intense light exposure for treatment of winter depression. *Psychopharmacology Bulletin, 26*(1), 3–11.

Wirz-Justice, A., Graw, P., Krauchi, K., Gisin, B., Jochum, A., Arendt, J., Fisch, H. U., Buddeberg, C., & Poldinger, W. (1993). Light therapy in seasonal affective disorder is independent of time of day or circadian phase. *Archives of General Psychiatry, 50*(12), 929–937.

Chapter 8

Terman, M., Terman, J. S., & Ross, D. C. (1998). A controlled trial of timed bright light and negative air ionization for treatment of winter depression. *Archives of General Psychiatry, 55*(10), 875–882.

Chapter 9

Burns, D. D. (1999). *Feeling good: The new mood therapy—The clinically proven drug-free treatment for depression.* New York: HarperCollins.

Greenberger, D., & Padesky, C. A. (1995). *Mind over mood: Change how you feel by changing the way you think.* New York: Guilford Press.

Westermeyer, R. (2004). *Kicking depression's ugly butt: Tried and true methods for outsmarting depression.* St. Louis, MO: Quick Publishing.

Chapter 10

Hedaya, R. (1996). *Understanding biological psychiatry.* New York: Norton.

Rosenthal, N. E. (1998). *St. John's wort: The herbal way to feeling good.* New York: HarperCollins.

Part III. Celebrating the Seasons

Chapters 14–17

Boorstin, D. J. (1983). *The discoverers.* New York: Vintage Books.

Cameron, I. (1974). *Antarctica: The last continent.* London: Cassell.

Cook, F. A. (1894). Medical observations among the Esquimaux. *New York Journal of Gynaecology and Obstetrics, 4,* 282–296.

Dewhurst, K. (1962). A seventeenth-century symposium on manic–depressive psychosis. *British Journal of Medical Psychology, 35,* 111–125.

Dickinson, E. (1924). *The complete poems of Emily Dickinson, with an introduction by her niece, Martha Dickinson Bianchi.* Boston: Little, Brown.

Eliade, M. (1965). *Experiences of the mystic light: Mephistopheles and Androgyne.* New York: Sheed & Ward.

Eliade, M. (1954). *The myth of the eternal return, or cosmos and history* (trans. W. R. Trask). Bollingen Series XLVI. Princeton, NJ: Princeton University Press.

Esquirol, J. E. D. (1965). *Mental maladies: Treatise on insanity.* New York: Hafner. (Original work published 1845)

Frumkes, G. (1946). A depression which recurred annually. *Psychoanalytic Quarterly, 65,* 351–364.

James, W. (1963). *The varieties of religious experience.* New York: University Press.

Jamison, K. R. (1989). Mood disorders and seasonal patterns in top British writers and artists. *Psychiatry, 52*(2), 125–134.

Jamison, K. R. (1993). *Touched with fire: Manic–depressive illness and the artistic temperament.* New York: Free Press.

Jones, J. R. (1966). *The man who loved the sun: The life of Vincent van Gogh.* London: Evans Brothers.

Manner, K. (Ed.). (1979). *Selected letters of Gustav Mahler.* London: Faber & Faber.

Marsh, M. (1976). *Philosophy of the inner light* (Pendle Hill Pamphlet 209). Pendle Hill, PA: Pendle Hill Publications.

Stone, I. (Ed.). (1969). *Dear Theo: The autobiography of Vincent van Gogh.* New York: Signet.

Wechsberg, J. (1972, March 18). Mørketiden. *The New Yorker.*

Winter Light: Life Beyond SAD

Bass, R. (1992). *Winter: Notes from Montana.* Boston: Houghton Mifflin.

Brown, L. (1976). *Weeds in winter.* New York: Norton.

Dickens, C. (1852). *Christmas books.* London: Thomas Nelson.

Hall, D. (1986). *Winter, in winter.* Hanover, NH: University Press of New England.

Henry, O. (1928). The gift of the Magi. In *The Complete Works of O'Henry* (pp. 7–10). Kingswood Surrey, UK: Associated Bookbuyer's Company.

Kullberg, M. (1993). *Morning mist: Thoreau and Basho through the seasons.* New York: Weatherhill.

Nelson, R. K. (1983). *Make prayers to the raven.* Chicago: University of Chicago Press.

Teale, E. W. (1965). *Wandering through winter.* New York: St. Martin's Press.

Thoreau, H. D. (1994). *Walking.* New York: HarperCollins.

Wallis, V. (1994). *Two old women.* New York: HarperPerennial.

Part IV

Peeke, P. (2000). *Fight fat after forty.* New York: Viking Penguin.

Peeke, P. (2005). *Body for life for women.* Emmaus, PA: Rodale Press.

APPENDIX A

Daily Mood Log

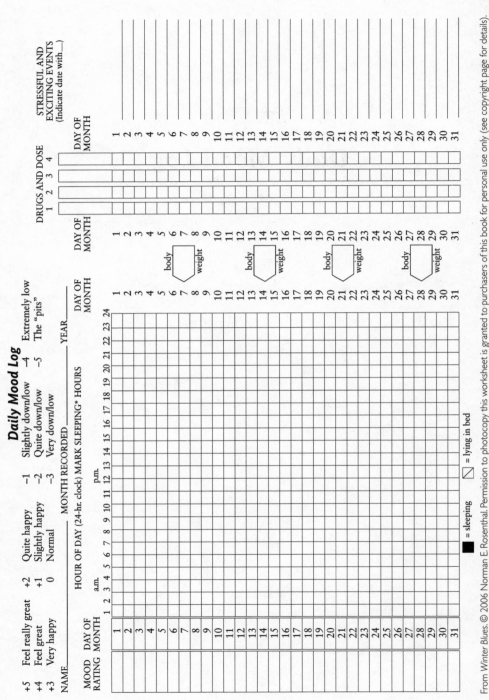

Daily Mood Log

+5 Feel really great	+2 Quite happy	−1 Slightly down/low	−4 Extremely low
+4 Feel great	+1 Slightly happy	−2 Quite down/low	−5 The "pits"
+3 Very happy	0 Normal	−3 Very down/low	

NAME _____ MONTH RECORDED _____ YEAR _____

HOUR OF DAY (24-hr. clock) MARK SLEEPING* HOURS

MOOD RATING	DAY OF MONTH	a.m. 1 2 3 4 5 6 7 8 9 10 11 12	p.m. 13 14 15 16 17 18 19 20 21 22 23 24
	1		
	2		
	3		
	4		
	5		
	6		
	7		
	8		
	9		
	10		
	11		
	12		
	13		
	14		
	15		
	16		
	17		
	18		
	19		
	20		
	21		
	22		
	23		
	24		
	25		
	26		
	27		
	28		
	29		
	30		
	31		

■ = sleeping   ▨ = lying in bed

DRUGS AND DOSE
1 2 3 4

DAY OF MONTH
1–31

STRESSFUL AND EXCITING EVENTS
(Indicate date with ___)

DAY OF MONTH
1–31

body / weight

APPENDIX B

Core Belief Worksheet

Core Belief Worksheet

Name: _____ Date: _____

Old core belief: _____

_____

- How much do you believe the old core belief right now? (0–100) _____
- What's the most you've believed it this week? (0–100) _____
- What's the least you've believed it this week? (0–100) _____

New belief: _____

_____

- How much do you believe the new belief right now? (0–100) _____

Evidence that contradicts old core belief and supports new belief	Evidence that seems to support old core belief with reframe

Should situations related to an increase or decrease in the strength of the belief be topics for the agenda?

Index

Fortunetelling, 201, 202. *See also*
    Cognitive distortions
French Revolution, 288
Freud, Sigmund, 191, 193, 243,
    272–273, 287
Friends, advice for, 247–251
Frost, Robert, 246, 298
Frumkes, Colonel George, 270–274
Full-spectrum light, 14, 128–129,
    131–132

Functioning, cognitive. *See also*
    Symptoms
  in chickadees, 76
  light therapy and, 122
  overview, 40–41
  when to seek medical help and,
    58–59
Funding of research, 307–308

G

Gabbard, G. O., 144
Garcia-Borreguero, Diego, 308
Gaskell, Charles Milnes, 237
Genesis, 289
Gender differences, 62, 74
Genetic transmission of SAD, 61–
    62. *See also* Causes of SAD
Giedd, Dr. Jay, 87
"The Gift of the Magi," 303
Gifts, in winter, 303
Gillin, Dr. J. Christian, 15, 308
Glacier, 295
Glod, Dr. Carol, 87–88
Goethe, Johann Wolfgang von,
    109–113
Golden, Dr. Robert, 115, 144
Gonyaulax polyhedra, seasonal
    rhythms in, 69–70, 71, 256
Goodwin, Dr. Frederick, 8, 308
Gorman, Dr. Chris, 136
Gould, Stephen Jay, 107
Graham, Kenneth, 303
Grandiosity, 105
Grenville, Anne, case history, 265–
    266

Great Year, 257
Greeks, 257, 265, 266, 267
Groceries, tips for buying, 317–319
Groundhog Day, 302
Guidelines for coping with
    November, 238
Guilt, 59, 182

H

Haiku, 304
Hall, Donald, 304
Halloween, 302
Halogen light, 119
Hamsters, 74–75
Han, Dr. Ling, 64, 308
Handel, George Frideric, 279, 280
Hanukkah
  history of, 257
  overview, 302
  planning for seasonal patterns
    and, 238–239
Hardy, Thomas, 288–289
Hawaii, light deprivation in, 67
Head-mounted light devices, 148–
    149f, 312
Headaches, 133, 134, 179
Hellekson, Dr. Carla, 20
Hemingway, Ernest, 279
Herbs, 178–181
Heritability of SAD, 61–62. *See also*
    Causes of SAD
Hesperian depression, 110
Hibernation, 73–74, 256, 297
Hippocrates, 3, 95, 108, 110, 264
History of SAD, 264–274
History of SAD research, 7–17, 111
History of seasonal time, 255–259
Holiday blues, 241–242
Holiday season
  case example of, 298
  history of, 257
  planning for seasonal patterns
    and, 238–243
  travel during, 240–241
Holte, Dr. Arne, 262–263
Houdin, Jean Eugene Robert, 147

Moon
cycle of, 255–259
influence of, 108–110
"Moral medicine," 269
"Moral treatment" of mood
disorders, 269
Mørketiden (murky times), 67, 261–262
Motivation
cognitive functioning and, 41
dopamine and, 218
to exercise, 171–172
stress management and, 182
Moul, Doug, 308
Mueller, Dr. Peter, 10, 12, 13

Mystic light experiences, 292–293
Myth of the Eternal Return, 257

N

Nasal passage dryness, 134, 135
National Alliance for the Mentally
Ill (NAMI), 314
National Depressive and Manic-
Depressive Association
(NMDA), 314
National Institute of Mental Health
(NIMH), 7–13, 28, 31, 32,
33, 36, 38, 41, 49, 56, 95, 97,
192, 260, 274, 307
National Oceanic and Atmospheric
Administration (NOAA), 170
National Organization for Seasonal
Affective Disorder (NOSAD),
187, 314
Natural light exposure
access to, 5
compared to light therapy, 151–152
poetry and, 289–293
Nausea, 134, 135, 179
Negative ion generators, 109, 183–185, 311
Negative ions, 109, 183–185, 185*f,*
188–189, 311. *See also* Positive
ions

Negative thoughts, 198–201, 204–206. *See also* Cognitive
distortions
Nei Ching, 187
Nervousness, 179
Neumeister, Alex, 308
Neurotransmitters, 77–79, 217–218
New Testament, 292
New Year, 239, 257
New Year's Eve, 298
New York Psychiatric Institute, 271
The New Yorker, 261
Newton, Sir Isaac, 279
Nicotine use, 45–48, 104
Night and day transitions, 70–72,
274
Nobel prize for medicine, 269–270
Nonseasonal depression. *See*
Depression, nonseasonal
Norepinephrine
antidepressants and, 218, 219*t,*
220
light therapy and, 80
overview, 78–79
Norpramin, 219*t,* 220–221. *See also*
Antidepressants
Northern Exposure, 148
Northern Light Technologies, 313
Norway, 261–263
Nottebaum, Dr. Fernando, 76
November, 226–236, 237–238
Nursing a baby, light therapy
during, 140

O

O. Henry (William Sydney Porter),
303
Oatmeal pudding, 325
Obesity, 37, 170
Obsessive-compulsive disorder, 161
October, 226–237
Oktoberfest, 302
The Old Man in Sorrow, 281
Omega-3 fatty acids, 180
Omelets, recipes for, 323, 330, 335
Optimism, 105

About the Author

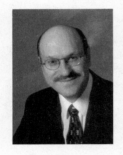

Norman E. Rosenthal, MD, an internationally acclaimed psychiatrist, first described seasonal affective disorder (SAD) in 1984 and pioneered its treatment with light therapy. During his long tenure at the National Institute of Mental Health, he published hundreds of scholarly articles, but is perhaps best known for his popular books, including *The Emotional Revolution* and *Winter Blues*. He is currently Clinical Professor of Psychiatry at Georgetown University School of Medicine, Medical Director and CEO of Capital Clinical Research Associates, and in private practice in Rockville, Maryland. Dr. Rosenthal and his work have been widely featured in the media, including on *Today*, *Good Morning America*, and National Public Radio. You can visit Dr. Rosenthal at *www.normanrosenthal.com*.